CranioSacral for Grief and Loss

"Diego Maggio expertly weaves a comprehensive exploration of CranioSacral Therapy and SomatoEmotional Release fundamentals in this book. His expertise is beautifully extended through a broad and exceptional range of interconnected material. *CranioSacral Therapy for Grief and Loss* stands as an indispensable resource for practitioners and anyone interested in the far-reaching foundations of CranioSacral Therapy and SomatoEmotional Release."

— TAD WANVEER, LMBT, CST-D, DIPLOMAT CERTIFIED BY THE UPLEDGER INSTITUTE INTERNATIONAL IN CRANIOSACRAL THERAPY AND AUTHOR OF *BRAIN STARS*

"Diego Maggio has created a masterpiece in the world of hands-on therapies, especially concerning CranioSacral Therapy. As a practitioner in the healing arts myself since 1971, *CranioSacral Therapy for Grief and Loss* exceeds any expectations that I had imagined. This is such an all-encompassing book. The depth and breadth Maggio delves into are a delight for the reader with an interest in the human energy field. He covers the physical, mental, emotional, and spiritual realms in an easily-accessible fashion. I highly recommend this book for anyone interested in the human condition and the therapeutic approaches to help elevate our shared experience of life on Earth as well as in making the world a touch better and then some."

— KENNETH KOLES, PH.D., D.SC., L.AC., PRACTITIONER OF CRANIOSACRAL THERAPY (CST) AND ORIENTAL MEDICINE

"In his book *CranioSacral Therapy for Grief and Loss*, Diego Maggio beautifully addresses grief and loss from a complete holistic perspective. Reading this book takes you on a journey through all aspects of the life cycle. His personal stories and deep emotions will have you re-experiencing your own story and life cycles, inspiring hope and healing. The depth and knowledge within these pages will entice you to revisit it more than once. I predict that each rereading will reveal a different layer of yourself on your path to wholeness. His in-depth knowledge and honoring of CranioSacral Therapy give the uncanny experience of feeling Dr. Upledger's presence."

— CAROL MCLELLAN, CMT, CST-D, CPO-D, INSTRUCTOR AT UPLEDGER INSTITUTE INTERNATIONAL

"*The Sky Above Berlin* (Der Himmel über Berlin) is a film in which angels wandering in the city observe people while listening to their thoughts. I remember a scene in which an angel enters a library, and so the people reading silently simultaneously gives voice to all the authors of the books. Diego Maggio may not be an angel, but in his book we find the same consonance of that library coupled with the strength of his thought, which transforms into a natural therapeutic gesture."

Thea Keber, organizational secretariat of
Cranio-Sacrale Upledger Italia

CranioSacral Therapy for Grief and Loss

Hands-On Techniques to Release Trauma Stored in the Body

A Sacred Planet Book

Diego Maggio, BSc (Hons), DO, CST-D
Translated by Giada Pianigiani

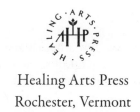

Healing Arts Press
Rochester, Vermont

Healing Arts Press
One Park Street
Rochester, Vermont 05767
www.HealingArtsPress.com

Healing Arts Press is a division of Inner Traditions International

Sacred Planet Books are curated by Richard Grossinger, Inner Traditions editorial board member and cofounder and former publisher of North Atlantic Books. The Sacred Planet collection, published under the umbrella of the Inner Traditions family of imprints, includes works on the themes of consciousness, cosmology, alternative medicine, dreams, climate, permaculture, alchemy, shamanic studies, oracles, astrology, crystals, hyperobjects, locutions, and subtle bodies.

Copyright © 2019 by Diego Maggio
English translation copyright © 2024 by Upledger Productions and Diego Maggio

Originally published in Italian in 2019 under the title *CranioSacral Therapy nel ciclo della vita: Ode alla vita* by BioGuida Edizioni
First U.S. edition published in 2024 by Healing Arts Press

All rights reserved. No part of this book may be reproduced or utilized in any form or by any means, electronic or mechanical, including photocopying, recording, or by any information storage and retrieval system, without permission in writing from the publisher.

Note to the reader: This book is intended as an informational guide. The remedies, approaches, and techniques described herein are meant to supplement, and not to be a substitute for, professional medical care or treatment. They should not be used to treat a serious ailment without prior consultation with a qualified health care professional.

Cataloging-in-Publication Data for this title is available from the Library of Congress

ISBN 978-1-64411-819-1 (print)
ISBN 978-1-64411-820-7 (ebook)

Printed and bound in India by Replika Press Pvt. Ltd.

10 9 8 7 6 5 4 3 2 1

Text design by Virginia Scott Bowman and layout by Debbie Glogover
This book was typeset in Garamond Premier Pro with Gill Sans MT Pro, ITC Legacy Sans, Frutiger LT Std, Arno Pro and Rival Sans used as display typefaces

To send correspondence to the author of this book, mail a first-class letter to the author c/o Inner Traditions • Bear & Company, One Park Street, Rochester, VT 05767, and we will forward the communication.

Scan the QR code and save 25% at InnerTraditions.com.
Browse over 2,000 titles on spirituality, the occult, ancient mysteries, new science, holistic health, and natural medicine.

CranioSacral Therapy is both a highly intuitive art form and a highly scientific method.

DR. JOHN EDWIN UPLEDGER,
CRANIOSACRAL THERAPY II: BEYOND THE DURA

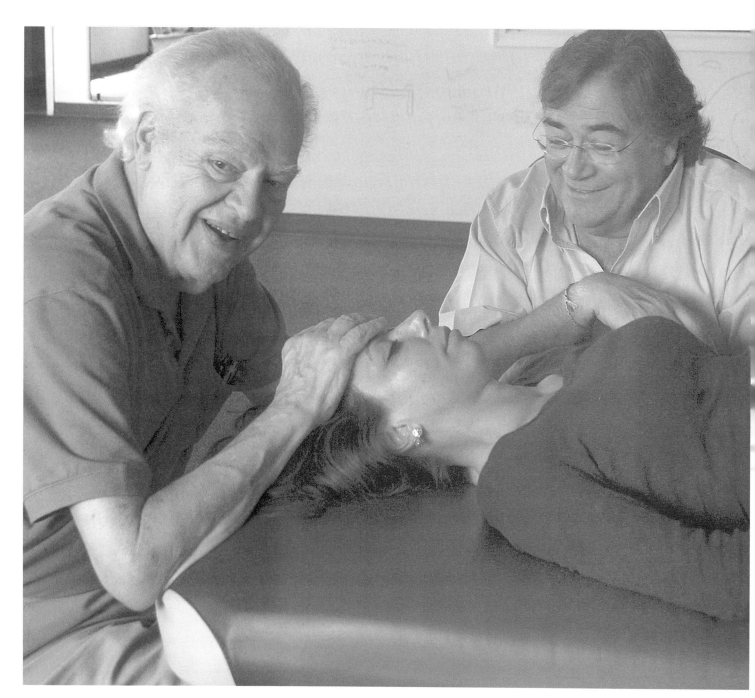

Dr. John E. Upledger and Dr. Diego Maggio

My thanks to

Dr. John Edwin Upledger (1932–2012), the man, the therapist, the Facilitator, the friend, who radically transformed my life and contributed with his own existence to transform the lives of thousands of other people who received, got to know, and learned CranioSacral Therapy (CST) and SomatoEmotional Release (SER).

John Matthew Upledger (1960–2017), to whom this book is dedicated. I consider him a role model for the determination he showed in every phase of his life, even the very last, and for the smile he always offered to others to infuse them with courage and gratitude to life. Ode to Life!

Dr. Patricia Quirini, who helped me translate my thoughts into didactic action with her essential working knowledge and her innate kindness and helpfulness.

Dr. Euro Piuca, who generously shared with me the results of his experience working with psychosynthesis.

Upledger Institute International, which allowed me to spread Dr. Upledger's therapeutic work worldwide and supported me in my role of CST and SER Instructor thanks to the quality and hard work of their team.

Last, but not least, a huge thank-you to Thea Keber for believing in me and encouraging me in this process. Since she had the honor to feel Dr. Upledger's touch, she could give me an active and indispensable support in the writing of this book, which I hope will contribute to making the world a touch better.

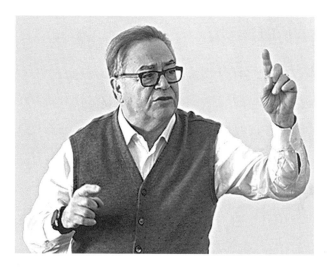

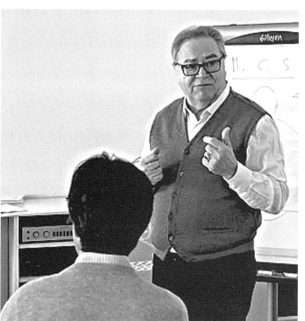

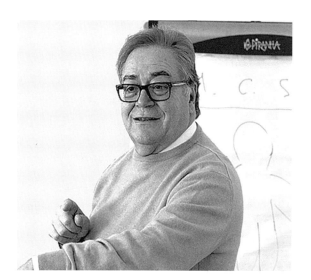

Dr. Diego Maggio teaching

Contents

PREFACE

Ode to Life   xv

INTRODUCTION

My Curriculum in This Life Cycle   1

CHAPTER 1

A Brief History of CranioSacral Therapy (CST)
and SomatoEmotional Release (SER)   9

CHAPTER 2

Life Cycle (*Cyclus Vitae*) Observations   17

CHAPTER 3

The Patient-Facilitator Relationship in CST   22

CHAPTER 4

Foundational Techniques:
A Synthesis of Knowledge   29

CHAPTER 5

Ego: Its Functions and Anomalies   46

CHAPTER 6

Biological Processes in the Life Cycle   54

CHAPTER 7

Separation and Loss: An Introduction   70

CHAPTER 8

Measuring Stressors:
The Holmes and Rahe Stress Scale   80

CHAPTER 9

Processing Emotions:
Using CST and SER for Integration and Release   91

CHAPTER 10

Constructive and Destructive Energy:
Harnessing Polarity for Transformation   103

CHAPTER 11

The Cerebral Hemispheres:
Connection and Harmonization   133

CHAPTER 12

Transformation:
The Concepts of Psychosynthesis   150

CHAPTER 13

Seats of Emotions: The Viscera and Meridians   172

CHAPTER 14

Small Deaths: Midrange Values on the Holmes
and Rahe Stress Scale   196

CHAPTER 15

Energetic Framework of the Human Body:
Assessing with the Vector/Axis System   207

CHAPTER 16

Chakras: Energetic Landmarks for
Mapping the Vector/Axis System   229

CHAPTER 17

CST and SER in Grief: Support for the Living   251

CHAPTER 18

Entropy and Syntropy:
Therapeutic Energy in CST and SER   279

CHAPTER 19

Major Stressors:
Critical Events on the Holmes and Rahe Stress Scale 297

CHAPTER 20

CST and SER in Death: Support for the Dying 309

CHAPTER 21

The Final Treatment:
The Origin of Techniques for Death and Transition 334

CHAPTER 22

Therapeutic Vibrations:
Harmonizing Energy Flow with Sound Frequencies 360

CHAPTER 23

Form of the Third Space:
Visualizing the Perception 381

CHAPTER 24

Mind-Body-Spirit Continuum:
Our Request to the Universe 405

CHAPTER 25

A Seven-Step Treatment for the Dying Process 421

CHAPTER 26

Ode to Life: Open-System Human Being 460

PARTING

Panta Rhei: **Everything Flows** 493

• • •

Acknowledgments 495

Notes 497

References 505

Figure Credits 517

Index 526

List of Exercises

Implementation of SQAR	30
Implementation of Arcing Technique	33
Implementation of the Significance Detector	36
Implementation of Therapeutic Imagery and Dialogue	39
Implementation of Balancing the Vector/Axis System	43
Self-Assessment Exercise	85
Polarity and Transformation Exercise	125
Direction of Energy Exercise	143
Self-Listening Direction of Energy Exercise	144
Meridian Emptying and Filling Technique	188
Energetic Visualization and Mobilization	221
Energetic Touch and Mobilization	222
Visualization, Assessment, and Mobilization of Vectors through the Chakras: Phase One	244
Visualization, Assessment, and Mobilization of Vectors through the Chakras: Phase Two	246
Nonverbal SER Technique	306
Personal Growth Exercise 1	322
Personal Growth Exercise 2	323
Technique for Respiratory Diaphragm Release	350
Technique for Thoracic Inlet Release	350
Perceiving Vibrations and Harmonizing Energy	375
Realigning Vectors Using the Third Space	397
Personal Growth Exercise: Understanding the Mind-Body-Spirit Continuum	454
Genealogical-Emotional Tree	466
Curriculum Vitae of the Vital Energy Continuum	470

A Note from the Editor

The author purposefully chose to include many voices from various types of authors throughout the text to allow you, the reader, to hear this array of theories, thoughts, and styles as if in conversation with friends or with several interesting people in order to both illuminate and enhance the topics at hand.

Throughout this book you will find a number of quotations, both long and short. Many of these, including several of the epigraphs that begin chapters and sections of text, are translated from texts originally in Italian or Italian versions of texts.

Quotations describing the techniques of CranioSacral Therapy (CST) and SomatoEmotional Release (SER) are included with the permission of Upledger Institute International.

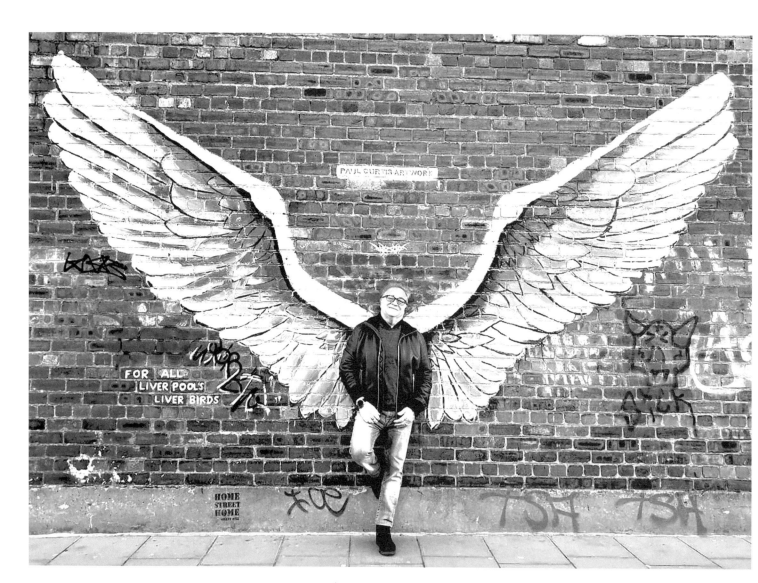

Dr. Diego Maggio in Liverpool

PREFACE
Ode to Life

I proposed the idea of this book after teaching a seminar titled "CranioSacral Therapy and Cyclus Vitae (Life Cycle): Separation, Death, and Loss" in 2018. That seminar itself was born from an explicit request made by John Matthew Upledger, son of Dr. John E. Upledger, the osteopathic physician who developed the practice of CranioSacral Therapy (CST). I was also inspired by my time spent learning from Dr. Upledger himself, who used to encourage his students to implement and develop CranioSacral Therapy with a sentence I will never forget: "We can make the world a touch better."

Though both the seminar and this book deal with topics like separation, death, and loss, they are meant to be an Ode to Life. You are probably wondering, *How is it possible to write (sing) an Ode to Life and, at the same time, address such topics?*

I can answer this question starting with the toughest subject—death, the great loss of losses. We do not experience death but indirectly. How, then, can we help someone going through the experience of death?

If we look to the biological evolution of our species, we see that we all have a cycle of time in which we are given the chance to revalue and complete some of what we might consider biological cycles, which trace the map of our entire Life Cycle, from birth to death.

In this complete and exclusive Life Cycle, many physical as well as emotional aspects interfere with our natural biological progression. Sometimes, they do it in so incisive a way that our biological functions change and accelerate, bringing us prematurely closer to the end of physical life.

Dr. Upledger told us, "CranioSacral Therapy is both a highly intuitive art form and a highly scientific modality." My favorite definition of art describes every aware gesture in our life as being a form of art. Therefore, in even one single instant of our lives, through intuition and/or experience, awareness becomes art.

This inference can help CST Facilitators understand and address the very delicate task of offering support to the dying and those around them, which CST teaches us can be accomplished by being present, warily and consciously listening to those who are going through this experience and, most of all, being grateful for the opportunity to assist and support the patient.

Even before that act, when we are simply contemplating the subjects of separation and death, we should remember that, as Dr. Upledger said, "The body is in an organized dysfunction; therefore, we have to disintegrate the dysfunction and ask it to reorganize." By bringing to our awareness the various reasons that frustrated—and are frustrating—our Biological Process, we will be able to evaluate what is inhibiting our well-being. In light of this awareness, we will also be able to work on destructive processes and modify and transform them into elements that can be useful for the constructive processes within our lives.

In this way, we can use Dr. Upledger's techniques and visionary genius to make "a touch better" both our own life and the lives of those who share a part of it with us, ask us for help, or are already part of our lives and need us to be there for them in situations of inevitable transformation of their Life Cycle.

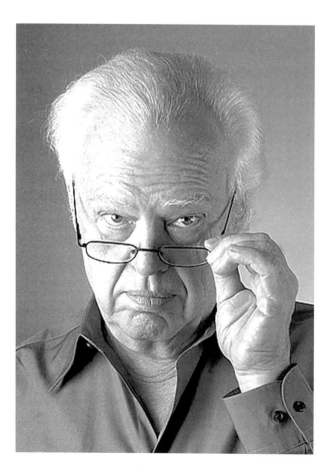

Dr. John E. Upledger

INTRODUCTION
My Curriculum in This Life Cycle

My name is Diego Maggio, and I am convinced that *everything happens for a reason.*

This concept is not so obvious until we truly realize, consciously and serenely, that even if sometimes the meaning of what we are living eludes us, everything gets clearer in time.

A proof of that is the life path I have followed to end up here, and today I expect my journey through life (and beyond) to continue as exuberantly as it has done so far. This does not mean it is and has been without obstacles and hard times or that I wish it would be, but only that I hope it continues to be overflowing with liveliness, always different and always new. If you think about it, it is the same for all of us.

Why all these premises?

Because it is fair that I introduce myself to the reader, and also because you will find among the chapters of this book several clinical observations about cases I was presented with. While you will find these cases under the title "Clinical Observations," I actually prefer to call the accounts of my encounters with some of my greatest teachers—my patients—"memoranda."

Anyway, it must be said that before these encounters, I had come a long way.

GOING THROUGH SEPARATION AND ABANDONMENT

I could say that, for me, everything starts with a separation culminating with a loss (which fits perfectly with the subjects of this book). At age seven, after the separation of my parents, I ended up essentially without a family. My mother remained in Italy, where I had been born, and my father left for Germany to live there and search for a job. At the time, neither of them was actually able to take care of my upbringing and basic needs.

Before turning eight, due to my mother's financial situation, I was urged to be "creative" in order to rustle up some money when she was unemployed. My creativity led me to knock on doors and sing a song to anyone who would open the door. Must I admit it? I enjoyed it!

I enjoyed seeing that people appreciated what I was doing and gave me their approval in the form of money I could bring home. To tell you the truth, the idea that I was actually asking for charity never crossed my mind. On the contrary, I thought my audience appreciated my singing skills.

My precocious artistic career was at some point interrupted because my mum brought me to an orphanage, where I lived until I was about twelve. But music always stayed in my blood and determined some of my most important choices later in life.

In the years I spent in the orphanage, I inevitably learned how to be independent, even on an emotional level, and to see life as something that can be turned upside down at any time. I figured that one must be ready to accept any change as a challenge worth the fight to face it and overcome it.

That mindset allowed me to take on almost enthusiastically the need to become an adult as soon as possible. It brought me to undertake singular adventures and experience new things that, at the time (the early 1960s), my generation was not generally experiencing.

LOSS AS OPPORTUNITY

Still following my passion for music, I chose to emancipate when I was a teenager, momentarily leaving behind my fragile family ties, aware that I could lose them for good. I set my mind on living my life . . . in the city of the Beatles!

It was 1966, the era of "flower power," the protests against the Vietnam War, and the motto "Make love not war!" I arrived in Liverpool mostly by hitchhiking—except for the route I traveled by train and ferry from the Gare du Nord in Paris to Victoria Station in London. Emotionally speaking, that journey was one of the most intense and important passages between two phases of my Life Cycle.

I believe it was because of the emotional excitement I was feeling that, when crossing the Channel from Calais on the French coast to Dover on the English coast, I was able to elicit the sympathy of the British official who was on duty on the ferryboat. He was issuing the permits to enter the country, and when he asked me why I was there at seventeen (a minor!) by myself and with no one waiting for me in England, I answered him confidently in my broken English, something like, "I am a student of English language and I go to Liverpool to see the Beatles." I probably sounded so bold and improbable that I amused the official into giving me a one-month residence permit.

I actually stayed in Liverpool for thirty years. I learned English by working during the day and going to pubs and discos at night. My first job was waiting tables. I then became a nightclub bouncer thanks to my black belt in karate. Leaving behind tens of jobs, either by my choice or my employer's, I always took the opportunities I was given. Thanks to the experience and mental elasticity I had developed in order to adapt to constant changes—even when they were forced on me—I participated in a wide variety of contests, with the intention of improving my working position. I ended up with an invitation from the prime minister, Margaret Thatcher, to a lunch offered by the historic Lancaster House. That happened on the occasion of the award ceremony for the best projects submitted to the "Fit for Work" contest about employment opportunities for people with disabilities, organized by the English newspaper the *Times*.

(CONSTRUCTIVE) LIFE CHANGES

My first contact with the world of therapists happened thanks to my first wife, Ann. When we got married, I was nineteen and she was about to enter the Children's Hospital of Liverpool as a pediatric nurse, having just concluded her apprenticeship. Through Ann's everyday work and the anecdotes she told me about it, I indirectly learned about hospital protocols, the occurrences of the night shifts in the wards, the best ways to take care of young patients and interact with their relatives, the importance of the therapeutic gesture, and, most of all, the importance of offering a smile to those who suffer and looking at them directly and empathetically, without ever losing the capacity for taking action. These were all things that Ann was able to master perfectly.

I had a son, Stefano, with Ann. I was barely twenty when I became a father. I could not have imagined it, but his birth started the greatest transformation of my life. I do not say that only because children obviously turn everyday life upside down. It was because the drive Stefano gave me through his life choices is why I am now an osteopath and a CranioSacral therapist and Instructor.

Through numerous life experiences together, my son became the catalyst of my professional career. It was thanks to him that I became aware of what I really wanted to do in my life, how I wanted to express myself, what the actual skills were that I could develop, and how I could find the means and the energy to start to transform my life all over again.

THE VISION BEGINS

My new life started thirty-five years ago when I enrolled twelve-year-old Stefano in the Southport Cycling Club of Merseyside, just outside the center of Liverpool. I wanted to take care of him and his physical well-being, so I answered a magazine ad placed by the British Cycling Federation. The ad announced the first course for "Soigneurs"—sports masseurs in cycling. That is how, on February 19, 1989, at the age of forty-one, I started a new profession as a sports masseur for the British Cycling Federation. From that moment on, I understood that manual therapy was to be my profession.

During my internship as a sports masseur, my teacher, Warren Hudson, who was also an osteopath, caused me to take interest in osteopathy thanks to his peculiar working method. The amount of study and work looked challenging, but the opportunity to attend the School of Osteopathy was given me once again by Stefano, although unconsciously, since he had decided to abandon competitive cycling for the love of young Hellen Edgerton, thus setting me free from the commitment to follow his sports activity.

That is when I started to learn this subject and enrolled at the Northern Counties School of Osteopathy, whose chancellor at that time was the renowned osteopath Harry Haws. On January 11, 1992, I obtained my diploma in osteopathy.

At the end of my studies in this field, while I was already working as an osteopath in my own clinic, an Irish colleague of mine, Mary Kennedy O'Brian, encouraged me to take part in the first CST seminar, which was about to take place in Edinburgh, Scotland.

MY FIRST EXPERIENCES WITH CRANIOSACRAL THERAPY

In that first CST seminar, I discovered a whole new world. I was immersed in so many different elements all melding together. It was a fusion between the art of therapy and science, between intuition and perseverance. It was exactly my way of seeing and living life.

After I completed the second level of CST, it was again Mary Kennedy O'Brian who presented me with the opportunity to participate in a therapy session with Dr. Upledger, physician, osteopath, acupuncturist, and founder of CST. The session was to take place in a hospital in Dublin, where we would have to treat one of Dr. Upledger's patients who was in a vegetative coma. The patient's name was Bryan. I did not need to be asked twice; having the chance to participate seemed like winning the jackpot to me, and more so because I knew that Dr. Upledger preferred staying in America and had not been traveling to Europe in the past years.

I met Dr. Upledger at the Beaumont Hospital of Dublin in 1994. I worked as his assistant for a week, side by side with him, his wife Lisa, Mary Kennedy O'Brian, and another colleague of ours, Brian Walker.

While I was assisting Dr. Upledger and participating in the treatments, I felt very awkward because the patient's body did not move at all except for the eyelids. I was used to working biomechanically, and I had only recently gotten to know CST techniques, which use a very light five-gram touch. Up until that moment I had not even implemented nonverbal dialogue with my patients. Therefore, I could not connect energetically with Bryan.

On the last day of our work, as we headed into the ward where Bryan was, we were welcomed enthusiastically by the other patients and the nurses of the ward. They were all extremely euphoric. In that moment, I thought Bryan must have awakened from the coma. And yet when I went and stood next to him and looked at him, he appeared to be in the exact same condition as he had been the previous days.

Dr. Upledger, on the contrary, actually saw some change. As he started to treat him, he asked, "Bryan, do you feel physical pain? If you like, blink once to say no and twice to say yes." Bryan blinked once.

I was getting goose bumps from emotion and surprise.

As the treatment continued, Dr. Upledger proceeded to ask Bryan, "May it be that you're sad we're leaving tomorrow?" Bryan then blinked several times and started crying. As he did so, I was treating him from the feet station, and I cried too.

That experience shook me. I realized that both Dr. Upledger and the patient had taught me that I would have been able to perceive the "voice" of people's souls if I had learned to touch their bodies with love.

On that last evening in Dublin, after we left the patient, I had the chance to speak with Dr. Upledger alone—and that occasion would definitively impact and revolutionize my perspective on reality in a way that I never could have even dared to imagine before. In the middle of our conversation, which was mostly made up of my questions to Dr. Upledger and his answers to me, he asked me very calmly and lightheartedly whether I remembered that we used to be friends in ancient Greece.

I had obviously heard about metempsychosis (the transmigration of the soul), but I had never considered it as an actual possibility. I certainly had never thought I would hear a physician and researcher such as Dr. Upledger talk about it in such terms. And yet he was talking about it very straightforwardly. In the rest of the time I would spend with him afterward, I would see how open his mind was to many other ideas, philosophies, theories, and experimentations.

Anyway, in Dublin I had to admit to him that, no, until that moment I honestly had never even taken into account the possibility of a previous life! Reflecting on his thought, I told him that if he believed we had been friends a long time before, then we could be friends again in the present time. And that is what happened in the next years.

. . . AND BEYOND

Dr. Upledger encouraged me to continue my studies in CST and SER, investigate these subjects further, and become an Instructor. In just one year I completed the whole didactic path, and in April 1995 Dr. Upledger himself asked me to stay in America and work at Upledger Institute International as an osteopath and CranioSacral therapist.

I was obviously flattered by his offer. I was not married anymore, and my son was now an independent adult, but after living thirty years in England I had the desire to go back to Italy, where I had been born. I therefore made him an offer of my own and asked him whether he thought it a good idea to found an Upledger Institute International in Italy, where there were no institutions authorized to teach his method, as opposed to other countries. He said yes.

To be honest, after all that time abroad, it was not easy to get used to the Italian environment again. Many changes had occurred during my thirty-year absence, including the rise of new social complexities and a shift to a bureaucracy that was much more complicated than the Anglo-Saxon one. Even the spoken language had become almost foreign to me, and I had trouble speaking fluently.

My good fortune, however, allowed me to meet many people who, either by helping me or by trying to undermine me, got me closer and closer to the realization of my project. I came into contact with so many people through the years that I would not be able to name them all without filling every page of this book. Thanks to them, I have never given up hope, and I transformed every input (whether it was negative/destructive or positive/constructive) into a further step toward my objective.

Anna Chiara Bosi, who later became an Upledger Instructor, was certainly one of the positive connections I had. Moreover, she was a speech therapist who had also undergone training in shiatsu, so it was through her that I got closer to the world of therapists practicing what in Italy is called the "well-being techniques."

We both moved to Trieste, my hometown, after living some time in Padua, the first city I had lived in after my return to Italy. It was in Trieste that I actually took a big leap forward—moving many more steps ahead in my Life Cycle—in the direction of what I am doing now.

EVOLVING

In the meantime, I continued to study and received the qualification to teach all the basic levels of CST and SER, plus some advanced specialized levels.

I also got my degree in osteopathy—a step that Dr. Upledger had suggested during our first meeting in Dublin, after I had introduced myself as a qualified osteopath. A couple years after moving to Italy, my dear British friend Philip Thomas, who is an osteopath as well, told me about a degree program in osteopathy at the Westminster University in London that was meant for professionals who had practiced at least within the last six years. I decided to take the chance I was given.

I was encouraged during this time by my second wife, Thea, who founded with

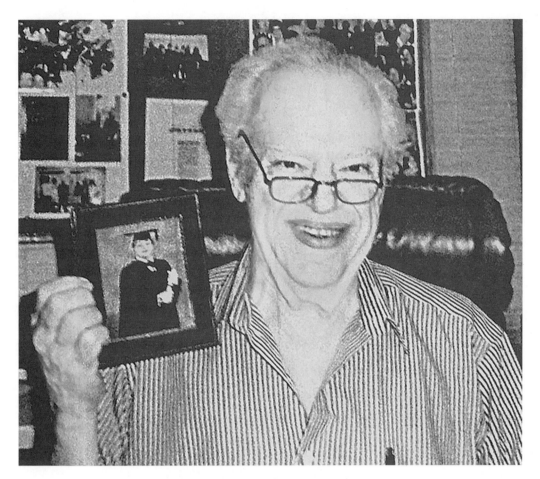

Fig. I.1. Dr. Upledger holding a photograph of Diego Maggio's graduation in 2008.

me Upledger Italia—Accademia Cranio-Sacrale in 2003 and still manages it today as copresident. More encouragement came from my student and friend Liana Bertolazzi, who worked in the research group led by Dr. Rita Levi Montalcini. I submitted my thesis, received my bachelor of science (with honors) degree at the age of fifty-nine, and went to England to attend the ceremony at Westminster University.

I sent the picture of my graduation to Dr. Upledger and my friend Philip Thomas, who put it on display in his living room. What moved me even more was knowing that the same picture was on Dr. Upledger's desk during the very last years of his life.

BETWEEN GRIEF AND REVELATION

At the end of his life, Dr. Upledger could remember very few people, and I was one of them. When he died, his son John Matthew asked me to create a new seminar for Upledger Institute International, which he was managing. The subject was peculiar.

It was supposed to be a seminar about loss, separation, bereavement, death, and abandonment.

It was an unusual topic for a CST seminar, and yet it was such a common theme in people's lives. I was reassured by the fact that this subject had been dealt with by a colleague of mine, but John Matthew explicitly told me that I needed to do something completely new.

As I was conceiving the seminar, John Matthew passed away too, after a long illness. He was always able to offer a smile to others up until the very last phase of his life. It was this unstoppable vitality of his that encouraged me the most to develop this seminar in a new modality, as he meant it to be. I tried to make it a chance to transform every single phase of people's Life Cycles in which loss, bereavement, separation, abandonment, or death occur into an Ode to Life, something we sometimes forget to express. CranioSacral Therapy helped me do that.

THE ENERGY CONTINUUM NEVER STOPS

Right now, as I am writing this book, I have just turned seventy, and I am well esteemed by many and disregarded by many others. I am currently pondering the possibility of teaching my seminar worldwide in all the Upledger institutes, and once again I am not alone in this reflection. I have the support of Upledger Institute International through Dawn Langnes Shear, Kathy Woll, and Alex Jozefyk, all of whom take care of its management, and the approval of my fellow Instructors.

I linger on the thought of sharing my joy serenely with my son and narrating my experiences to Dante and Luca, my amazing grandchildren, reminding myself not to feed my Ego. What is yet to happen will surely amaze me—for better or worse—since anyone who lived and is living knows that in each and every moment reality can be more incredible and fruitful than any fantasy. It can overcome any conceivable boundary over the course of one, a hundred, or a thousand Life Cycles, transforming at each step what we think is permanent.

CHAPTER 1

A Brief History of CranioSacral Therapy (CST) and SomatoEmotional Release (SER)

The diseases that escape the heart devour the body.
HIPPOCRATES OF KOS

In order to understand Dr. Upledger's work and get to know SomatoEmotional Release (SER), a further evolution of CranioSacral Therapy (CST) and also the greatest innovation in the field of manual therapies, a brief historical background is needed.

THE DEVELOPMENT OF CRANIOSACRAL THERAPY

Dr. Upledger (1932–2012) was a physician and acupuncturist known all over the world for being the founder of CST. He started his studies analyzing the work of Dr. Andrew T. Still (1828–1917), who is considered the father of osteopathy, and continued his research in the field of cranial osteopathy by developing the theories of Dr. William G. Sutherland (1873–1954) to prove their validity.

It is perhaps best to start with some of Dr. Still's fundamental concepts that fascinated Dr. Upledger so much:

- The body is a unit.
- Structure and function are interconnected.
- The body is a self-corrective mechanism.

Dr. Still's osteopathy practice took into account the entire skeleton except for the skull, which he considered to be a compact bony structure. Dr. Sutherland, on the other hand, upon observing a disarticulated skull model, proposed that all the cranial bones could move, not just the mandible, as was commonly believed. Dr. Sutherland

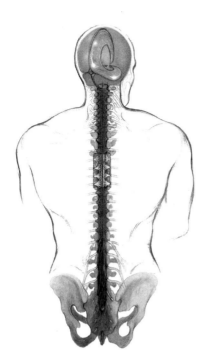

Fig. 1.1. The craniosacral system

undertook research to demonstrate this theory, and in 1931 he published an article about it, titled "Skull Motion." He was opposed, however, by the majority of the medical and academic world of the time, exactly as had happened to Dr. Still before him and would happen to Dr. Upledger after them both.

More than forty years after the publication of "Skull Motion" (more precisely, from 1975 to 1980), Dr. Upledger undertook research to demonstrate the validity of Dr. Sutherland's theory about the movements of the skull. The University of Michigan gave him the responsibility of leading a team of twenty-two other researchers for that purpose. At the end of this research, not only did Dr. Upledger establish that cranial bones move, but he, along with the other researchers, found vascularization, innervation, and connective tissue supporting their claim.

That was only the first step. From that moment on, Dr. Upledger revolutionized Dr. Sutherland's field. Once Dr. Upledger had proved that the skull has its own movement, he could show the results of his studies in the scientific academic world and explain why, through his discoveries, it was possible to develop cranial osteopathy. He continued to develop this field, including both theoretical studies and practical implementation, until it took shape as a new manual therapy, which he called CranioSacral Therapy.

It is necessary to make a short but essential clarification about CST in order to help those who study manual therapies understand why this method has been presented as an innovative technique since it came to life. As an example, let us analyze Dr. Sutherland's perspective on the sphenoid bone.

Dr. Sutherland was convinced that the sphenobasilar joint is a symphysis and, consequently, that all the lesions the sphenoid might be subjected to would be primary lesions. Dr. Upledger noted that histologically this joint is actually a synchondrosis until between fourteen and eighteen years of age. Thereafter the spheno-occipital complex fuses as one bone, but it still has inherent mobility due to the make up of bone, which allows for movement. Therefore, not all the lesions of the sphenoid can be primary; some of them must necessarily be secondary. Even just knowing this fact allows any therapist's work to be more focused, precise, and effective.

Dr. Upledger also introduced other new therapeutic concepts and techniques to enrich his work, including the following:

- the "Pressurestat Model," a theory that illustrates a mechanism behind the circulation of cerebrospinal fluid through the semiclosed, hydraulic craniosacral system, helping to explain its palpable, rhythmic expansion and contraction. This theory was useful in the development and teaching of CST, and current physiological knowledge has helped to revise this theory with additional mechanisms for what we feel in the body in regard to movement in the craniosacral system. The application of CST remains the same, we just have further understanding of the connections between CST and health of the body.
- the "Direction of Energy," a technique that allows you to harmonize the energy vibrations that are present in the body.
- the noninvasive five-gram palpation during treatment.

Nonetheless, on several occasions Dr. Upledger described his theories while mentioning Sutherland's model as an example, and that is not by chance. As the enlightened therapist he was, Dr. Upledger was in fact perfectly aware that citing the model of another physician in order to develop and surpass it can be a way to induce other researchers to do the same. In time, other people would feel encouraged to mention his own model while working to transform and develop it as well. This is what we see today with new theories being developed as science has learned more about the functioning of the craniosacral system and the brain.

Dr. Upledger wanted to give others the chance to develop theories by studying and researching models, both in allopathic medicine and through various holistic techniques. His intentions were always to create a new paradigm that could be shared and spread to help people's well-being.

After the foundation of CST had been laid, Dr. Upledger helped develop another and even more peculiar innovation in the field of manual therapies. Since he was a researcher but also, and more importantly, a therapist, he had ample clinical observations, which eventually brought him to consider and identify a new fundamental component of therapy. Keeping in mind that everyone manages emotions differently, Dr. Upledger noticed that his patients' individual emotional responses had a great influence on their physical bodies. Working from this observation, he developed a new therapeutic approach: SomatoEmotional Release.

THE DEVELOPMENT OF SOMATOEMOTIONAL RELEASE

SomatoEmotional Release is the natural evolution of CranioSacral Therapy. It serves as a key to open the door of our consciousness in our path to well-being and as an aid to address and solve several problems and dysfunctions that are otherwise hard to treat.

Dr. Upledger proposed that therapy sessions devoted to working on the whole body (physical and emotional) could help patients deal with emotional issues more efficiently than sessions devoted to separate parts and dysfunctions. His clinical experiences confirmed his theory, inspiring his pioneering work in the release of somatic and emotional issues. He called this form of therapy SomatoEmotional Release (and we will mostly call it by its acronym, SER, for reasons of brevity).

SER is a process that helps identify and release the emotional component connected with the residual effects of an underlying trauma and the symptoms it provokes. In addition, the technique is used as a means to promote cooperation between patient and therapist, with the objective of bringing maximum improvement to the patient's state of health with each treatment.

SER is based on the direct, noninvasive palpation techniques of CST, including the listening techniques and the techniques to perceive the craniosacral rhythm (CSR). It seeks interaction with the patient in a welcoming context and without any mediation of external means. Its implementation is carried out through simple CST procedures that can give immediate comfort to the patient and allow the therapist to have a different approach. In fact, the therapist should be able to understand the patient's verbal signals as well as nonverbal signals transmitted by the patient's body, even when a patient has difficulty with oral communication, like in the case of sensory and/or neurological deficit. This particular type of approach can be adopted even in preverbal pediatric contexts and when language barriers constitute an obstacle between therapist and patient.

In his research to develop and refine SER, Dr. Upledger went through neuroscientist Paul D. MacLean's triune brain model and took into account its main components (neural network, reptilian brain, limbic system, and neocortex), the reticular activating/alarm system (RAS), the temporomandibular joints, and the functions of the trigeminal nerve within the RAS. He analyzed all the emotional stimuli and the various cerebral areas they involve. He studied atomic particles and quantum physics.

He elaborated the concept of Energy Cysts to connect physical and emotional trauma. He considered the different aspects of trauma, including the environmental context. He drew upon his knowledge of Carl Gustav Jung's analytical psychology and Roberto Assagioli's psychosynthesis. And he examined perception and reasoning (problem-solving) skills through the concepts of learning, memory, thought, and social psychology derived from Fritz Perls's theories of Gestalt psychology.

Let us stop here with what might appear to be a mere list of the studies carried out by Dr. Upledger, since it is more useful to introduce a tool that can help all therapists treat patients on their paths toward self-healing. In fact, we are now going to analyze the main concept that SER is based on: discovering how emotions can transform the body, contribute to disease or healing, preserve health, or weaken the organism.

CST, SER, AND ENERGY CYSTS

In order to understand how the body might react to physical or emotional trauma by retaining its memory in tissues on a cellular level, we must explore the subject of Energy Cysts. They are, as described by Dr. Upledger, spots where entropic energy, which is disorganized energy (see the second law of thermodynamics), gathers in tissues, creating obstructions in the flow of energy. Energy Cysts develop in people's bodies after physical and/or emotional trauma, which can have its origin in pathogens, viruses, spiritual issues, et cetera. The emotional component connected to trauma inhibits the correct flow of vital energy, often affecting the craniosacral rhythm by changing its optimal symmetry, quality, amplitude, and rate (SQAR) and therefore also the craniosacral system.

Basically, Energy Cysts influence the individual's entire homeostasis. Homeostasis is the natural tendency common to all living organisms to reach relative stability, both in the internal chemical and physical aspects and in behavior. This dynamic regime normally continues over time through self-regulating mechanisms, even when the external conditions change.

CST and SER help dissipate (release) Energy Cysts, which are identified initially through various assessment techniques, such as the Significance Detector and Arcing, which allow the CST and SER therapist to perceive/detect the Energy Cysts in the patient's body.

Once detected, the Energy Cyst can be treated through touch. After perceiving the fascial restriction where an Energy Cyst is located, for example, the practitioner may notice that the craniosacral rhythm appears to stop. This is the signal of the Significance Detector, which indicates the presence of emotional trauma connected to pain or dysfunction. At this point, the Facilitator can start a dialogue with the patient, a technique Dr. Upledger called "Therapeutic Imagery and Dialogue."

This particular dialogue is a conversation with the patient's Higher Self—or "non-conscious" or "Inner Physician," as Dr. Upledger defines it in his book *Your Inner Physician and You.*

An Energy Cyst can often release during the implementation of the assessment methods, as the Facilitator's hands "listen" to the fascial modification occurring in the patient's organism. The detection of fascial restrictions leads to the identification of the organs or physiological systems that are suffering and therefore gives the Facilitator the chance to treat them accordingly.

In other cases, it is necessary to empathize with the patient through an unconventional type of language. One of these languages, and its respective techniques, is based on sensory integration, which involves the five senses.

Facilitators can choose the method to use, relying on their own perception of the signals received from the patient's Inner Physician. During the treatment session, most people experience visualizations and others experience bodily sensations, taste memories, olfactory memories, auditory perceptions, et cetera. Sound, for example, is considered a universal language, and that is why it is one of the possible languages used with the techniques described in this book.

Let us try to imagine Energy Cysts as physical spots in our organism, located on one of the energy channels, such as the meridians of traditional Chinese medicine, or within one of the organs of the physical body, such as the liver or spleen.

Just like a stone dropped into water, an Energy Cyst emits circular concentric waves with a point of origin. The vortex the Energy Cyst creates can spread in the organism from the inside to the surface of the body. An analogous phenomenon that might come spontaneously to mind is the visual perception of wave propagation. It is possible to draw a parallel between the vortex of waves from the Energy Cyst and the diffusion of electromagnetic and sound waves (you will find a scientific explanation of these concepts later on in this book). The vortex created by the Energy Cyst interferes with the normal energy flow. Its waves have a movement, an amplitude, and an intensity of their own, and they are linked to various frequencies.

Let us take the case of sound, the most adequate language to dialogue with the patient's non-conscious. The therapist might detect dissonant vibrations created by Energy Cysts and their vortexes in the overall harmony of the patient's organism or, even better, identify the organ or physiological system that sounds disharmonic in the dysfunction.

To go a little more into detail, here are the precise characteristics of Energy Cysts as provided in the study of CST and SER:

- They are found in the patient's head or body in correspondence to one of the lines of the energy vectors.

- Within the vector/axis system (the energetic framework of the person), the vector line along which an Energy Cyst is located allows us to identify a certain organ or physiological system that is suffering.
- The cause for the suffering of that organ or system is attributable to the consequences of a physical and/or emotional trauma.
- Trauma causes anomalous symptoms that can be detected in a specific area of the physiological system, altering the entire homeostasis of the individual.

PREPARING TO LEARN

When Dr. John E. Upledger wrote the study guide for his first class on CranioSacral Therapy, he chose to quote various authors, using these quotes as aphorisms to introduce the "new world" within which the therapists would delve. It was his desire to help therapists understand that in order to study, understand, and practice his method, they would have to cross a new frontier, using a particular "pass," which if it had been printed would have had the inscription: "Be willing to change their minds about their certainties and always keep an open mind."

In fact, Dr. Upledger knew that in this new world of CranioSacral Therapy there would be no place for those who were not willing to change the view that they had of themself before proposing to clients the change that leads to self-healing. Rather than subtracting from their existing knowledge or skills, keeping this open mind would serve to build upon them.

Dr. Upledger began his study guide by citing Stephen R. Covey (1932–2012), the American educator and entrepreneur, and the book Covey published in 1989 that made him famous all over the world, *The 7 Habits of Highly Effective People: Powerful Lessons in Personal Change:* "Each of us tends to think we see things as they are, that we are objective. But this is not the case. We see the world, not as it is, but as we are—or as we are conditioned to see it."[1]

Dr. Upledger then proposed the concept of a "belief system"—a frame of reference based on a feeling of certainty. He cited Tony Robbins (1960–), author, motivational trainer, and expert in neurolinguistic programming, who teaches about the theory of the six basic needs of a person, and who facilitated his own self-healing from a pituitary gland adenoma: "Remember, as long as you believe something, your brain operates on automatic pilot, filtering any input from the environment and searching for references to validate your belief, regardless of what it is. . . . People with beliefs have such a strong level of certainty that they are often closed off to new input."[2]

Dr. Upledger defined his educational seminars as experiential, saying that the "efficiency factor" of his trainings was due to providing knowledge of the subject and also a conscious action that would, in time, lead to wisdom.

BETWEEN ART AND SCIENCE: THE VITRUVIAN MAN

CranioSacral Therapy is both a highly intuitive art form and a highly scientific modality.

Dr. John E. Upledger,
CranioSacral Therapy II: Beyond the Dura

The *Vitruvian Man* (fig. 1.2 below), by Leonardo da Vinci, represents the union of art and science. This masterpiece seems a visual depiction of Dr. Upledger's statement given above.

The man in this image is contained within two geometrical figures, the circle and the square, which the Greek philosopher Plato said were "perfect" shapes. These geometrical structures surrounding the image of the man represent creation: the square stands for Earth, and the circle stands for the universe. The man's relation to the two figures is absolutely proportional, symbolizing the perfect nature of the creation of man in harmony with Earth and the universe.

The name *Vitruvian* was given to this image as a tribute to Vitruvius, an architect and writer of ancient Rome who is considered to be the most famous architecture theorist of all time.

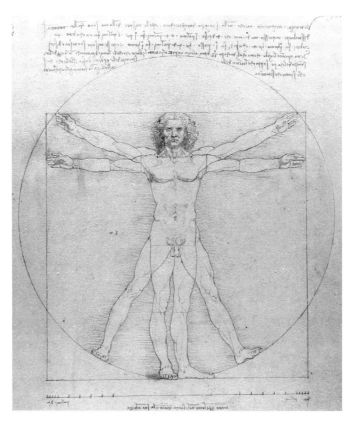

Fig. 1.2. *Vitruvian Man,* by Leonardo da Vinci

CHAPTER 2
Life Cycle (Cyclus Vitae) Observations

The soma is a vehicle and an organ of intellect and soul.

PLATO, *PHILEBUS*

Human beings are open systems, energy units undergoing a constant cycle of exchange with the environment in an effort to maintain homeostasis. The human organism as a whole includes all types of structures, from the subatomic particle to the anatomical and physiological unit. Its potential manifests itself throughout the entire Life Cycle, from birth to death.

As described in chapter 1, the holistic concept of the human body elaborated by Dr. Andrew T. Still fascinated Dr. Upledger, who expanded and developed Dr. Still and, after him, Dr. Sutherland's subject, further exploring the potentiality of the human body as an open system and its energetic balance inside the existential Cycle of Life, to the point of creating a new manual therapy—CranioSacral Therapy (CST).

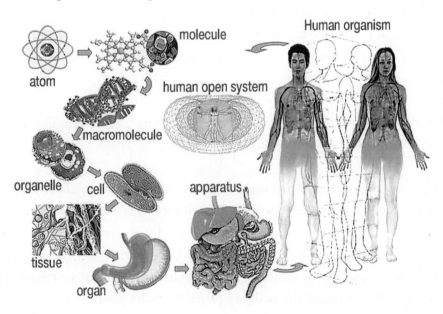

Fig. 2.1. From atom to human being: an introduction to the Life Cycle

Dr. Upledger was the first physician to introduce the concept of a physical dysfunction being fed by an energetically destructive component. On this premise, he built a new therapeutic approach that is complementary to CST—SomatoEmotional Release (SER).

EURYTHMY OF SOMATOEMOTIONAL RELEASE

This path through known scenarios toward unknown destinations starts from an examination of the peculiarities of SER and the complementary and mutual nature of its connections with CST.

The first points of this discourse are the methodology and the objective of SER. In order to examine them, it is necessary to understand the process that allows an interaction between therapeutic methods—with CST being the preferred methodology—and the interaction between the Facilitator and the person being treated.

SER works as a support to the functionality of the organism within the relations between the physiological systems of our bodies. For instance, it acts upon the central parasympathetic nervous system, inducing relaxation and therefore acting upon the fascial restrictions and tensions. It helps the patient with pathologies that affect both organs and functions through:

- promotion of closeness and listening between the Facilitator and the patient
- promotion of lower levels of anxiety
- restoration of psychophysical well-being
- resolution of psychosomatic disorders
- reduction of clinically relevant symptoms
- rebalance and restoration of the abilities of the central, peripheral, and autonomic nervous systems
- faster resolution of functional deficits and physical pain
- identification of the emotional aspect connected with a pathological event
- detection of autonomic nervous reactions

Upon evaluating the emotional component associated with the physical trauma, the Facilitator implements SER through specific techniques that are meant to assess and release physical impediments caused by an emotional trauma—the Energy Cysts. In fact, clinical observation and experience suggest that Energy Cysts sometimes manifest themselves as an anomalous or distal symptom consequent to an impairment of the patient's physical ability to dissipate trauma and thus pain.

SER uses specific whole-body assessment techniques that allow us to identify and then neutralize Energy Cysts and the symptoms connected to them. You will find later in this book a more detailed examination of some of these evaluation techniques, such as the Significance Detector (connected with an image, thought, or unsolicited sensation), Arcing, and Therapeutic Imagery and Dialogue.

The principles and the practice of the dialogue between the Facilitator and the patient, the integration of postural assessments, the introduction to the theory of vectors as applied and connected to the analysis of the energetic framework of the body in the vector/axis system, and the interactive relationship between various techniques and functional evaluations are all elements that meld into a eurhythmic synthesis giving birth to SER.

The techniques and assessment methods of SER are meant to recognize and treat the somatic manifestations connected to the emotional part of the physical trauma. They are based on the same knowledge and training that are needed when dealing with the craniosacral system, its morphofunctional organization, and the methods used to restore functionality on a systemic/homeostatic level.

SER can lead to a correct clinical analysis of the patient, which is a fundamental requirement for choosing the most adequate therapeutic option. It also allows the Facilitator to train in the type of approach that is effective within the therapist/patient relationship to acquire the proper level of control in the treatment process. In SER, the technical implementation of neurobiological notions highlights the key role of multidisciplinarity in the advancement of knowledge about functional restoration.

In order to improve SER communication abilities, and consequently guarantee the efficiency, adequacy, and safety of the assistance the patient receives, the Facilitator must take into account not only Jungian psychology—the activity of the unconscious in particular, which is defined as non-conscious in the context of SER—but also Gestalt psychology, or the psychology of form, and Assagioli's psychosynthesis psychology, which considers human personality as an all-inclusive concept. The Facilitator must also convert the concepts of each approach into manual therapeutic gestures. The process of listening to the patient and acquiring information about them occurs both verbally and through the aptonomic language of touch. This certainly determines a higher level of humanization in treatments and improves the Facilitator's competencies, technical skills, behavior, and therapeutic action.

Through the deeply layered methodology of SER and the listening and understanding of the body language of CST, the complementary reciprocity of Facilitator and patient is offered both as an incentive to their cooperation and as a tool for the individual who is in pain to get the best from the therapy.

SER AND THE APTONOMIC TOUCH

The term *aptonomy* derives from two Greek words: *hapsis,* "touch," and *nomos,* "rule." We know that touch is the foundation of sensory perception and is experienced through contact and tactile sensitivity, exactly as we know that touch is the sense connected to the skin and the surface of the body. It is sometimes defined as "the most ancient sense" for its ability to establish a type of knowledge that is extremely deep and immediate.

For instance, touch is essential in the first deep cognitive contact between a mother and her newborn baby. It maintains its importance during the whole Life Cycle for its function in recognizing closeness, affection, relationships, and especially respect, attention, and care when dealing with elderly or ill people.

Noninvasive touch allows us to consider individuals through their bodies, but even more through their corporeality, which is expressed by sensations, feelings, and emotions. SER is actually the technique to rely on when it is necessary to manage those sensations, feelings, and emotions, while always remembering to use the correct approach toward the patient.

Another important observation is connected to the role that the skin plays in touch and somatic reactions when the external environment and the inside of the human organism are interacting. There are substantial proofs indicating that touch is involved in the functioning of the immune system and skin is involved in the expression of immune response. Some evidence suggests that the immune system, the nervous system, and the endocrine system are physiologically integrated.

Current research in neuroscience has made a fundamental conceptual turn. It is clear that mind-body functions are regulated by chemical agents and neurotransmitters that influence the immune system and consequently the other systems of the organism. Among these substances are the neuropeptides (endorphins), which carry out a key role in the complexity of the hormonal balance. Neuropeptides (endorphins) are distributed unevenly within the nervous system and are closely connected to opioid receptors.

A high level of endorphins provokes alpha brain waves connected to states of serenity, pleasure, and relief from pain. It has been speculated that an increase in the release of endorphins and other opioid peptides that provoke euphoric sensations, often perceived in the alpha state of consciousness, activates the immune system and its functioning. Other strong connections have been found between the immune system and behavioral and sleep patterns, circadian rhythms, nutritional factors, and stressful experiences. It has been proved that the central nervous system—and any factor that is able to alter it—can influence the functions of the immune system and the structural interactions of synapses within neuronal connectivity in relation to the psycho-neuro-immune functionality of the ventricular, cerebrovascular, cerebral, reticular, and endocrine systems.

The dorsal horn of the spinal cord is a key area for sensory and tactile information since it is here that this kind of information is processed. This is the first synapse of the central nervous system. Tactile stimulation, such as the touch (palpation) used in CST, is able to encourage the production of neuropeptides. The latter send messages to the hypothalamus and immune system, which in turn activate the healing process and the limbic system, starting the cyclical connection between the endocrine and the immune systems.

The connections between the approach of SER, our knowledge about the complex integrated network of chemical and cellular mediators constituting the systems and apparatuses of human organisms, and the manual techniques implemented in CST to control the treatment process allow patients to enhance the efficiency of the homeostatic response of their own organism and increase their level of awareness about their own health.

CHAPTER 3

The Patient-Facilitator Relationship in CST

True empathy is always free of any evaluative or diagnostic quality.

CARL RANSOM ROGERS

Up to this point we have introduced CST and SER and highlighted how, through these methods, the morphofunctional organization of the craniosacral system can be elaborated and developed through some of its connections to physiological systems and apparatuses and the emotional sphere. At the same time, we have indicated how it is possible to enhance the processing of sensations connected to the symptoms of physical and emotional functions on a systemic level. This process fosters the patient/Facilitator relationship and raises the patient's level of awareness about their body.

We must not fail to note that the origin of the gesture starting the therapeutic action, just like at the origin of any technique adopted to help the patient, lies in the Facilitator's adoption of the correct attitude in the therapeutic approach to the patient. The correct approach allows us to empathize—without sympathizing—in order to establish a constructive therapeutic synergy.

Given that CST is a holistic mode of treatment, it is clear that it is meant to search for the primary cause, or the secondary ones, that have produced the symptom(s). This technique offers support and facilitation to the patient's well-being in any phase of their Life Cycle, from the intrauterine phase to the end of existence, passing through every possible condition, such as discomfort, disease, old age, coma, et cetera.

As stated before, the peculiarity of CST is the palpation (using the five-gram touch) through which the therapist listens to the person's body. This kind of touch must be subtle, receptive, open, purposeful, patient, and present in the listening of the body and corporeality.

The Facilitator's active listening is a necessary condition to facilitate human self-corrective and self-healing mechanisms. The Facilitator operates within the constant training of the correct approach toward the patient, observing mainly four key principles:

Maintaining impartiality: understanding the motivations of each structure

Avoiding judgment: never judging

Being present: giving attention (*I am here for you now*)

Not feeding the Ego: the Ego is only a temporary structure of childhood; we avoid giving it energy in order to form an authentic empathetic relationship with the patient

By following these four key principles, the Facilitator can start a synergistic and empathetic relationship with the patient and create a common space in which individual personalities do not intervene, a neutral area that Dr. Upledger called the "Third Space," where the patient and the Facilitator's non-consciouses—or Higher Selves or Inner Physicians—meet. *Third Space* is no-man's land, space without judgment, where all is one, empathy reigns, and healing takes place.

Dr. Upledger encouraged Facilitators to trust their own hands and let them be their eyes in the therapeutic action or facilitation. Trusting the hands and constant training of the attitude build the correct approach that allows the Facilitator to acquire the ability to communicate with the patient on all levels—verbal or nonverbal, conscious or non-conscious—through intentional touch.

This attitude shows that the correct mental approach during the treatment can support the facilitation and the solution of issues such as separation, loss, bereavement, and death.

CONSCIOUS VS. NON-CONSCIOUS

The term *non-conscious,* as Dr. Upledger adopted in his development of his manual therapy, is used in SER to define any physical, psychological, or spiritual process that is unconsciously described by the patient.

In the relationship between patient and Facilitator, the most important moment in the treatment is represented by the Third Space, which emerges thanks to what Dr. Upledger called melding (blending); it is the starting point for the Therapeutic Imagery and Dialogue between one conscious/non-conscious Higher Self and the other.

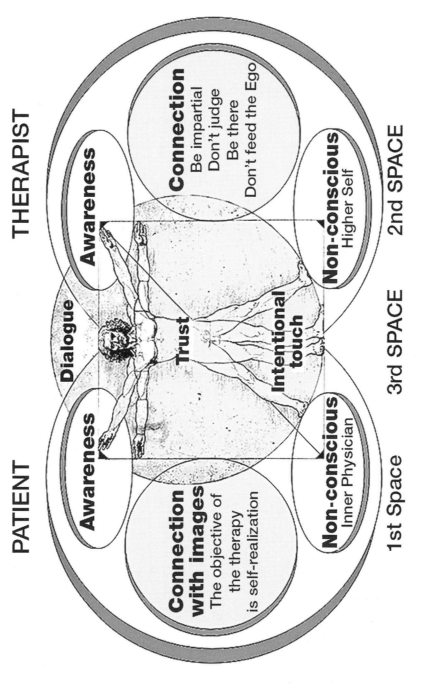

Fig. 3.1. The Third Space in the patient/Facilitator relationship. Third space is no-man's land, space without judgment, where there is melding and empathy and the healing takes place.

RELATIONSHIP OF CONSCIOUSNESS AND NON-CONSCIOUSNESS FOR FACILITATOR AND PATIENT

	Facilitator	Patient
Conscious	Awareness of one's own abilities, knowledge, skills	Need for treatment because of a concrete issue or as a preventive measure
Non-conscious	Intuitive listening; trust in one's hands and their wisdom	Ability to become aware of both the problem and its causes

The body is a unit. In the dialogue between the Higher Self of the Facilitator and the Higher Self of the patient, the Facilitator can communicate with every structure, function, system, or cell and thus support the patient in every situation, condition, or phase of their Life Cycle.

When facing an existential and universal subject, such as an experience of separation, loss, and/or bereavement, the fundamental objective is to always consider all the structures and functions involved in the treatment. It is possible for the Facilitator to support the patient in the transformation process toward a constructive phase through the activation of all the self-balancing mechanisms of the body, melding conscious and non-conscious (mind-body/psyche-soma).

Facilitators must always keep in mind that the reality that emerges during the treatment is the patient's and not their own. Facilitators also should avoid proposing or indulging ideas and perspectives that are antithetical to the patient's vital functioning, trying to debunk the widespread but erroneous doctrine that postulates that *positive = favorable* and *negative = unfavorable*. Only in this way can we face scenarios of separation, small deaths, bereavement, and loss.

THE FREEDOM OF PURE LISTENING OF THE BODY

Freedom of listening means reaching a degree of awareness that makes it possible to listen to the voice of the Higher Self through the conscious/non-conscious dialogue between Facilitator and patient.

The need to place the welcoming and therapeutic gesture in the panorama of the Facilitator's competencies and the therapeutic process is very much felt by many health care professionals and demanded by manual therapists. The sense of touch is essential not only to carry out technical procedures that require great skills but also to establish a contact with our patients. That is especially true when touch becomes a method to acquire information, and even more so when it is also therapeutic.

Nowadays, health care professionals are no longer the mere product of an exclusively subjective medical management of a body-object. They are individuals who, just like the patients, start a dialogue to achieve a therapeutic alliance based on teamwork. Hence our wish is to share a type of knowledge able to improve the competencies of Facilitators and improve the awareness of those who receive the treatment.

Nonetheless, touch is only the vehicle. Ultimately, it is awareness that heals. As Frank Ostaseki wrote, "If the gesture expresses awareness, the physical contact will have transforming effects."[1]

In fact, the aptonomic contact offers an emotional confirmation to individuals and allows them to build basic levels of confidence. This produces a series of positive/constructive physical and emotional phenomena, which can even change one's ability to respond to diseases and, at the end of the Life Cycle, to live the dying process.

GESTURE AND ACTION

When speaking of the significance of the healing act, it is important to reflect upon the two elements constituting it: the gesture and the action. They both imply a contact, but *gesture* has a communicative quality, whereas *action* consists of the series of movements that give shape to the healing practice.

The Facilitators who implement the healing act seem to have two specific needs:

- the scientific basis or rationale, which is the ethical basis of this contact *(Does it produce positive effects? Why?)*
- the definition of the procedure or the protocol needed to discuss it, to repeat it, and to communicate it *(What does it consist of? How is it done? When should it be done?)*

In CST, the choice of an efficient, describable, repeatable, communicable, and recordable gesture is based on the operative rationale, which comes not only from a scientific need but also from the ethic necessity to give the individual the best possible intervention. In SER, the quality of the contact is determined more by personal and individual characteristics. The choice of the modality relies on the Facilitator's individual knowledge, professionalism, and motivation.

For this reason, a specific training on this subject is fundamental. I am convinced that for professionals working closely with loss and death, it is extremely useful to reflect upon the healing action and to share their reflections with each other. This promotes the circulation of information and actions within a group of people that also includes patients and their caregivers.

This path was designed to allow those who already know CST and SER to get familiar with concepts such as death and transition from both the Facilitator's and the patient's point of view. They also learn a further tool of analysis, approach, and evaluation that can help them choose the most adequate gesture in the phases of each individual's Life Cycle in which separation, bereavement, and loss has occurred or is occurring.

It develops through the description of manual techniques that are needed to help the terminally ill and those who suffer any of the so-called small deaths, such as divorce, loss of job, change of residence, and so on.

Our intention therefore is to further analyze and develop CST and SER techniques, highlighting the importance of a multidisciplinary approach to enhance the therapeutic alliance in which teamwork is essential to share a kind of information that is as fundamental as training and study.

The relationship that is thus created is able to:

- enhance the patient's comfort, emotional state, and well-being
- address a specific symptom, such as pain, stiffness, et cetera
- provide the contribution of complementary methods, such as the energetic rebalancing

OBJECTIVES

The objectives we should aim for in our training are:

- to acquire awareness about the aptonomic value of the gesture and the action when working with terminal patients and people suffering from the emotional stress caused by a severe or small loss
- to highlight that the healing quality of the gesture lies not solely in the technique but also in the "way of being" and that it plays a very specific role for health care teams when the patient cannot be cured—because even in that case, there is still plenty that can be done
- to learn how to master one's own emotions in the face of events involving death or envisaging it
- to learn how to accompany the patient in the processing and acceptance of a negative event

⁂ CST-CENTERED VISIONS ⁂

Commenting on the topics of this chapter, my observations cannot but concern a Facilitator's gestures as the natural and aware manifestation of their knowledge, competencies, and technical skills.

Since the facilitating gesture of CST and SER expresses the Facilitator's way of being and way of addressing real-life scenarios, throughout this book I would like to present you with the interpretation of some images that emerged from my non-conscious to my conscious awareness. I cannot help but give my interpretation of these images from the perspective of a Facilitator (for fun, but not without a reason). After all, I have always thought that the awareness of the gesture that is expressed in the therapeutic action can be compared to an art form that "synthesizes intuition, science, and knowledge," to paraphrase Dr. Upledger's words.

Let's start with a work by Dalí.

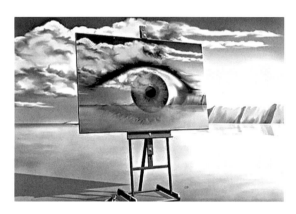

Fig. 3.2. Reproduction of *An Eye with a View,* by Salvador Dalí

Dalí is considered one of the greatest painters of the surrealism movement. In *An Eye with a View* (fig. 3.2), he combined the means of perception (the eye) with the object of the perception (in this case a landscape), putting one into the other as if subject and object were separated elements united into one new identity. At the same time, he took these elements out of context, depriving them of their original identity.

What is the analogy with SER?

Conscious and non-conscious exist in the same reality, but individual perceptions can differ even when the same reality is observed. We must try to create a bridge, a melding, connecting different perceptions in order for them to communicate between each other in a new, transforming identity.

CHAPTER 4
Foundational Techniques
A Synthesis of Knowledge

There is something magical in rhythm; it even makes us believe that we possess the sublime.

JOHANN WOLFGANG VON GOETHE,
MAXIMS AND REFLECTIONS OF GOETHE (1908)

This chapter describes some of the techniques employed in CST and SER. It is meant to introduce their development through a functional implementation to address issues involving separation, bereavement, loss, and death when the patient's problem requires it.

SQAR: LISTENING TO THE CRANIOSACRAL RHYTHM

SQAR stands for *symmetry, quality, amplitude,* and *rate,* which are four qualities of the craniosacral rhythm (CSR) we can evaluate. A SQAR evaluation assesses the overall functionality of the craniosacral system, which in turn expresses the functionality of the body. We can use the SQAR evaluation to find evidence of a problem (or the residue of a problem that was solved) and to assess the overall vitality of the paravertebral muscles, and more specifically the innervation of their tissues.

The CSR is the physiological movement of the craniosacral system. The CSS is a physiological system and therefore regulates various activities in the organism and interacts with other physiological systems, such as the respiratory, cardiovascular, endocrine, and immune systems. Our cerebrospinal fluid supplies the central nervous system, removing toxins and waste metabolites and protecting everything that is contained in the cranium. It is produced by plasma and enters the system through the choroid plexuses in the subarachnoid space of the ventricles. It flows between the arachnoid mater and the pia mater and is constantly reabsorbed through the arachnoid granulations.

Implementation of SQAR

1. Evaluate through palpation, placing one's hands on specific areas of the body. These areas are called "listening stations," and there are four main ones:

- dorsums of feet (top part of foot above the arch)
- anterior surface of the thighs
- shoulders
- three cranial vault holds (see figure 4.1 below).

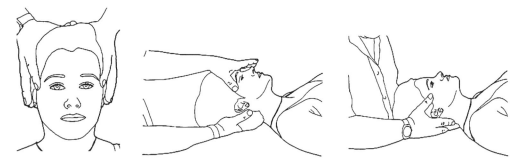

Fig. 4.1. The three cranial vault holds

2. Use the listening stations to perceive the symmetry, quality, amplitude, and rate (SQAR) of the craniosacral rhythm. Any anomalies in the SQAR indicate less-than-ideal functionality of the craniosacral system.

Note: There are also secondary listening stations—heels, superior anterior iliac spines, and the ribs—that can be evaluated.

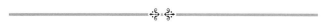

Definitions

S = Symmetry: The physiologic movement of paired and unpaired bones. If the external and internal rotation of paired bones or the flexion and extension of unpaired bones are not symmetrical, we are probably facing a dysfunction caused by fascial and/or emotional issues.

Q = Quality: The vital force expressed in the patient's body through the vigor of the CSR. It changes according to the individual's physical and emotional state.

A = Amplitude: The ability or inability of the CSR to cover the complete range of physiological movement. It is possible to have symmetry but lack amplitude, another signal of fascial and/or emotional dysfunction.

R = Rate: The number of seconds that are necessary to complete the physiological movement of the CSR. Normally the CSR rate ranges around six to eight cycles per minute. If the cycles per minute are less than six, a chronic issue may be occurring; if they are more than eight, we may be in the presence of an inflammatory state.

Clinical Notes

At the beginning of a treatment session, I often carry out an initial SQAR assessment in order to get an overall picture of my patient's possible dysfunctions.

Not all the dysfunctions I might detect in a patient's body are primary lesions, but I take note of each of them. If I still have some time left in the session after treating the primary lesions, I use it to treat the secondary lesions I found during that first SQAR assessment.

ARCING TECHNIQUE

The wounds of the Spirit heal, and leave no scars behind.
GEORG WILHELM FRIEDRICH HEGEL,
PHENOMENOLOGY OF SPIRIT

In CST, Arcing is the most useful assessment method to find Energy Cysts—and consequently the primary physiological dysfunction. This evaluation tool can be implemented by placing the hands on various parts of the patient's body—or keeping them at a close distance to it. It allows us to locate the vibrations produced by Energy Cysts and draws the Facilitator toward their center.

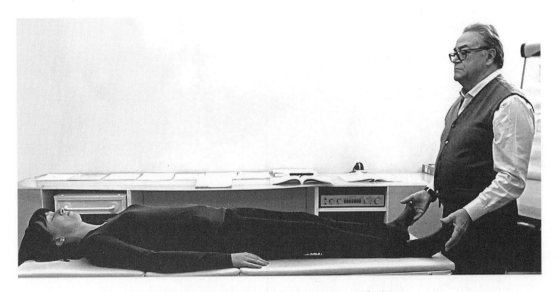

Fig. 4.2. Evaluation with the Arcing technique

Arcing requires the therapist to sense the energetic waves of interference produced by an active lesion, which tend to be superimposed over the normal subtle physiological motions of the body, organs, tissues, and energies. Practitioners then trace these waves to their source by manually sensing the arcs they form. When arcing is used, the source of the waves is considered to be the core site of the underlying problem or lesion, which may actually be some distance from the location of the patient's symptoms. Usually the active lesion is disruptive to gross physiological activities, as well as to more subtle energy functions and patterns.

Active Lesions: Energy Cysts

The physical/physiological effects of the Energy Cysts depend mainly upon their power—the amount of energy they contain—and their location in the body. Energy Cysts can contribute to the reinforcement of spinal cord segments, for example, causing a reinforced segment syndrome (facilitated segment syndrome).

Energy Cysts can be identified in many ways. Sometimes it is enough to analyze the painful area indicated by the patient, but it is important not to rely exclusively on this method since the patient could be experiencing referred pain or the dysfunction of a secondary node.

Each Energy Cyst produces vibrations with a different intensity; it can range from the parameters of the heartbeat at its peak to the parameters of the craniosacral rhythm at its minimum rate. The vibration of an Energy Cyst is generally about forty to sixty cycles per minute.

The Energy Cysts perceived by the Facilitator through vibrations represent active lesions. There are other types of lesions that can be perceived through touch (palpa-

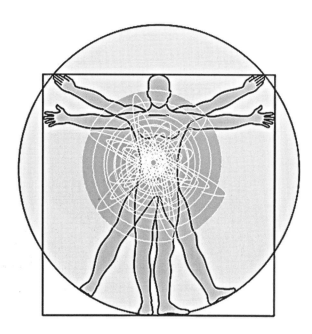

Fig. 4.3. Energy Cyst and the vibrational field

tion) but are residual or chronic, not active; these inactive lesions might be perceived as fascial restrictions.

The Energy Cysts that are discovered thanks to the Arcing technique are not the answer to the physiological problem. In fact, they are just the signal the body gives to indicate that it is necessary to start searching for the possible causes of the dysfunction.

Implementation of Arcing Technique

1. At the start of the treatment session, Arc (that is, use the Arcing technique) to locate any Energy Cysts, placing your hands symmetrically on the soles of the patient's feet or the patient's hips or shoulders or using one of the cranial vault holds (see fig. 4.1 on page 30).
2. Treat the patient according to the information received through the vibrations you perceive.
3. After the treatment, Arc again to evaluate whether the Energy Cyst you located was successfully dissipated, in which case no vibrations will remain. If Arcing detects any residue of the disorganized (entropic) energy, the treatment must be repeated until the organized (syntropic) energy is restored.

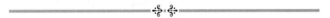

Clinical Notes

In CST treatments, the Facilitator does not focus primarily on the patient's symptoms but rather searches for the cause(s) that generated those symptoms.

When a patient comes to my office with a painful and contained symptom, I never treat the symptom immediately, but I look for its cause or causes. Therefore, I use the Arcing technique either after SQAR or straightaway.

To do this, gently place your hands symmetrically on the head, then the thoracic inlet, the inferior costal margins, the pelvis, the thighs, and finally the feet of the patient. At each area of examination, allow your hands to passively move with the inherent body motion of the patient. If the arcs your hands are feeling are symmetrical, there is no problem. If the arcs are not symmetrical, envision the nucleus of the arcs and determine their intersection point. That point is the location of the restriction or lesion. Place your hands in as many positions as you need to precisely locate the area of dysfunction.

The energy vortex emanated from the nucleus of an Energy Cyst draws me to the nucleus itself, allowing me to locate it in a specific spot of the patient's body. Once I have located one or more Energy Cysts in the patient's head or body, I treat the person through the Direction of Energy (see chapter 11) or a local fascial release. If the Significance Detector indicates something (as described below), I use the SER technique of the Therapeutic Imagery and Dialogue (see page 37).

SIGNIFICANCE DETECTOR

When the heart speaks, the mind finds it indecent to object.

MILAN KUNDERA,
THE UNBEARABLE LIGHTNESS OF BEING

Significance Detector is the name Dr. Upledger gave to the phenomenon of perceiving an abrupt interruption of the craniosacral rhythm.

The Significance Detector is the key to accessing a patient's non-conscious voice. One of the Facilitator's abilities must be to detect the subtle sensations of the body through palpation, such as by listening to the pulsation of the CSR. When we place our hands on the patient's body to listen to the CSR, and the CSR appears to stop voluntarily, we have experienced the Significance Detector, and we are in contact with the patient's non-conscious.

The Unsolicited Image

The Facilitator often uses the Significance Detector technique in order to access what is called an "unsolicited image," meaning a thought, sensation, or memory that emerges from the patient's non-conscious in that precise moment. An unsolicited image is useful for starting the Therapeutic Imagery and Dialogue.

Significance Detector vs. Still Point

When the Significance Detector occurs, the Facilitator may have the impression that the CSR has met a solid obstruction. This is unlike what happens with the Still Point, another CST technique in which the CSR seems to stop its pulsation softly

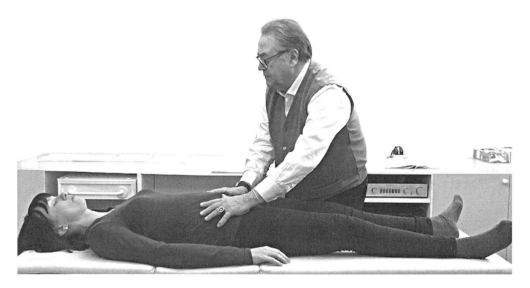

Fig. 4.4. Evaluation with the Significance Detector

and gradually. In the Significance Detector, the perceived halt of the CSR occurs spontaneously in the patient; with the Still Point, the perceived interruption of the CSR occurs solely after a solicitation.

We must note here, that the CSR does not actually stop in either a Still Point or a Significance Detector. In both cases, it is perceived to stop. But from the clinical point of view, when a person goes into a Still Point, we no longer perceive or palpate the craniosacral rhythm (CSR). What is experienced as a Still Point may not be a single mechanism but different phenomena manifesting as a Still Point, and the experience of stillness may be experienced on different levels. With a Significance Detector, once again, we perceive through our palpation and blending, the absence of the CSR. But measurably, even though the CSR continues, there are many other changes happening within that seeming "stop." There is measurable chaos, perhaps reflecting the changes happening within the body during a Significance Detector: in the CSS, in the fascial system, in the energetic systems, and accompanied by shifts in awareness from conscious to non-conscious experience.

Thus, the perception of the stoppage of the CSR with the Significance Detector differs from the perception experienced with the Still Point, mainly because the perceived interruption is very abrupt in the first case and gradual in the second case.

SIGNIFICANCE DETECTOR VS. STILL POINT

Significance Detector	Still Point
The CSR appears to stop abruptly	The CSR appears to stop gradually
The CSR can appear to stop in any phase of the cycle	The CSR slows before appearing to stop
The CSR appears to stop autonomously, with or without an external solicitation	The CSR slows before appearing to stop only with an external solicitation
The CSR appears to stop with the patient's self-correction or discovery	The CSR attempts to win the resistance of the Facilitator's solicitation

Significance Processes

Any factor causing the perception of an abrupt interruption in the patient's CSR is extremely important, and the Facilitator needs to find out what provoked it. The phenomenon of the Significance Detector indicates that something meaningful is occurring in the patient, either consciously or on a level of consciousness that is close to awareness. This phenomenon occurs in correspondence with different types of psychological and/or emotional events and plays a key role in the Facilitator's evaluation and work.

The Significance Detector could manifest itself in the patient for several reasons, such as:

- a body position allowing the dissipation of an Energy Cyst or facilitating SER
- the reemergence of a meaningful symbol or image
- a key word said during the dialogue
- the memory of a conversation that addressed a critical topic
- other factors bearing a particular importance to the patient's emotions

The Facilitator also can employ the Significance Detector to determine when the patient's physiological reactions are crucial in the therapeutic process.

By virtue of the nature of their role, Facilitators might offer their presence when a patient decides to address a terrible image or memory. But it is necessary to be mindful of the importance of empathizing rather than sympathizing with the patient, particularly in situations that could evoke the Facilitator's emotional involvement. In this way, patients can make their own discoveries instead of being given ready-made answers.

Implementation of the Significance Detector

1. Place your hands on one of the main listening stations of the patient's body, where it is possible to perceive the CSR and connect with it. Be sure to keep your hands symmetrical and parallel.
2. If you perceive what feels like an abrupt interruption of the CSR while treating an Energy Cyst, you may immediately start the Therapeutic Imagery and Dialogue (see page 39), keeping your hands in the position for treatment.

Note: If you are in an inconvenient distal position and cannot easily start the Therapeutic Imagery and Dialogue when the Significance Detector occurs, you may change your position and put your hands on the diaphragm of the thoracic inlet. That can make it easier to be more connected in the conversation and to enhance the attention, respect, and acceptance that should be given to the patient.

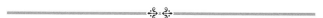

Clinical Notes

When I have to treat a person who has come to my office for the first time, I always ask myself whether that person wants to receive a strictly manual and physical treatment or intends to address their emotional connection to their condition through dialogue.

The Significance Detector technique allows us to identify what the person's choice is. Even if the patient initially wants to be treated only physically, it does not exclude the possibility that an emotional release might occur anyway at some point of the treatment. Similarly, a treatment that is solely emotional might later bring us to a type of work that is mainly physical and manual.

Only through the Significance Detector can we be directed toward the correct approach. If I do not perceive any obstruction in the CSR when placing my hands on the patient, I mainly focus on the manual aspect of the therapy. On the other hand, when I detect the perceived interruption of the CSR, I immediately invite the patient to start a Therapeutic Imagery and Dialogue.

As a patient manifests emotions during the dialogue, it must be noted that the Facilitator's hands are always placed on the physiological dysfunction in order to perceive fascial modifications and, especially, the dissipation of the entropic energy in the patient's body as the dialogue develops.

THERAPEUTIC IMAGERY AND DIALOGUE

What is truth? A difficult question; but I have solved it for myself by saying that it is what the "voice within" tells you.

MOHANDAS KARAMCHAND GANDHI
(MAHATMA GANDHI)

We can consider imagery to be the symbolic language of the non-conscious. The symbolism of the imagery can be concrete or abstract, and its definitions can translate into mental images, sounds, smells, sensations, and/or other perceptions emerging from the non-conscious to consciousness.

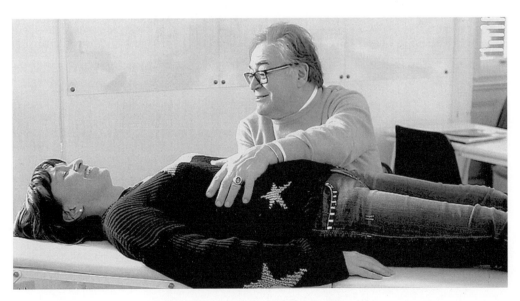

Fig. 4.5. Therapeutic Imagery and Dialogue

The Facilitator may use the patient's imagery as a tool to foster the healing process, and that is why we call this technique Therapeutic Imagery. Therapeutic images can disclose themselves spontaneously as voices of the patient's non-conscious, or they can follow the Facilitator or the patient's conscious solicitation. If they are used effectively, therapeutic images can facilitate the healing process on very different levels of consciousness.

When we establish a contact and a dialogue through therapeutic images, we are encouraging the non-conscious to become conscious. To start a significant dialogue between the patient's non-conscious and consciousness is an essential step toward growth, awareness, integration, and healing.

Solicited and Unsolicited Images

The Therapeutic Imagery and Dialogue can be initiated with a patient when:

- the Significance Detector occurs (the CSR appears to stop) and a spontaneous and unsolicited image emerges in the patient's consciousness
- an image is solicited in order to communicate with the patient's non-conscious

This book addresses specific subjects, such as loss, separation, bereavement, small deaths, death, and abandonment, that strike a chord with all of us because of our personal experiences. It is easy therefore to understand how the Facilitator can make use of the solicited image with a person who is asking for help in facing such a situation. Through the solicited image, the patient is encouraged to access the sphere of awareness, inviting their Inner Physician—or Guide or Higher Self, if you prefer—to dialogue with the different levels of consciousness.

Dialogue

When a patient indicates that they have encountered an image but cannot interpret or explain it, the Facilitator can gently start the dialogue by asking questions such as:

- Does your Inner Physician know the problem?
- Does it want to share its knowledge about the problem?
- Does the problem have a purpose?
- If it does have a purpose, what is it?
- What can be done to make the problem not necessary anymore?
- Is there a lesson to learn?

This dialogue can continue until it is clear what needs to be done, and by whom, in order to make the patient's problem, which has been found thanks to the voice of the patient's non-conscious, not necessary anymore in its current form.

Afterward, the Facilitator must negotiate an agreement between the patient's non-conscious and consciousness, searching for a constructive resolution that can be accepted by both sides and result in the patient's growth and integration. The dialogue entails a negotiation between the parts, or subpersonalities, involved in the problem. The Facilitator facilitates the negotiation as these parts, arising from the patient's non-conscious, emerge to consciousness. The parts are asked to cooperate by participating alternately in the dialogue until it is possible to find a solution to the problem that is acceptable for all of them.

Objectives

The main objective of the Therapeutic Imagery and Dialogue is to achieve the maximum well-being for the patient. This is achieved through the maximum connection via blending and melding between the therapist and the patient, as well as between them and the universe.

More specifically, the Facilitator's purpose in Therapeutic Imagery and Dialogue is:

- to allow the outflow of the energy connected with the destructive emotion that has compromised the person's well-being and ability to make use of positive/constructive resources
- to learn how to perceive the voice of the non-conscious when it emerges through the Significance Detector
- to be able to facilitate the dialogue between conscious and non-conscious
- to become familiar with the language of the non-conscious (concrete and abstract symbolism)
- to identify the different types of energy connected with emotions (either syntropic/constructive or entropic/destructive)
- to facilitate the transformation of destructive energy into constructive energy
- to enhance the positive resources that can emerge even from scenarios of separation and/or loss, transforming the destructive scenarios into a constructive potential for the present and future of the individual

Implementation of Therapeutic Imagery and Dialogue

In order to effectively start the Therapeutic Imagery and Dialogue, it is extremely helpful to use the Significance Detector at the beginning of the session.

1. Place your hands on one of the four main listening stations (e.g., on the skull or shoulders) or anywhere else on the body, keeping them symmetrical and parallel. Make an assessment and decide what your approach will be.

2. Induce relaxation through CV4/Still Point and other relaxing techniques.
3. Try to connect with the patient.
4. Solicit imagery through intention by addressing the Inner Physician, Higher Self, Guide, et cetera.
5. Facilitate dialogue between the different levels of consciousness. Use the dialogue as a therapeutic tool. Identify the conflict, and try to negotiate an acceptable solution for the inner discordance.
6. Express your gratitude for the opportunity to communicate with different levels of consciousness.
7. End the session with a plan of action in order to acquire a better understanding of everyday life. Say goodbye with a smile, lightening the atmosphere after the hard topics that were addressed, and, if it is appropriate, laugh with your patient!

Clinical Notes

If the Significance Detector occurs while I am treating a patient's physical dysfunction, I start the Therapeutic Imagery and Dialogue.

I have noticed that patients often want to speak while a physical dysfunction is being treated. Consequently, I learned to perceive the negative charge hiding behind their words and to understand that those words are only the tip of the iceberg. They signal the entropic energy feeding the dysfunction and its destructive potential.

The entropic energy can be a sign of the Significance Detector as well. If my non-conscious is open to welcome the patient in that moment, it perceives the anomaly of the physical dysfunction on different, subtler levels.

If I am in a distal position from the patient's head (the knees, for example), I get closer. In my experience, patients feel better taken care of if they can see my face while I work. It is also useful to me to be able to observe their face and notice their facial expressions as they speak or during pauses and silence. Sometimes I receive meaningful signals from their non-conscious, even through such simple expressions as smiles, laughter, tears, lip quivers, or frowned eyebrows, which may indicate I can start developing a dialogue.

WORKING WITH THE VECTOR/AXIS SYSTEM

The mathematical concept of vector comes from the intuitive idea of a physical quantity (such as displacement, velocity, and acceleration) with a magnitude and a direction in the three-dimensional space.

EDOARDO SERNESI

Everybody recognizes the term *vector* as a concept of mathematics—just think of the Cartesian coordinate systems we study at school. Dr. Upledger found inspiration in this concept when he defined the characteristics of the vector/axis system in the human body.

In physics, a vector is a quantity with a **magnitude** (length), a **direction** (indicated by the arrow), and a **point of application** (if we consider the point of application, we can say that the vector is *applied*.)[1] Dr. Upledger taught that these concepts can be adapted to the human body to evaluate the individual's energetic framework in a functional way and guide CST treatments.

Dr. Upledger defined the vector system as the energetic framework of the human body. Each vector traces the path of energy flow through a person's body. As a system, the vectors trace the energetic map of the body.

When the system is adequately energized, there is a magnetic attraction between the physical body and the vectors. An interruption, bending, or misalignment of a vector is an unmistakable signal of lack of melding between the physical body and the energetic framework and the inevitable occurrence of dysfunctions, such as Energy Cysts, that can keep interrupting the organization and integrity of the body.

We could imagine the vector/axis structure in the body as the bed of a river and its tributaries. As long as each watercourse follows its direction and does not exceed its capacity, the river flows as usual; if any external factor causes the water to deviate from its normal flow, the river itself begins to shift and change.

As we will see later, events such as the small deaths (e.g., trauma, dysfunctions, Energy Cysts, passive or chronic lesions, etc.) contribute to interruptions of the vital energy continuum and cause an energetic imbalance in the vector/axis system, modifying the entire energetic framework of the body.

In the human body, the energetic framework can reflect the functionality of the physical framework and vice versa. For example, in the case of osteopathic lesions (dysfunctions involving the functionality of the bony structures that constitute the physical framework), a vector/axis system that is not correctly aligned could inhibit the readjustment of the bone framework or replicate the lesions after its restoration, preventing any long-lasting resolution.

How to Visualize the Vectors

The energy lines of the vectors can be visualized in many different ways depending on individual intuition and visualization skills, which can vary according to each person's way of imagining, perceiving, and visualizing.

The Facilitator can visualize vectors even without touch, though it is important to remember that, in CST, the hands are the Facilitator's eyes.

Therefore, there are two distinct methods to visualize/perceive a person's vectors: exclusively on an energetic level or through touch. For example, Dr. Upledger used to visualize vectors as shining lines that could either stay inside the patient's body or exit its physical boundaries. Other people perceive these lines as lines of different colors, or pencil marks on the body, or wooden or metallic threadlike beams within the body.

To understand how the visualization of vectors takes place, we can use an analogy with the meridians and parallels of Earth, imagining them straightened and applied to the body. By standing or lying down with the body straight, hands at the sides, and legs straight, a person creates crossings of horizontal and vertical straight lines. Now imagine that inside the body, at the two ends of the horizontal lines, other vertical straight lines go downward in each upper and lower limb, following a central path inside it. The intersections of these lines form ninety-degree angles. That is a basic mapping of the vectors (see fig. 4.6).

Vectors usually have a movement, an energy force, and a direction of their own. For this reason, we can say that they either align with an axis or diverge from it; therefore, they can also be considered in relation to their axis. The combination of direction and energy force forms the vector/axis system.

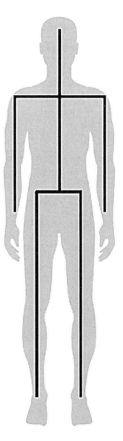

Fig. 4.6. Diagram of the vector/axis system of the human body

Perceiving and working with the vector/axis system requires Facilitators to have confidence in their abilities to expand their own sensory boundaries. Very often Facilitators limit or block their intuition and ability to visualize. To address this self-limitation in the experimentation and expansion of their limits, they must try to contact a part of themselves that is often relegated to a subaltern space of the awareness: the ability to imagine and confidently follow intuition, transforming it into action. You cannot imagine the universes you could discover by training to follow this advice.

If Facilitators have difficulties in visualizing the vector lines, they can rely on the perception of the vector/axis system through palpation. The listening station that is commonly employed to perceive and assess the vector/axis system is the feet. From this vantage point, it is possible to perceive and follow the vector lines of the body and, at the same time, perceive their possible interruptions and modifications in relation to their axis.

Objectives

What are the therapeutic objectives of working with the vector/axis system?

- To evaluate the energy framework (the vital energy continuum) of the individual
- To realign the vectors to their axes
- To reestablish and foster a balanced energy flow in the organism

Implementation of Balancing the Vector/Axis System

When we perceive a vector deviating from its axis—that is, an energetic misalignment—we must bring the vector back to its correct position. A misalignment of a vector or any interruption of its energy flow can be caused by an Energy Cyst. Therefore, it is necessary to locate the Energy Cyst, find the cause(s) that generated it, dissipate it, and restore the energy flow.

1. Start the evaluation by placing your hands on the patient's insteps, keeping them symmetrical.
2. Visualize the vectors within the vector/axis system. Assess the alignment and the flow of energy.
3. Realign the vectors to their axes, removing the cause of the misalignment.

Note: To align the vectors to their axes, we can employ body mobilization techniques or other techniques meant to restore the correct position of the vectors, as Dr. Upledger explained in *SomatoEmotional Release and Beyond*.

Clinical Notes

When I assess a patient's state of health on a physiological and functional level, I also observe the physiological and energetic entirety of the individual; therefore, I always assess the conditions of the vector/axis system.

I generally use the first part of a session, at the same time that I assess the SQAR of the craniosacral rhythm, to evaluate the vector/axis system as well. An assessment of the functionality of this system helps me develop the appropriate method of treatment.

Even when the work I need to do mainly concerns the emotional side of the physical dysfunction, I could not go on without considering the vector/axis system and its state. The vector/axis system indicates the impoverishment of vital energy caused by destructive emotions and the consequent inability or difficulty of the organism to restore physical functionality.

❖ A CST-CENTERED VISION ❖

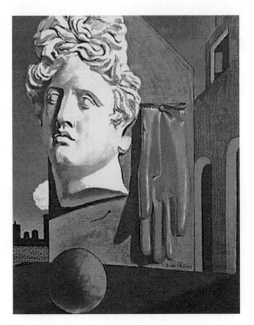

Fig. 4.7 Reproduction of *The Song of Love,* by Giorgio de Chirico

The Song of Love, by Giorgio de Chirico (fig. 4.7), sets forth a new poetic of space, portraying an existence that goes beyond the sensible appearance of empirical reality (making it a metaphysical painting).

In CST, the art of Facilitators is the ability to evoke the most hidden and still images and sensations from the patient's non-conscious. First through the Significance Detector and then through the Therapeutic Imagery and Dialogue, archetypes manifest themselves and retrieve their own meaning in order to give it back to the patient's consciousness, thus becoming a sort of "song of love" for the patient's healing.

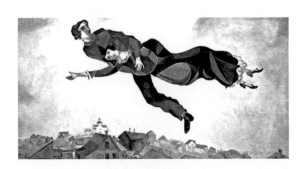

Fig. 4.8 *Over the Town,* by Marc Chagall

Over the Town (fig. 4.8) was inspired by a surreal short story written by the painter Mark Chagall himself.

Just as Chagall's short stories and dreamlike images defy the laws of physics and portray the emotions of inner landscapes, SER reveals the patient's inner landscape through the Therapeutic Imagery and Dialogue and explores the dimension of the Higher Self, searching for healing in an exclusive space that is devoted to the meeting of the patient's and Facilitator's Higher Selves.

CHAPTER 5

Ego

Its Functions and Anomalies

More the knowledge lesser the ego, lesser the knowledge more the ego.
ATTRIBUTED TO ALBERT EINSTEIN

The Ego is one of the biggest enemies of a correct Facilitator/patient approach. In fact, the Ego is only a need of human psyche. In humans, its function is temporary; it belongs to childhood because it is a childhood defense mechanism. Not giving energy to the Ego means not giving energy to reductive, shallow, and self-centered feelings and ways of reasoning.

Our goal in life should be to follow our Higher Self, since our existential needs and our adult relationships cannot be fulfilled through the childish modalities and defense mechanisms that belong to the Ego. Our connection with our Higher Self can exist only if we are trained not to feed the self-referential and selfish energy of the Ego in its various manifestations.

For example, a correct attitude for a CST and SER Facilitator involves relying on *self-confidence,* which is very different from being self-referential, and activating *receptive mindfulness,* an activity that belongs to the Higher Self, instead of control, an activity that belongs to the Ego.

The Facilitator's task therefore is to eradicate all the nourishment of the Ego and, as an adult act of love, to let trust take root in the ground of life, whatever happens in it. Not feeding the Ego is one of the main conditions for communicating with the patient's Inner Physician or Higher Self. Only under this condition are we able to transform any shallow or self-referential attitude when dealing with feelings and personal experiences.

By indicating in his texts the key points of the correct approach between Facilitator and patient, Dr. Upledger provided us with a powerful tool for not feeding the Ego. As described in chapter 3, these points include:

- maintaining impartiality
- avoiding judgment

- staying present and mindful
- not feeding the Ego

It may look like the Ego has an important role in our personalities, especially when we need to prove our real skills, abilities, and knowledge. Only self-confidence, however, is able to fulfill our constructive resolutions since it operates at the service of truth and the consciousness of the Higher Self.

As soon as Facilitators understand how not to feed their own Ego, they are able to establish an authentic and healthy relationship with their patients. This translates into a therapeutic alliance and encourages patients to let the voice of their Higher Self be heard.

In this way, through a communication between Facilitators' and patients' Higher Selves, patients start to respect themselves, to trust themselves and their ability to achieve self-realization constructively, and to become aware of their ability to independently activate thoughts and gestures that can lead them to well-being in an honest and transparent process.

THE NON-CONSCIOUS VS. THE EGO

During his studies to develop the key principles of SER, Dr. Upledger found many similarities in the psychological theories of analytical psychology, Gestalt psychology, and psychosynthesis. These theories regard the self as the psyche in the entirety of conscious and unconscious components.

Dr. Upledger was a physician, an osteopath, and an acupuncturist, not a psychologist. With SER, he did not want to create a complementary method used only by psychologists and psychotherapists. Since the principles of CST and SER consider the human being as a whole, Dr. Upledger used concepts taken from psychotherapy mainly to develop the analogies he found when treating his patients with SER. This work allowed him to gather all information that could help a Facilitator determine the different levels of manual therapy treatment.

This is how Dr. Upledger introduced the concept of the non-conscious, which encompasses all that can constitute an obstacle for the patient's healing process or passage between different phases of the Life Cycle. It communicates to the Facilitator through the emotions that are stored in the patient's body and cause physical symptoms.

The patient's non-conscious also includes the voice of the Inner Physician, which holds the solution to remove the symptoms and indicate the causes that provoked them.

Bringing the voice of the non-conscious to the patient's awareness, SER presents the patient with a way to connect with the Higher Self or Inner Physician and consequently to have a wider vision of their own and others' inner potential.

Dr. Upledger found this proposition to be the most correct and coherent in the mediation between SER and the psychological theories that do not put the Ego at the center of human psyche and consider the human being as a whole. In his vision, this whole is made of different parts that are contained in a single unit, which is greater than the mere psyche.

Let's now examine some of the theories Dr. Upledger incorporated in his vision.

EGO IN CARL GUSTAV JUNG'S ANALYTICAL PSYCHOLOGY

In Jung's analytical psychology, or Jungian psychology, the Ego is regarded as the central complex of consciousness, the element that is necessary to the individual during early childhood to develop the child's identity.

Jung regarded the development of the Ego as an indispensable phase in the growth of newborn babies; it helps them overcome the detachment from their mother's breast, experience the first step toward self-awareness, become aware of the difference between subject and object, and develop the knowledge of what they are not in order to understand what they are.

Nonetheless, the Ego is also a complicated element of the human psyche and, as such, is extremely malleable and colonizable. When the unconscious invades it with its contents, and when complexes find a space from which to control it, the Ego can be manipulated and become insecure. (Note that Jung talked about complexes as psychoemotional blocks with a very high energy charge rather than as pathological phenomena.)

The Ego is often run by complexes (e.g., power complexes or complexes that develop around money, sex, prevarication, etc.) and is attracted to what is accessory for the person and not what is essential to their nature. When the Ego is controlled by the unnecessary, it loses its primary function, which is essential only in childhood to become aware of one's own identity. At the same time, it inhibits the development of intentionality and decisiveness, which are indispensable elements for adults to achieve the main objectives of their lives.

When he gave his definition of Ego, Jung thought it was essential to distinguish it from the self. To him, the self was actually an overarching reality that must absolutely not be confused with the Ego. The only way to make the presence of the Ego plausible in an adult is to recognize a conscious relation of subjugation to the self.[1] He noted:

> In the center is a virtual nucleus I call the self, which represents the totality or sum of conscious and unconscious processes. This is in contradiction to the Ego or partial self, which is not conceived of as being in contact with the unconscious elements of the psychological processes.[2]

EGO IN FRITZ PERLS'S GESTALT PSYCHOLOGY

In Gestalt psychology, when the Ego is addressed in its negative meaning, it is identified in connection with a syndrome called "egotism." Egotism represents a condition of isolation in which individuals are desensitized, do not empathize with others, do not experience diversity and the unexpected anymore, and do not perceive themselves in relation to the stimuli coming from the external environment.

In the perspective of Gestalt psychology, the Ego is essentially necessary only during childhood to discover and express individual identity. Egotism transforms and turns upside down the main function of the Ego, which is connected with growth and child development. It obstructs evolution, preventing the discovery of diversities that make the individual exit isolation and come into contact with the external world. Egotism tends not to discover the external environment but rather tries to subdue and subject it to its needs, interrupting or resisting spontaneity.

The condition created by egotism consists of an insufficient differentiation between individual and environment and an ineffective communication between internal and external world. In Gestalt psychology, it is considered a lack of convergence between the organism/individual and the self.

Gestalt psychology recognizes a positive function of egotism as well, and it is expressed through touch, interaction, and a constructive dialogue with the self. In the contact with the self, egotism loses its negative characteristics if it begins an empathetic relationship with the external environment, developing a self-sustaining and self-promoting position.

Fritz Perls defines the all-encompassing function of the self through an image: the inner world of the individual as a figure stretched toward the changing world but retroflexed toward the individual.[3]

EGO IN ROBERTO ASSAGIOLI'S PSYCHOSYNTHESIS

Assagioli includes the Ego in both the evolutional and involutional disorders of individual identity. In the first case, the Ego creates conflicts between egocentric tendencies—which belong to the part of the human being that feeds on the attention we receive—and altruism, or the will to achieve the common good. In the second case, the Ego imprisons individuals inside themselves in an inner conflict made merely of desires and instincts that aim only to be satisfied and consequently lose all relations with the external world.

According to Assagioli, since the Ego is part of all human beings, it must have a positive function. This function intervenes when the Ego is moved by self-preservation instincts in an objectively hostile environment that can be dangerous for the individual's psychophysical safety. This case implies a certain attention toward the external reality, not only toward oneself, as well as an observation of the outside.

Similarly, in the life of each human being there are situations in which the Ego can assume a predominant role in one's identity. That is made possible by the egocentricity that the Ego inspires but does not dominate, and by egoism, which is inspired not only by the Ego but also ruled by it completely. With egocentricity, the individual's identity develops a neurotic subpersonality that is based upon fear and uneasiness and distances the person from the others. With egoism, individuals identify themselves with a narcissistic, strong, and dominant subpersonality whose need to satisfy itself becomes essential, sometimes to the point of destroying everything in its way in order to reach the object of its desires.

One exercise individuals can do for their own personal growth, as proposed in psychosynthesis, is to recognize the Ego, downsizing its role when it influences personal development negatively, and to strive for transformations that bring self-improvement and the search for the common good.

> *Now individuals will face another, superior task—to discipline themselves and choose goals that can coincide with the well-being of others and the common good of mankind.*
>
> ROBERTO ASSAGIOLI

According to Assagioli, the Ego, or personal self, persists from childhood to old age, whereas the contents of individual personalities and subpersonalities change completely, just as the physical body is constantly changing the material it is made of while still keeping the same organic unity.

In his analogy between the physical body and human psyche, Assagioli observed a fundamental divergence. Unlike the human body, whose biological functions are all automatically balanced, the psyche is not characterized by a spontaneous balancing and coordination of all its functions. In fact, it is constantly torn apart by the conflict between its constituent parts.

Through psychosynthesis, Assagioli provided a scheme, a transformative model, to bring a harmonious and inclusive synthesis of all the parts of human psyche and remove the conflicts among them every time they represent an involution instead of an evolution. Assagioli's model can be employed through the function of will, an essential element to achieve an evolutional transformation of the individual into the synthesis that is the most helpful in facilitating a harmonious relationship with one's own self.

In order to allow the personal self, identified by the Ego, to blend with the transpersonal self (the Higher Self or spiritual self) into a neutral, harmonious synthesis, the will must identify the motivation and objectives of each part to achieve a constructive synthesis.[4] Describing the two forms of the self, Assagioli (with coauthors) wrote:

> The objectives of the personal self are egocentric. In Maslow's terms, they are aimed at the satisfaction of needs and desires. The spiritual self is oriented toward the outside [altruistic] and does not ask nor desire anything *from* the outside. It is not hard to see the difference.[5]

CHARACTERISTICS OF THE EGO AND OF THE HIGHER SELF

Table based on the work of James Hollis as shared in a 2006 interview with Amy Edelstein, "Cos'è l'ego? Intervista a James Hollis su Jung" found on Arianna Editrice website.

The Ego	Analogy in the Higher Self
The Ego aims to serve itself.	The Higher Self aims to serve others.
The Ego seeks acceptance from the outside.	The Higher Self seeks inner authenticity.
The Ego sees life as a competition.	The Higher Self sees life as a gift.
The Ego wants to preserve itself.	The Higher Self wants to preserve others.
The Ego looks to the outside.	The Higher Self looks to the inside.
The Ego notices any lack.	The Higher Self notices abundance.
The Ego is mortal.	The Higher Self is eternal.
The Ego is attracted by lust.	The Higher Self is attracted by love.
The Ego looks for wisdom.	The Higher Self is wisdom.
The Ego enjoys rewards.	The Higher Self enjoys the journey.
The Ego causes pain.	The Higher Self heals.
The Ego rejects God.	The Higher Self embraces God.
The Ego tries to be filled.	The Higher Self is whole.
The Ego is me.	The Higher self is us.

Clinical Observations

The episode I am going to tell you about shows how counterproductive it is for Facilitators to feed their Egos.

I had just come back to Italy, and to continue my work I was relying on a physician friend who let me use his office and treat his patients once a month.

I felt I needed to show my abilities as a therapist to prove to my friend that I would do anything in order for the treatments on his patients to be successful. Therefore, when he introduced me to one of them and told me that no one had been able to solve his problem, I accepted the opportunity to treat him in a sort of God complex, feeling as if I was being invited to a sumptuous meal.

As soon as the patient entered the office, I noticed that he had a bit of a limp. I obviously did not ask him anything about it since I was convinced that I would certainly understand what was causing that gait, deal with it, and miraculously solve it. The patient told me that he was there because of his back pain. I made him lie down on the therapy table and, misled by the impression I had when I first saw he had a limp, confirmed in my mind that he had a short leg syndrome.

Once I had assessed the lack of symmetry between the malleoli, inebriated by my supposed evaluation abilities, I stubbornly avoided asking the patient for further information about his asymmetry. I started implementing osteopathic and CST techniques, overlooking the correct approach that should be employed by any good therapist during a treatment.

As time passed, the treatment did not seem to improve nor modify anything. I was getting more and more frustrated, and the more I frustrated I got, the more I yanked on the patient's leg, hoping for it to finally become longer. It was awful!

At the end of the session, I had obviously not achieved anything, and I was almost on the verge of blaming the patient for my failure. Worn out by my vehemence, he told me that he had contracted poliomyelitis when he was a child, which was the reason for his asymmetrical limbs.

I could not explain to you how I felt. Needless to say, that patient never came back for other treatments. Still to this day, after more than twenty years, every time we run into each other he changes direction or crosses to the other side of the street so that he does not have to speak to me.

I was feeling guilty about what happened, and I realized that it was my Ego that carried out the treatment in my place. So one day when I saw him walking in the street, I decided to approach him and ask him how he was doing. He was probably shocked, and maybe scared that I would volunteer to treat him again, so he kept walking. Trying to leave me behind, he told me from a distance, "I've never been better in my life, thank you!"

❧ A CST-CENTERED VISION ❧

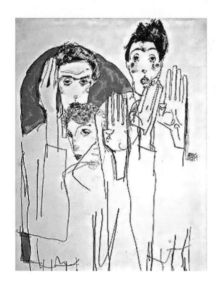

Fig. 5.1. *Seers,* by Egon Schiele

Egon Schiele's *Seers* (fig. 5.1) is a double self-portrait. In this and others of his self-portraits, Schiele did not try to define his identity but rather decided to portray the extraneous side of the "I." His self-portraits often show an image projected outside of itself, as if a double with altered features had come out from a mirror.

In exactly the same manner, the Ego deforms us. It creates a barrier and distances us from the others until we are strangers even to ourselves and our deepest essence, the Higher Self, is eradicated from us.

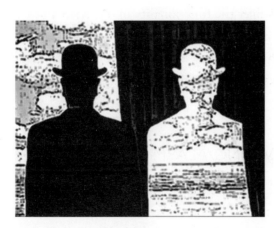

Fig. 5.2. *Reproduction of Transfer,* by René Magritte

In René Magritte's *Transfer* (fig. 5.2), the figure of the man on the left appears to have moved aside to allow us to see the landscape behind the curtain, making us understand to what extent our perception can be altered.

On a craniosacral therapeutic level, we could interpret the painting as the overall perspective on reality hidden by a partial vision—the vision of the Ego. It also is possible to find its meaning in the desire to let the clear part of ourselves emerge, penetrating the heavy curtains of the Ego with the consciousness of the Higher Self.

CHAPTER 6

Biological Processes in the Life Cycle

Experience is not what happens to a man; it is what a man does with what happens to him.

ALDOUS HUXLEY, *TEXTS AND PRETEXTS*

Our biological life starts from the moment the ovum is fertilized and ends with clinical death. The latter can occur naturally or be abruptly caused by an event that does not allow the organism to "pass away" naturally.

Between birth and death, our lives develop throughout the succession of numerous events. Some of these events may endanger the functionality of our RAS and are therefore usually defined as being negative. In this text, however, such events will instead be considered destructive, which means they essentially are traumas—and we will later see why. The destructive events in our lives can affect our physical, emotional, and spiritual well-being.

THE RETICULAR ACTIVATING/ALARM SYSTEM

The reticular formation is a neurological structure shaped like a net and located in the brain stem. Much of the input and output of the brain passes through this formation. It is connected with the limbic system (which supports the information linked to our emotions and five senses) and so influences our emotional systems. It also plays a role in the control of the autonomic nervous system, reflexive movements, balance, consciousness, attention, and the sleep-wake cycle.

This mass of nerve cells and fibers is connected with the limbic system, the reptilian brain, and fundamental structures such as the olfactory bulbs, the thalamus, the hypothalamus, the hippocampus, and the amygdala, which we will analyze later. The reticular system therefore influences every other system of the human body, from the cardiovascular system to the gastrointestinal tract, from the endocrine system to emotional response.

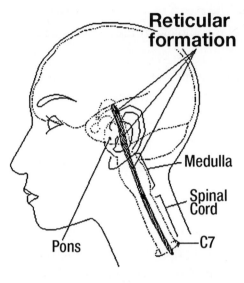

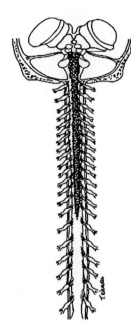

Fig. 6.2. The brain stem and spine

Fig. 6.1. Reticular formation in the brain stem

The reticular system is strongly affected by changes in stress levels. In a fetus, it can be affected by the mother's emotional stress. It is said to keep stressors in its memory and recognizes similar ones, accumulating them. Think of the common psychological reaction to bereavement in which a superposition between memories of previous situations of grief can be observed; this is the reticular system's stress memory arising. Some who believe in reincarnation think that even the memory of the stress of previous deaths could be recovered.

The RAS is activated when the reticular system detects a danger that needs to be faced or avoided—that is, situations that provoke fear or the fight-or-flight response. Its activation is a response to the information the reticular formation transmits. The RAS involves the trigeminal nerve (cranial nerve V) and, consequently, the temporo-mandibular joints, which are fundamental for survival. We will later analyze these structures as well.

THE INFLUENCE OF DESTRUCTIVE EVENTS

The aim of this section of the book is to understand what phases of the Life Cycle within our personal Biological Process were characterized by experiences and events involving separation and/or loss, what kind of influence they currently have upon us, and how they could affect our future. Then we can learn how to transform the negativity that destructive events generated in our bodies and minds, sometimes even enabling ourselves to transform the entropic energy connected with the traumatic event and change our future for the best.

To do this, we first need complete awareness of the events that carried a destructive significance. We then must revisit the period of our Biological Process in which they occurred.

We often may assume that a particular negative event did not affect us in a destructive way, or that it occurred so long ago that we can just forget about it. Even more frequently, we think that events we regard as positive cannot be considered stressors or cannot have a destructive component. In fact, even positive events can be stressful, with their destructive effect hidden by their apparent and contingent positivity.

Let us take one possible case scenario within the Biological Process of the Life Cycle—conception—and the very different developments that can evolve from it.

This event is obviously part of our biological parents' experience, and it allowed for us to be here now in this particular phase of our Life Cycle. Imagine the following scenario.

A woman finds out that she is pregnant, and a man is told that he will become a father in about nine months. According to specific implications and premises, such as physical, emotional, and social conditions, the discovery of this occurrence envisages different possibilities. Both the woman and the man could rejoice enthusiastically, but one or both of them also could panic because they do not want the responsibility of being parents and eventually might even spiral into depression.

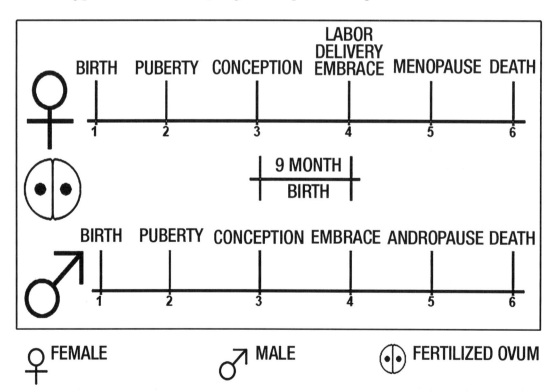

Fig. 6.3. Biological Process in the Life Cycle

In the second hypothesis, which we could define as a negative scenario, two very different and distinct phases of the Biological Process of the Life Cycle are involved: One is conception; the second is the beginning of new lives after the ovum is fertilized (the child's and those of the parents).

For the woman and the man who are now becoming parents, if one accepts the new phase of life but is rejected by the other person, the consequence might be the future development of an emotional trauma. For the fertilized ovum, the imprint connected with the negative emotion of the rejection occurs in the form of Cellular Memory. Such occurrences in Cellular Memory could negatively affect the development of the fetus.

The sense of abandonment provoked by rejection is an imprint that could even affect future choices in the development of the individual, whether parent or fetus. In the different phases of their Life Cycle, individuals could actually reiterate that abandonment by rejecting the people around them or searching for situations that force them to face abandonment again. This happens because they have internalized rejection as a lesson learned and, even unknowingly, recognize it as a known situation, as opposed to other scenarios involving acceptance and positive reception.

Clearly, right now I am analyzing only the negative aspects since I want to underline how emotional factors can affect the Life Cycle in the present, even when they are connected to events that occurred a long time ago. We will see later how we can find opportunities to transform our open system as human beings, if we have not been able to do it yet.

For our objectives, we must not forget that our organism has a Cellular Memory. Some health issues or disorders can be connected to specific phases of our Biological Process, whether they are underestimated or clearly meaningful, and whether they are quite old or recent.

CELLULAR MEMORY AS FEEDBACK

We have mentioned Cellular Memory, a subject that should be analyzed in depth with much more than a few lines. Discussion of this topic implicates many other fields in a sort of chain reaction, but since we cannot go too much into detail here, we are going to provide you with the very basics. The following paragraphs will highlight some of the concepts, topics, aspects, and disciplines that address the influence of stress (trauma, traumatic change of state) on Cellular Memory.

Epigenetics

The term *epigenetics* comes from the Greek prefix ἐπί (*epi*), "over, around," and γεννητικός (*gennetikòs*), "concerning the heritage of one's family." It is a relatively recent branch of genetic research analyzing changes that affect the phenotype without an alteration of the genotype. Therefore, it studies "unstable" heredity, which constitutes the response to intrinsic and environmental stimuli. It also makes the organs quickly adaptable to physiological and environmental changes through modifications that vary gene expression without requiring any kind of alteration in the nucleotide sequences of DNA.[1]

Arthur Riggs defined epigenetics as "the study of mitotically and/or meiotically heritable changes . . . that cannot be explained by changes in DNA sequence."[2]

Sir David Charles Baulcombe, a geneticist and professor of botany at the University of Cambridge, said about epigenetics, "DNA is central—epigenetics is an important side show to the DNA. . . . Traditionally we thought that genes encoded proteins—but we now know that they also specify regulatory RNA. It provides a molecular memory of our past experience. Stress is particularly important—probably all forms of stress including physical and psychological."[3]

About epigenetics and molecular correlations involved in the homeostatic process, the Treccani *Enciclopedia della Scienza e della Tecnica* states:

Current research is identifying the kinds of external signals able to induce a state of emergency in epigenetic activity and the molecular mechanisms that are connected to it. Moreover, more and more researchers are convinced that the key to understand the evolution of species and populations lies in the study of environmental influences and developmental systems. Research on epigenetic heritage and phenotypical plasticity allows room to the role of environment in evolution, and both fields of study seem to lead to ecological evolutionary developmental biology . . . focused on the relationship between genetic information and environmental information.[4]

Psychoneuroendocrinoimmunology (PNEI)

PNEI is the discipline that studies mutual correlations between the psyche and biological systems in a given environment. PNEI focuses mainly on bidirectional correlations between psyche, nervous system, endocrine system, and immune system. It was born as a result of studies about stress and developed in the 1930s thanks to Hans Selye, founder of the study of the neurobiology of emotions. His work allowed researchers to discover the functions of neuropeptides, the molecules able to connect the psyche, the immune system, the endocrine system, and the nervous system.

The functions and interconnections of neuropeptides were later studied by American neuroscientist and pharmacologist Candace Pert (1946–2013), who even worked with Dr. Upledger. For now, we just need to know that she proved the existence of opioid receptors, the cellular binding sites of endorphins in the brain.[5]

Character-Analytic Vegetotherapy

This field analyzes the neurovegetative system and the autonomic system from the anatomical and physiological point of view (vegetotherapy) to identify the possible physical location of psychological disorders (character analysis). It was promoted by Austrian psychiatrist and psychoanalyst Wilhelm Reich (1897–1957), who was Freud's student in Vienna and spent a big part of his life in the United States, where he died. He was one of the most important forerunners of PNEI. The research he conducted in the 1930s about orgone energy and the social role of sexuality became so well known that it overshadowed the other fundamental principles of his theories. One of these principles is the concept that we now call "holism," which he defined as the "functional unity of mind and body." This basic idea was developed by his most famous disciple, Alexander Lowen, who introduced a specific approach called "bioenergetic analysis" about a decade later.[6]

Bioenergetics

Alexander Lowen's approach led to the creation of many schools of bioenergetic theory and practice. Bioenergetics assesses the personality of the individual on an energetic level, connecting work on the body to work on the mind. The objective of bioenergetics is basically to help people solve their existential and relational problems, enhancing each individual's innate ability to feel pleasure and joy of living. As Indian philosopher Osho said, "Happiness is a birthright." The same principle can be found in the U.S. Declaration of Independence of 1776, which states that the "pursuit of Happiness" is an inalienable right. Bioenergetics is still used today to intervene effectively on muscular tensions and stress, improving the overall well-being and functionality of the individual.[7]

Auxology

Auxology is a branch of medicine that studies a limited period of the Biological Process (physical growth from birth to the age of twenty years) through a multidisciplinary approach that includes various medical specializations and some different disciplines, such as economics, sociology, anthropology, hygiene, human factors, ergonomics, et cetera. The objective of auxologic studies is to use specific protocols and measurements to determine the different possibilities of the individual's growth and development in relation to environmental variations. Among the factors considered essential in auxology we find genetic, endocrine, nutritional, socioeconomic, environmental, psychological, and stress factors.[8]

Entelechy

The term *entelechy* was coined in ancient Greece by philosopher, logician, and scientist Aristotle (384–322 BCE), who proposed a particular philosophical perspective on reality that considered the development of all organisms and living beings as the pursuit of an inherent, innate objective. In this view, all organisms develop according to their own intrinsic law, which is meant to realize their peculiarities and the expression of their potential through action.

The development of entelechy has continued through the ages:

Neoplatonic philosophers (third century) partially shared the Aristotelian conception. They talked about the form of bodies as longing to immanence, not only for transcendence, as Plato believed.

G. W. Leibniz (1646–1716), German philosopher, scientist, logician, theologian, diplomat, jurist, and historian, recovered entelechy by introducing the philosophical metaphysical concept of monadology, which concerned substantial forms of being he called "monads." Monads are essentially eternal, inseparable, and individual "spiritual atoms." They obey their own laws, do not interact, and individually reflect the entire universe in a harmony prearranged by the Supreme Monad—God. They are organized in temporal space and work autonomously but synchronously.

J. W. von Goethe (1749–1832) proposed for entelechy the archetype of the plant, an ideal vegetal and biological model that manifests itself through tangible exterior signs during the evolutionary developmental phases and adapts progressively to different environmental conditions.

H. Driesch (1867–1941), German philosopher and biologist, revived the term *entelechy* to indicate the vital force that he believed to be intrinsic in embryos and responsible for their development. This was in contrast with the mechanistic theories of his time, which regarded them as "machines."

C. G. Jung (1875–1961) developed the concept of entelechy in analytical psychology through what he called the "individuation process." He believed that all individuals are born with a particular nature and/or vocation. The discovery of one's own nature is essential for all individuals, and it can be encouraged through their actions and lifestyle, with the purpose of getting closer to the fulfillment of a harmonious realization within their Biological Process and the maximum goal of their Life Cycle. The individuation process usually starts during the fourth decade of life. It occurs in people who separated and emancipated successfully from their parents, reached an adult sexual identity, and obtained a certain degree of independence through their work. For Jung, individuation is the fulfillment of psychic completeness and integration.[9]

SomatoEmotional Release can contribute considerably to support the individuation process through visualizations and the Therapeutic Imagery and Dialogue technique.

Circadian Rhythms

Under normal conditions, the whole organism, as well as each single cell, has a regular rhythm, which can be affected by numerous factors of different magnitude, such as the rotation of Earth and the consequent succession of light and darkness. Even one single living cell can change its own form, location, concentration, and activity over the course of only twenty-four hours. Biology, and chronobiology in particular, addresses the fascinating and currently unsolved issue of the identification of mechanisms that allow specific cells to accurately measure the twenty-four hours of the biological rhythm in the human organism.

The rhythm that characterizes the whole organism is always the combined result of different rhythms. In fact, it is determined by the specific rhythms of each cell of the body.

One of the main factors determining circadian rhythms in living organisms is the succession of light and darkness, which synchronizes them according to the requisites of adaptation and environment. Even environmental factors, such as the availability of raw food materials and outdoor temperature, are periodical and hence have a rhythm of their own. Humans and social animals also are synchronized with the rhythms of the other members of their own group. In our civilization, social signals prevail over physical environmental stimuli since misleading factors, such as electric lighting, substitute the natural succession of light and darkness. Therefore, circadian rhythms can be subjected to strong oscillations, whether collective or individual. However, that does not mean that there is no precise organization in human physiological functions, whether we consider the major ones, such as blood circulation and breathing, or less obvious ones, such as cell division (mitosis).

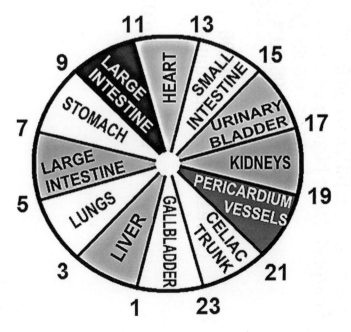

Fig. 6.4. Circadian rhythm—our biological clock

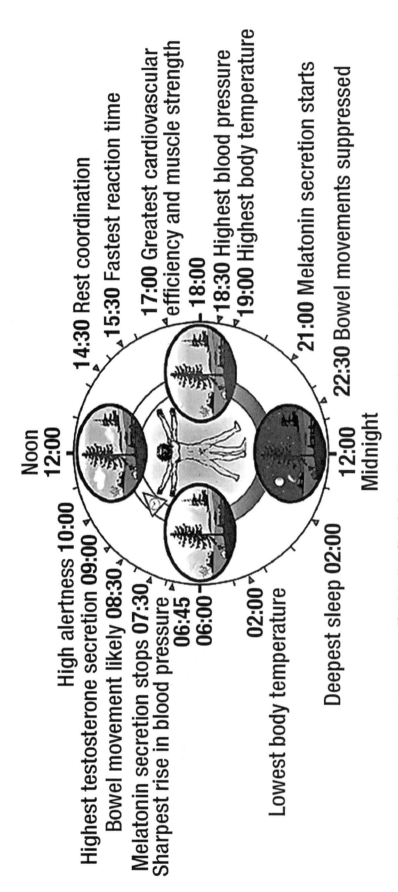

Fig. 6.5. Circadian rhythm—the inner clock of the human body

Calculation and mental activity are characterized by a clear circadian periodicity as well, even though the rhythm of cerebral waves (alpha, beta, gamma, etc.) is ultradian, which means that it has a shorter frequency than the circadian rhythm. In addition, different geophysical cycles respond to circatidal, circannual, or other rhythms.

Each organ of the human body has its peak of activity in a specific phase of the circadian clock. In this phase it is particularly easy to detect the dysfunctions connected to that organ or the systems it belongs to. However, the circadian system and its chronological organization of the physiological processes controlling the whole organism continue to work perfectly as long as the individual is young and healthy.

With age, the periodic structure of circadian rhythms is altered. Consequently, some rhythms anticipate or delay their distribution in the twenty-four hours; others reduce dramatically the oscillation of their amplitude.[10]

It also is true that civilized humans nowadays measure time mainly according to behavioral, social, and emotional signals.

MacLean's Triune Brain

American physician and neuroscientist Paul D. MacLean (1913–2007) took an interest in the functioning of the brain with regard to its correlations with self-preservation, adaptability to the environment, and reactions to the "internal environment" of the human being, meaning the emotions. He divided the brain into three fundamental anatomical areas:

- reptilian brain
- limbic system (or mammalian brain or paleomammalian brain)
- neocortex (or neomammalian brain)

Each of these structures is said to regulate specific functions, called "operators."

The reptilian brain is connected to the primary, innate needs and instincts of human beings. The reptilian operators are isopraxic (behaving in the same way and mimicking), specific, sexual, territorial, hierarchical, temporal, sequential, spatial, and semiotic. On the anatomical and functional level, it is similar to the brain of reptiles and structurally represents the most ancient part of the brain, which developed about 500 million years ago. In addition to the regulation of reflexive/involuntary activities, it manages instinctive functions that are necessary for survival, such as the choice of territory and its defense and the fight-or-flight instinct. Anatomically, the reptilian brain in the human organism involves the diencephalon, the midbrain, and the initial part of the cerebellum.

The limbic system is connected with emotions. Its operators are emotional: phobic, aggressive, protective (child care and maternal instinct), loving, and playful. It is

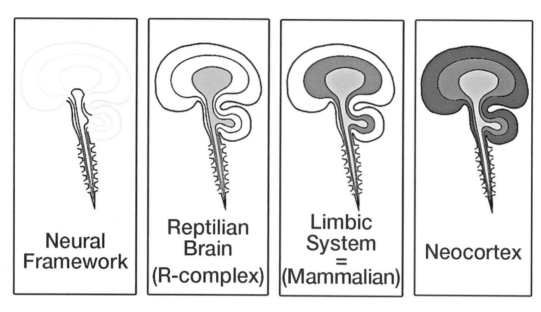

Fig. 6.6. Diagram of MacLean's triune brain

more recent than the reptilian brain, dating back to 300 million to 200 million years ago. This part of the brain is more flexible than the reptilian brain and manages emotions, such as anger and fear, as well as self-preservation in the form of nourishment and protection from the dangers of the external environment. The anatomical location of the limbic system in the human organism mainly involves the olfactory bulbs, the septum pellucidum, the fornix, the hippocampus, the amygdala, the anterior cingulate cortex, and the mammillary bodies.

The neocortex is connected with the operators that belong specifically to human beings. These are the functions separating human beings from other species: holistic, reductive, generalizing, causal, binary, and emotive. It is the most recent of the three brain structures, and it is believed that it developed 200 million years ago in human primates. It is the area in which critical thinking, language, adaptability, learning, and long-term planning develop. Reflection, logical thinking, abstract thinking, ideas, inventions, and imagination come from this area as well. In the human organism, the neocortex is the largest part of the cerebral cortex and is made of neural materials.

Each portion of the triune brain affects human behavior. Though they all differ on a structural and chemical level, they interact and cooperate between each other.

In human life, traumatic stimuli (stress) can alter the functional balance of the three aspects of the brain. The separation—the lack of integration—between the functions of the triune brain allows individuals to feel something external in their own thoughts, as if they were experiencing something independent from their will. Consequently, they react to the stimuli by enhancing or diminishing the hierarchical subordination between one structure and the other, which can result in the modification of the heritage of behavioral dispositions in the species.[11]

LIVING ORGANISMS

Describing the "biological universals" that define living organisms, Italian philosopher and historian Pietro Omodeo wrote: "'Living' indicates a cellular open system delimited by a selective border, traversed by self-regulated flows of matter, energy, and information, which allow it to reproduce and evolve through generations, adapting to changing environments."[12]

In the most commonly accepted definition, all living organisms must own some general biological characteristics, among which are the following:

Evolution: They advance, develop, and transform through their own evolutionary ability because they can vary the set of genes constituting the DNA (either the individual DNA or that of their group, the genotype) or characteristics, such as morphology and growth, and the biochemical and physiological characteristics (phenotype).

Order: They have a given structure.

Code: They contain information/instructions about their structure and functions.

Growth and development: They can grow autonomously because they are able to reproduce and give birth to new organisms that are similar in their development and have the same ability to reproduce.

Energy: They assimilate and transform energy and give it back to the environment since they are thermodynamic systems.

Sensitivity and mobility: They can respond to external stimuli.

Regulation: They maintain autonomously their homeostasis.

We have already encountered the concept of homeostasis, and we will see some of its other aspects in the next chapters. We now want to provide a more detailed definition of what it means from the *Treccani Encyclopedia*:

> The ability of living things to maintain the value of some internal parameters around a preestablished level, continuously disturbed by various external and internal factors. The ordered set of subsystems that make up the human organism is responsible for a network of control systems, whose simultaneous intervention regulates the flow of energy and metabolites, so as to keep the internal environment unchanged or almost unchanged, regardless of changes in the external one. The self-regulation of

living organisms is a fundamental concept of modern biology, formulated at the end of the ninteenth century. by the French physiologist C. Bernard.

The disturbances mentioned above can be either objective (physiological or environmental in origin) or subjective (emotional and/or traumatic in nature).

One of the objectives a Facilitator must pursue is the conservation of a constant physical/organic/psychoemotional/adaptive balance (homeostasis) in the individual and the greatest possible enhancement to facilitate the passage to known and/or unknown phases of the Life Cycle.

EVOLUTION AND CELLULAR MEMORY

In individual development, the determining factors for evolutionary growth are many, as are the scientific and medical disciplines that examine them. Let us see some of these disciplines, at least those that can help us widen our comprehension of the complexity and subjectivity of the homeostatic balance and the continuity of evolution in every person within their Life Cycle.

Biology and Natural Science

Biology, the science that studies physical, chemical, and emergent processes of the phenomena that characterize living beings, and natural science, the study of the physical, chemical, and biological aspects of Earth, the universe, and all life forms, including humans, see evolution as the phenomenon of growth and development that changes the state of all living organisms until their specific functions stop. For human beings, the phenomenon of evolution lasts as long as the activity of their Biological Process within the Life Cycle—from birth to death, passing through maturity. Nevertheless, there is a heritage that does not die with the death of a single organism. Rather, it survives as genetic and Cellular Memory, determining the evolution, modification, and transformation of all the organisms. In human beings, such heritage can take on a configuration that is either direct (the genetic heritage of the offspring) or indirect and transverse (connected to environmental influences and/or the interaction with accidental factors and/or contamination), and it causes variations detectable both diachronically (over time) and synchronically (at the beginning and at the end).

Quantum Theory

As discussed earlier, our Cellular Memory holds generational memories, which are the memories connected to experiences of trauma and stress that were passed on by previous generations. The mechanisms that provoke the emergence of Cellular Memory in relation to a common experience, not a personal one, act through neural paths that are activated by a known stimulus, either identical or similar to the one contained in Cellular Memory, and reiterate the reaction that was previously experienced. Just as known neural processes induce our organism to reiterate an emotionally negative/destructive pattern in reaction to physical and/or emotional trauma, it is possible, once the origin is recognized and acknowledged, to similarly create and activate neural processes in order to reprogram the reaction and determine a transformation in the original behavioral pattern—from destructive/negative to positive/constructive.

Quantum physics analyzes another aspect of Cellular Memory: collective Cellular Memory, which is considered as an energy field generated by individual Cellular Memories. In 1900, Max Planck theorized that energy is made of invisible particles of matter that he called "quanta." Albert Einstein later confirmed Planck's thesis with his theory of the photoelectric effect. French physicist Alain Aspect then developed the theory with his work on the double-slit experiment, quantum tunneling, and wave-particle duality. Quantum phenomena were applied in physics, chemistry, and medicine. Biologists observed and identified the superposition of quantum states and the tunnel effect in many biological processes. We know today that quantum events are determining factors for heredity since the genetic code is written in quantum particles, and quantum genes code the functions of all living beings.

Commenting on Johnjoe McFadden and Jim Al-Khalili's 2014 book *Life on the Edge: The Coming of Age of Quantum Biology*, clinical developmental psychologist Piero di Giorgi wrote:

> All the information stored in memory is "entangled" (which means that it remains connected but nonlocalized in a communication that becomes virtually eternal) and constitutes a single quantum wave.
>
> Memory has a quantum foundation and quantum events have a holistic nature. That means that memory derives from a quantum entanglement process. Each fragment of information is connected to all the others simultaneously. If memory is holographic and constitutes a single quantum field, all the information and the events keep superposing unconsciously with similar probabilities until new information comes to interact with the unconscious memory and the set of memories is holographically diffused and activates a "decoherence," causing the superposition of different states to collapse in one single state and give us normal macroscopic perceptions—that face, that object, that idea. The superposition of states that correspond to many classic configurations—one for each fluctuation—is reduced to that single act of consciousness. The consciousness is the critical point where the state superposition collapses into classic states. It is clear that, by resorting to the unconscious, the role of emotions and emotional life for memory and consciousness is crucial.[13]

Clinical Observations

One of my patients once contacted me to ask whether CranioSacral Therapy could be useful to help him get rid of a sense of sickness he was going through. He did not display any physical dysfunction, but he was experiencing lethargy, a lack of willpower, and an overall sense of dissatisfaction. All of this was occurring despite the fact that he had a job he liked. Since he very much enjoyed the everyday satisfactions and contacts that came with his job, he did not care about not earning much from it. The interactions he was able to have through his job actually made him feel socially fulfilled. He was curious, did not lack intellectual stimuli, loved to spend time outdoors, and loved meeting people, but he did not disregard some occasional time by himself. He exercised and alternated physical activity with moments of reflection. He did not use medication or need it.

I invited him to lie on the therapy table and used the SQAR assessment. I immediately perceived a lack of vitality. His rhythm was still average, but it was clear he was fatigued. I worked with the meridians, trying to revitalize them, and with the solar plexus chakra.

During the treatment, the patient told me he was starting to sense a strong heat inside all of his body, which made him feel more in connection with himself. We started the Therapeutic Imagery and Dialogue and he immediately visualized the color green. This brought me to the heart chakra, but I simultaneously felt drawn toward the third ventricle. I moved to his head and followed the attraction, which brought me to the center of the head, exactly where the third ventricle of the brain is located. On an emotional level, CST considers the third ventricle to be the "heart of the brain." If it is dysfunctional, it can be recognized as the cause for sadness and depression. For this reason, as I was connecting with the third ventricle, I asked the patient what he was thinking about. That is how I came to know that when he was younger he suffered a traumatic brain injury during a sports activity. Although he recovered physically, I had the impression that a latent sense of fear of physical death had remained inside him. I talked to him about it, and he told me that after the accident he had made the decision to live in the moment, with no projects for the future, and to welcome only short-term situations into his life.

When the first treatment took place, the patient was forty years old and did not have any vision of his future. He did not think he wanted to accomplish any new project or get involved with other people. Other treatments followed, and I worked on his heart and all the organs and systems involved in depression, sadness, and fear (limbic system, compression/depression triad, reticular system, pericardium, lungs, kidneys). Something changed in the patient's attitude;

he gradually started to feel the need to get involved in both short-term and long-term projects for his future.

The perceptions he had experienced about a possible interruption of the vital energy continuum (caused by the shock of the accident that had occurred when he was young) had been held by his Cellular Memory and created a paradox effect: A fear of death was preventing him from fully living the phases of his Life Cycle. He was not aware of this specific memory held by his non-conscious, but it made him boycott any decision envisaging a future realization, obstructing any situation of constructive growth and delaying the natural cycle of his Biological Process.

Now the patient has two children. He recently told me that they made him discover he was born to be a father and that being with them and watching them grow is the greatest thing in the world for him. He has never suffered from apathy again. He still has the same job, but he widened his hobbies and took an interest in gardening, which he enjoys with people who share with him the joy of seeing nature develop throughout the different seasons. Now he does feel fulfilled.

CHAPTER 7

Separation and Loss

An Introduction

Remember that everyone you meet is afraid of something, loves something, and has lost something.

H. JACKSON BROWN JR.,
THE COMPLETE LIFE'S LITTLE INSTRUCTION BOOK

Stress resulting from separations and/or losses is detectable not only in situations that are objectively painful and unfavorable but also in favorable situations that are expressly sought by the individual. Numerous examples could be mentioned, but it will be enough to discuss a couple of them. Our first example of a sought and favorable situation concerns one of the possible phases of a woman's Life Cycle, childbirth. After delivery, the mother experiences happiness for having her newborn child. However, since the child has been sheltered in her womb for months during pregnancy, birth also represents the separation from the fetus, which means that the mother will not be able to perceive her child's movements inside herself anymore.

Another example is the scenario of two emotionally connected adults deciding to move in together by mutual agreement. The event in itself is sought and positive, but the change in pace of life and the abandonment of previous houses and personal contexts may cause emotional stress, upsetting the individuals involved in the relationship.

Ordinary life situations, such as separation and loss, may be experienced in different or even opposite ways by different people and are not always attributable to positive and negative concepts or models. This premise introduces one of the most significant concepts of this book: A trauma factor (stressor) does not always consist of a destructive event, and a trauma does not always have a destructive outcome.

SEPARATION AS LOSS

Loss can be either objective or subjective. When the mind processes a separation as a loss, that separation is experienced as trauma. Instead of fading, the trauma is fed by the emotional component that is associated with it, impressing on fascial and Cellular Memory and generating an Energy Cyst.

Objective Loss

Events objectively involving separation and loss are those that seem to reflect objective reality the most. Among the most common we can mention are the death of a loved one; birth in its connotations of separation and loss (abandonment of the mother's womb); biological losses, such as the loss of a limb or part of it, an organ, or an embryo or fetus; separation from a partner, friend, relative, or pet; loss of a meaningful object, a job, a house, money, or financial security; and the anticipatory grief over the unexpected and impending loss of one's life (e.g., being diagnosed with a degenerative and/or irreversible disease).

Subjective Loss

Subjective loss is the state of consciousness induced by the external world after an objective loss. It is perceived through the senses or any kind of emotional, psychological, or sentimental state of mind. Subjective experiences include the way we perceive the concept of death/loss of life; the experience of grief following the loss of a loved one; the perception of a specific life situation/scenario involving any kind of lack; the loss of social, religious, or political identity; and detachment from a specific group.

"Small Deaths": Rites of Passage

These are the phases of passage from one specific condition to another within the Biological Process of the Life Cycle. They are characterized as the group of biological and transformative events and difficult passages that constitute the fundamental changes of life. They follow one another, combine in different spatiotemporal stages, shape our entire existence, and evolve through signs, manifestations, and causes that will lead to physical death through a logical and/or natural process.

The "Loss of Losses": Death

The idea of death is a speculative concept since it is an objective fact that death does not exist for the living. Living beings do not experience death directly. We only know the fear of death and its different modalities, from the so-called natural death to suicide (labeled sometimes as negation of life or as a solution to life), including euthanasia, or assisted suicide.

> ## THE FACILITATOR'S OBJECTIVES IN SITUATIONS OF SEPARATION AND/OR LOSS
>
> As we will see throughout this book, one of our objectives is to train our ability to distinguish the different types of energy that are connected with individual emotions and actions/situations, and in particular syntropic (organized and constructive) energy and entropic (disorganized and destructive) energy.
>
> As we have seen, separations in the Life Cycle, whether objective or subjective losses, can be experienced as trauma. With that concept in mind, Facilitators can see that patients seeking a treatment might be:
>
> - individuals who need to address/readdress their personal experiences of separation and/or loss
> - individuals who complain of a physical symptom that actually may be connected with a recent or past loss
>
> In either case, the Facilitator's aim is to dissipate the destructive energy, helping patients acquire awareness about their own difficulty and the possibility of transforming the (entropic) destructive energetic potential into (syntropic) constructive energy, to the advantage of their present and future life path.

Separation and Loss in the Biological Process

We are now going to examine some events of the human Biological Process, deliberately interpreting them in their connection to separation and loss. This quick analysis can help us train our ability to detect the aspects of our experience that may be considered negative, while we also get used to recognizing another fundamental aspect, the transformative potential.

Birth: For the newborn, separation from a warm and safe environment; for the mother, loss of the sense of exclusive biological connection with the fetus.

Puberty: Loss of sexual innocence and hormonal quietude; meaningful change in the emotional side of the personality; essential change in physical identity.

Conception: Loss of the fetus through miscarriage or abortion necessitated by serious physiological dysfunctions in either the mother or the fetus; rejection following the refusal of maternity or paternity; as connected to the difficulty/impossibility of conceiving, a possible loss of self-esteem, and the redefinition of one's own identity.

Labor/delivery: Loss of the intimate inner contact with the fetus; in the case of forced induction or cesarean section, potential loss of both self-confidence and the confidence in one's ability to carry out a biological function.

Embrace: The first sensory contact through tactile and olfactory recognition is inevitably followed by the first removal of the newborn from the embrace.

Menopause: Loss of fecundity, loss of libido, loss of bone density, thinning of the intervertebral discs, loss of elasticity in the tissues, possible loss of memory, et cetera.

Andropause: Loss of psychoemotional balance involving either the loss or the increase of libido and erotic fantasy, thinning of the intervertebral discs, possible loss of memory, et cetera.

Death: Even experienced indirectly, death brings fear of losing the continuum of life, fear of pain, fear of the unknown, and fear of losing earthly situations or material and emotional possessions.

LOSS AS A CONSEQUENCE OF POSSESSION AND BELONGING

Science, literature, and philosophy abound with studies and theories on objective and subjective loss. However, in order for a situation/scenario of loss to occur, there must be a prior experience, or at least some kind of perception, involving possession, attachment, or belonging to someone or something.

For example, within the studies on the first phases of the Biological Process, we find scientists such as British psychologist, psychiatrist, and psychoanalyst John Bowlby (1907–1990), who dedicated his life to the study of the psychological conditions of the individual. He focused especially on the first part of childhood. This included the moment of the first detachment (separation/loss) from the intrauterine physiological condition as well as the sensory detachment (recognition followed by removal from the mother's breast, body, or embrace) and emotional detachment (removal from the parent's vital space). He thus elaborated the theory known in the scientific world as "attachment theory," described in his trilogy *Attachment and Loss*. According to Bowlby, attachment is "an adaptive need accompanying the individual from the cradle to the grave, influencing the development of personality since the first days after birth, with an impact also on the relationships established later in life. Depression, anxiety, and similar conditions in adults can therefore be connected with experiences such as a painful separation from the mother figure (or from the caregiver) that occurred during childhood."[1]

In order to elaborate his research and support this theory, Bowlby gave particular attention to ethnology and biology, with specific reference to the studies of Konrad Lorenz and Harry Frederick Harlow. Afterward, Bowlby gained international fame, especially for his studies on the psychological conditions of children without a family or familial care.

To say it in a very simplistic way, the trauma of delivery and birth—in the context of separation from the mother's womb—constitutes the normal and necessary condition to guarantee the conservation and genetic heritage of our species.

Nonetheless, from an epigenetic point of view, the way traumas and stress affect each individual's life is extremely important, particularly if we focus on childhood trauma. Some studies have revealed that individuals who experienced specific difficulties during either early or late stages of childhood show significant epigenetic variations.

EPIGENETICS AND TRAUMA

Epigenetic variations caused by trauma and never adequately addressed manifest themselves during an individual's entire adult life. In addition, they can be transmitted to future generations, just like traumatic factors involved in the Biological Process of one's Life Cycle. In fact, resorting to a speculative simplification, we could conclude that the completion of pregnancy through the phases of labor and delivery may cause excessive stress (anxiety, fear, pain, etc.) since it adds to contextual stress—meaning the stress that might be experienced due to very specific cultural and social conditions, or to a situation of emotional abandonment/rejection, or to a context of poverty and conflict. This may even be attributed to stress experienced in the same situation on a generational level, especially if the situation brought a person to a particularly traumatic and/or unresolved outcome that remained impressed in cellular and genetic memory.

As Simone Gardini, cofounder and CEO of biotechnology company Genome Up, writes:

> What we are is not already inscribed and enclosed in our "genome." On the contrary, as it was proven time and again, it is determined by a "process of dynamic interaction between the genome and our environment." The experiences in the environment of everyday life could actually be able to shape genetic activity through "epigenetic modifications," which would mean that the relations between genotype, phenotype, and environment are governed by similar molecular processes.[2]

A study carried out by an international group of researchers indicated that gene expression in a newborn child is extremely different from gene expression in an elderly person, and that gene expression is constantly evolving through the Life Cycle. In particular, the researchers found that aging was associated with "silencing" genes with a protective function. The director of the research group, Manel Esteller, noted that epigenetic lesions, unlike genetic ones, are reversible through modification of DNA "methylation" schemes (an epigenetic modification that alters the accessibility of DNA without changing its underlying sequence), and this can occur even with just a change of lifestyle, such as diet.[3]

Starting from embryonic development, and during all the stages of development of the human Biological Process, epigenetic mechanisms are activated via molecular and enzymatic pathways, thereby altering the molecular transcription of DNA or RNA through methylation. And as Gardini states:

> Highly stressful events such as grief, abuse, disease, or trauma can mark the body as well as the mind, especially when they are endured by children and adolescents. Nonetheless, the effects of these traumas may also be inherited, thus affecting the physical and psychological health of descendants with issues such as psychiatric pathologies and developmental disorders. The occurrence of such instances was proved by a study, carried out by a research group of the Tufts University School of Medicine of Massachusetts and then published in *Translational Psychiatry,* which confirmed that vulnerabilities in children can be connected with their parents' epigenetic alterations.[4]

Therefore, with our DNA sequence we also inherit the epigenetic quality of RNA, which influences the Biological Process of our Life Cycle on both neurobiological and behavioral levels. This epigenetic quality can be altered, transformed, and improved through the dissipation of a contingent or past trauma.

SIGNIFICANT LOSSES IN THE BIOLOGICAL PROCESS

Grief is usually associated with losing a person or a meaningful relationship, but it actually has much wider connotations. Grief is also related to phases following the so-called small deaths (note that the meaning and value of this term does not coincide with Reich's definition of orgasmic energy). For example, an individual might experience grief immediately following the arrest of a personal plan, the renunciation of an objective, the occurrence of a new disability, a negative change in lifestyle, and so on.

Later we will explore the stages of grief as defined by Swiss psychiatrist Elisabeth Kübler-Ross, who followed the studies carried out in this field by Bowlby and other psychologists and psychotherapists.

Right now, however, our concern is to underline that when dealing with grief—meant as the condition following a traumatic or stressful event connected with any kind of loss—rationality often fails to properly address the psychological and emotional state experienced by the individual, regardless of the amount of time they take to process it. Not processing the stages of grief after a traumatic abandonment or loss could compromise or prevent the natural passage from one phase to the other within the Biological Process of one's Life Cycle.

As discussed in chapter 6, entelechy holds that all organisms develop according to their own intrinsic law, which is meant to realize their peculiarities and the expression of their potential through action. A traumatic occurrence in a life path can block or delay the development that is meant to eventually bring a person toward this accomplishment. Similarly, the study of epigenetics tells us that the experiences in the everyday environment are able to shape the activity of genes through epigenetic modifications. Cellular Memory, therefore, can retain the negativity connected to a traumatic loss and the grief for that loss, thereby affecting the vital energy continuum.

Nonetheless, our thoughts and actions can intervene and transform negativity. Even though we often believe that we are not able to overcome the harshness of a certain phase of our Biological Process, or to preserve our vital energy continuum, we can realize that we have the means to recognize, address, transform, and dissipate trauma, past or present. We can realize whether the emotion that is connected with the trauma is our own or has been induced, and thereby we can become aware of both its physical and emotional destructive manifestations and causes.

Clinical Observations

A woman in her thirties booked an appointment with me because of her persistent cervical pain. Before coming to my office, she had already been treated several times with different kinds of therapies, but she had never received any benefit from them. Then she was treated with CranioSacral Therapy while on vacation, and the results had positively surprised her. Once she was back from her holiday, she came to me, since we lived in the same city.

Even after examining her medical history from the occurrence of the first symptoms eight years before, I found nothing during my first evaluation that allowed me to identify what was causing such persistent pain. I treated her with both CST and osteopathic methods, but I could not find the reason for her pain. I asked her whether she had received any dental or orthodontic treatment, but her answers did not give me a better understanding of the situation.

During the second session, I started to work mostly with techniques meant to alleviate the tension of intracranial and spinal membranes. Something did not add up, and I was led to believe that her pain had to be connected with some past trauma and the emotionality connected with it, but I could not gather what it might be.

The young woman still wanted to continue with the CST treatments because her pain had faded a little after the first two sessions, and she was feeling much more reassured and stronger in dealing with it.

The mystery unveiled itself in the third session. She burst into tears and told me that she had had an abortion ten years before in Italy, where it was not then legal. She had become pregnant during a vacation in which she had occasional unprotected sex with various people. For this reason, she did not know who the father was. She believed that it was not possible to talk about it with her parents, so she felt completely alone and destabilized and decided to have an abortion.

She never addressed nor processed that loss. She told me that afterward she started to feel as if she didn't "belong with myself" anymore. Two years later the cervical pain started.

She came back several times. She also started seeing a psychologist, saying that she finally felt she had the will and the strength to "fix some personal stuff," partly because cervical pain was not tormenting her anymore.

A young man came to my office complaining of persistent, though not disabling, lumbar pain. He immediately told me he knew the cause of his pain. He had been a ballet dancer since a very young age and was now a professional in classical and contemporary dance. I checked his vector/axis system and found it misaligned. I recalled Dr. Upledger's description of his own work with a ballet dancer, so I enthusiastically thought that I could similarly solve my patient's lumbar pain.

After some treatments, his pain diminished a little but did not disappear.

I thought it was because I did not have the same skills as Dr. Upledger. He used to say, "The best therapist is the patient," and I had decided to treat this patient for a biomechanical dysfunction, trusting what he had told me himself. What was I missing?

I checked his vector/axis lines again and was brought in the direction of the third chakra. I investigated further and evaluated the spleen and liver meridians, but I still could not understand.

The patient was always talking during the treatments about his experience as a dancer, from the very beginning to when he entered the corps de ballet of the Teatro alla Scala in Milan, Italy. As if by intuition, while I was assessing the energetic quality of his meridians, I told him I once had seen a ballet at the Mariinsky Theatre in Saint Petersburg. At that precise moment, his attitude changed completely and he suddenly looked sad. He told me he had always had the ambition to dance in the corps de ballet of that theatre, and the feeling for him was like "a nail in my back." I rarely had patients describe their symptoms with such clarity. The problem was that he was not tall enough for the selective standards used to choose the dancers at the Mariinsky.

Although he had been able to obtain a prominent position as a dancer of the Teatro alla Scala of Milan thanks to his technical and artistic skills, the suffering that had come from the impossibility of being chosen for the Russian corps de ballet had always stayed inside him.

What he was going through was grief due to losing the chance to achieve a specific personal and professional plan. The dance world had welcomed and taken care of him to the extent of making him direct all his plans for the future toward that environment, and then he had been "abandoned."

❧ A CST-CENTERED VISION ❧

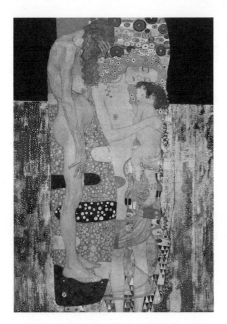

Fig. 7.1. *The Three Ages of Woman*, by Gustav Klimt

The subject of Klimt's *Three Ages of Woman* (fig. 7.1) is a symbolic reinterpretation of the three stages of a woman's life—childhood, maternity, and old age. The image can perfectly illustrate the Biological Process of an individual on both a physical and an emotional level.

The three figures ostensibly show very different complexions. The old woman has marked skin and a curved posture, as if to symbolize the weariness of her existence; the young woman has white and smooth skin and shows her protective force by holding the child; the little girl has pink cheeks and innocently enjoys her rest, trusting her mother's embrace completely. It also can be noted that the little girl is in the foreground, representing life as it starts to develop, which means the beginning of the Biological Process. The central section is occupied by the young woman, who represents fecundity with her embrace, whereas the old woman on the left, symbolizing the final part of the Biological Process, is almost fading into the background, as if she belongs to a different dimension of life.

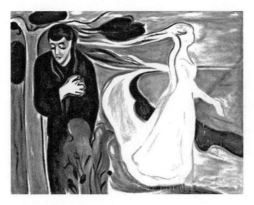

Fig. 7.2. *Separation*, by Edvard Munch

Edvard Munch's *Separation* (fig. 7.2) expresses the emotional bond that stays inside the individual after a separation, represented here by the female figure's hair flowing behind her. Munch commented on his own painting with the following words: "He doesn't really understand what is happening. Nonetheless, even when she has disappeared, he feels the thin threads of her hair wrapping around his heart, which bleeds and burns like an incurable wound."[5]

The image represents what in this therapy we call a small death, a traumatic event due to objective or subjective separation/abandonment/loss that causes a blockage in the vital energy continuum.

CHAPTER 8

Measuring Stressors
The Holmes and Rahe Stress Scale

Change is the process by which the future invades our lives.
ALVIN TOFFLER, *FUTURE SHOCK*

In order to delve into the subject of measuring stressors, it is essential to keep in mind that we are analyzing any situation that generally implies change, more specifically a type of change that follows an event involving separation and/or loss.

Within the Life Cycle of an individual, such occurrences might be labeled "psychosocially stressful events," "stressing agents," "life events," or "stressors." Whether they are ordinary or extraordinary, positive or negative, destructive (traumas) or constructive (evolutionary changes following the loss of a known situation), they become determining factors for the social and individual existential readjustment that is necessary and sometimes inevitable.

Many therapists and psychotherapists have studied these events (the stressors) in relation to their patients' different physical and emotional reactions. After many years and the analysis of thousands of cases, they summarized the results of their research in various rating scales to assess the impact of stressors on individuals.

Two psychiatrists in particular, Thomas Holmes and Richard Rahe, wrote an article in 1967 about the correlation between the effects of traumatic factors in life events and some diseases. It was based on their clinical experience and research conducted on more than 5,000 patients. The outcome of their research was summarized in a scale, best known as the Social Readjustment Rating Scale (SRRS), and sometimes called the Holmes and Rahe Stress Scale.

THE HOLMES AND RAHE STRESS SCALE

Rank	Event	Life Change Units
1	Death of a spouse or partner	100
2	Divorce	73
3	Marital separation or separation from partner	65
4	Jail term	63
5	Death of close family member	63
6	Personal injury or illness	53
7	Marriage	50
8	Fired at work	47
9	Marital reconciliation or reconciliation with partner	45
10	Retirement	45
11	Change in health of family member	44
12	Pregnancy	40
13	Sex difficulties	39
14	Gain of new family member (birth, marriage of son or daughter)	39
15	Business readjustment (mergers, failures, etc.)	39
16	Change in financial state	38
17	Death of close friend	37
18	Change to a different line of work	36
19	Change in number of arguments with spouse	35
20	A large mortgage or loan	31
21	Foreclosure of mortgage or loan	30
22	Change in responsibilities at work	29
23	Son or daughter leaving home	29
24	Problems with in-laws	28

THE HOLMES AND RAHE STRESS SCALE (*cont.*)

Rank	Event	Life Change Units
25	Outstanding personal achievement	28
26	Spouse begins or stops working	26
27	Begin or end school/college	26
28	Change in living conditions	25
29	Revision of personal habits	24
30	Trouble with boss	23
31	Change in work hours or conditions	20
32	Change in residence	20
33	Change in school/college	20
34	Change in recreation	19
35	Change in church activities	18
36	Change in social activities	18
37	A moderate loan or mortgage (for a car, a fridge, etc.)	17
38	Change in sleeping habits (more/less hours of sleep, jet lag, etc.)	16
39	Change in number of family get-togethers	15
40	Change in eating habits (quantity, quality, meal time)	15
41	Vacation	13
42	Christmas*	12
43	Minor violations of the law (parking violation, official warning, etc.)	11

*Christmas is in the original scale but could presumably be replaced with any major holiday.

In this scale, Holmes and Rahe listed forty-three common stressors and gave a value for their impact on an individual's emotional sphere using what they called "life change units" (LCUs). These LCUs represent the impact of a particular event on people when they are forced to make changes and reorganize their lives because of it.

There are certainly many more stressors in addition to those listed by Holmes and Rahe, and other therapists use different scales, though there are many similarities. There are stress assessment scales meant to be used with children and adolescents, thus taking into account their specificity and different kinds of collocation, evaluation, and measurement.

Different stressors may occur together, in which case their respective ratings in the Holmes and Rahe Stress Scale must be added together. The total of the sum indicates the condition of the individual and the probability for said individual to develop an "adjustment illness."

For the purposes of CST, it is essential to remember that unsolved traumatic events may be associated with active lesions and manifest themselves as Energy Cysts inside a person's body. The more that traumas are ignored, misunderstood, or underestimated and consequently remain unsolved and accumulated, the more the defenses of the organism weaken, creating a breeding ground for adjustment illnesses.

In Holmes and Rahe's evaluation, the likelihood of developing an adjustment illness in relation to the sum of the LCUs is summarized as follows:

- from 100 to 150 LCUs = 30% likelihood
- from 150 to 299 LCUs = 50% likelihood
- more than 300 LCUs = 80% likelihood

PATHOLOGIES CONNECTED WITH STRESS

One of the most well-known pathologies caused by situations of intense and prolonged stress is post-traumatic stress disorder (PTSD). It is not an actual disorder but rather a traumatic syndrome leading to a serious clinical picture and demanding psychotherapeutic attention.

Dr. Upledger addressed PTSD cases. One of his studies was an experimental research project in which he treated Vietnam War veterans with a combination of CST and psychotherapy. That project subsequently gave birth to Dr. Upledger's Intensive CST and SER Treatment Protocol, which is still being used in the Upledger Institute Clinic in Florida and in some other international branches of the institute (including the Italian one). Dr. Upledger also discusses the implementation of CST and SER in cases involving PSTD in his book *Cell Talk:*

> Another area in which this work has proven remarkably beneficial is in Post-Traumatic Stress Disorder (PTSD). We have worked with all types of victims of violent crimes, from rape to attempted murder. We also have worked with children

who have been abused and/or have been victims of satanic-cult rituals. We have worked intensively with PTSD-disabled Vietnam War veterans. They have all done well.

The factor that all of these cases seem to have in common is residual of consciousness energy from the perpetrators of the violent acts, or simply from the energy fields of the location, such as those present on some battlefields. When the therapist blends with the PTSD patient, the practitioner can locate this destructive area within the consciousness energy field and help the individual identify it also. Working together, it seems that the constructive energies of patient and therapist are able to expel the destructive energy. During the time of expelling, the unwanted consciousness energy field is often visible to the therapist and patient (we often use multiple therapists for one patient during this process). Once the destructive consciousness energy has been expelled, the patient can respond very quickly to counseling and/or other therapies to which there had been no reaction before.[1]

As Dr. Upledger makes clear, PTSD is a type of pathology that can affect not only combat veterans but also adults and children who have experienced traumas such as:

- bullying, mobbing, stalking, persecutions
- dire poverty
- war, terrorist attacks, guerrilla warfare
- an episode or a series of episodes of violence (sexual abuse, bullying, torture, harassment)
- extreme events (earthquakes, fires, floods, etc.)
- significant objective and subjective losses and separations
- bereavement (that was not processed or was only partly processed)

Fortunately, people do not always develop PTSD when these or similarly difficult occurrences take place. Therefore, most individuals involved in events such as these display only temporary emotional reactions, which may be painful but do not constitute a structured PTSD. According to Matteo Simone:

Trauma can be considered from two different points of view. When addressing its "objective" aspect, the assessment regards mostly the intrinsic gravity of the event. For example, torture and abuse are painful experiences that are unbearable for anyone, and as such they are to be considered objectively traumatic.

On the contrary, the "subjective" dimension must be evaluated taking into account the subject over the event itself. In this case, it is imperative to focus on the way a specific individual processes the traumatic event. There are no two people who feel and react to a trauma in exactly the same way. What is harmful for one person may be stimulating for another.

Stress symptoms can be fought by removing and/or alleviating the causes of stress, but trauma is essentially a fracture. It is related to the loss of contact with oneself, one's family, and the surrounding environment. A loss such as this is often hard to recognize since it develops over time, very slowly.[2]

OTHER STRESS ASSESSMENT SCALES

There are several stress assessment scales. Most of them are normative and also address the psychosocial factors caused by stress, consigning the items (stressors) with specific values. Normative scales follow the technical foundation of the Holmes and Rahe Stress Scale, which nowadays is still the main normative tool in this field. Therefore, they also attribute relevance to the stressors according to their social context. Some normative scales focus on specific sectors (e.g., work-related stress, caregiver stress, or the stress connected with specific dysfunctions, disabilities, pathologies, etc.).

There are also subjective stress scales, which indicate several stressors but leave a certain autonomy to the subject, who is supposed to determine, assess, and quantify the effect and relevance of each stressor in that particular moment of their life.

In addition to the Holmes and Rahe scale, among normative scales assessing nonspecific perceived stress, another one that is very well known is the Perceived Stress Scale (PSS), created by American psychology professor Sheldon Cohen and later adapted and modified several times. The Interview for Recent Life Events (IRLE), a stress assessment scale created by Eugene Stern Paykel and collaborators that comprises sixty-one stressors (eighteen more than the Holmes and Rahe scale), is quite well known as well. Another quality scale is a PTSD self-assessment questionnaire created by the psychiatry department at the University of Siena, Italy, which includes eighty-seven questions, divided in two parts to create a comprehensive assessment.

Self-Assessment Exercise

Here we have the first of some brief self-assessment exercises that are integrated in the book to give you the chance to proceed gradually and consciously as we analyze the peculiar transformative process of CST.

Below you'll find the list of stressors 31 to 43 on the Holmes and Rahe Stress Scale. These stressors are those that affect the Life Cycle of the individual less critically than the rest.

Instead of using Holmes and Rahe's LCU (life change unit) rating scale, we propose the following alternative.

1. Choose three stressors from the table below that apply to you and write them down.

HOLMES AND RAHE STRESSORS: 31 TO 43

Rank	Stressor	Mark 3 stressors that apply to you
31	Change in work hours or conditons	
32	Change in residence	
33	Change in school/college	
34	Change in recreation	
35	Change in church activities	
36	Change in social activities	
37	A moderate loan or mortgage (for a car, a fridge, etc.)	
38	Change in sleeping habits (more/less hours of sleep, jet lag, etc.)	
39	Change in number of family get-togethers	
40	Change in eating habits (quantity, quality, meal time)	
41	Vacation	
42	Christmas	
43	Minor violations of the law (parking violation, official warning, etc.)	

2. Rewrite each of the three stressors using specific key words that apply to you (for example, "change in eating habits" might become the key word "diet") and put them in the stressor column of the table that follows (see the sample table).
3. Write in the middle column a name or adjective to define a negative feeling or evaluation that you associate with each stressor (for example, diet = deprivation).
4. Write in the third column a word describing a positive emotion or evaluation that you associate with each stressor (for example, diet = health improvement).

SAMPLE TABLE

Stressor	Negative Emotion/ Evaluation	Positive Emotion/ Evaluation
Diet	Deprivation	Health improvement

SELF-ASSESSMENT

Stressor	Negative Emotion/ Evaluation	Positive Emotion/ Evaluation

---

A BRIEF DISCOURSE ON STRESSORS

It is easy to deduce that each stressor may assume a negative connotation in relation to other factors, such as:

- the period of life in which it occurs
- its emotion-related components (objective, subjective, social)
- the presence or occurrence of other stress factors at the same time
- the life change that is forced upon the individual in order to address and overcome stress
- emotions that connect this stressor to other similar stressors experienced in the past and/or to the difficulties endured in order to deal with them (even if each of these stressors had a very different impact by itself)

Let us take as a model the example of a stressor previously proposed (See sample table above).

We have used the word *diet* to summarize stressor 40 of the Holmes and Rahe Stress Scale. *Diet* should have a neutral connotation (if we rely strictly on the definition of the word), simply and generically indicating the way an individual eats (their eating lifestyle). However, the term *diet* often is employed to define a change in everyday nutrition. If this change has a therapeutic objective, which means the objective of correcting specific medical conditions, it also could imply that the clinical picture of the individual is not ideal. In this case, stressor 40 could go side by side with a stressful event/scenario that is much more traumatic, such as the diagnosis of a health issue that demands a diet in order to improve or be solved.

Changing our eating habits also modifies the rest of our lifestyle, on both a personal and a social level. We are deprived of the freedom of not thinking about how much we eat or what we eat. Nonetheless, a change in our nutrition, even when it is forced on us, causes us to be more aware of and give more attention to the quality of our daily food intake. Thus, not only can it improve our health, it brings us to a new state of awareness.

Epigenetic studies and research have observed that nutrition is one of the factors that causes the increase, reduction, and modification of the signals on the DNA surface and on the histones, influencing over time the way DNA is read. Professor Alessandro Fatica notes, "For example, some foods increase the production of methyl groups, favoring the DNA methylation. Consequently, what we eat can influence the epigenetic state of our cells, thus changing the gene expression, and pass it onto the next generation."[3]

We have discussed, although only superficially, some aspects and negative and/or positive implications that may emerge when analyzing a single stressor (number 40, in this case) among those listed in the Holmes and Rahe Stress Scale. Therefore, it is no wonder that in a more in-depth personal analysis of the meaning of a specific stressor, each of us can interpret that stressor differently and give it a more positive or a more negative connotation according to our own experiences.

Clinical Observations

A woman in her fifties came to my office complaining of an interscapular pain referred to the sternum area. The patient felt a "dull ache" that had been persisting over a long period of time. She described the symptom as a recurring sensation of lack of breath due to dorsal pain. She thought it could be a cardiac problem, even though the results of the several tests she had undergone contradicted that idea.

During my physical examination of the woman, I detected a strong tension in the rhomboid muscles and a lack of the proper fascial mobilization in the respiratory diaphragm. After the first session, the restriction of the rib cage had released slightly. When she came back for the second session, she told me that after the initial relief following the treatment she had not observed improvements. In fact, when I assessed that area again, I found that the area of restriction persisted, just like the patient's pain.

I started treating her using the Significance Detector and subsequently employed Therapeutic Imagery and Dialogue. During the dialogue, the topic of vacations came up. When I asked her to talk about it in more detail, the patient told me that she had not gone on holiday for some years due to events that had changed her lifestyle and imposed that limitation. In fact, the company she owned with her husband had gone bankrupt, not for their inability to manage it but because of a bureaucratic setback.

She and her husband then had to start from scratch, but after a while her husband fell into depression, so she had to find the courage to address the situation with abnegation, taking over for her husband and accepting the responsibility of two jobs. Willing or not, she unfortunately felt overwhelmed by that situation, especially because she could not ask for or find comfort at home.

Sometimes this kind of situation just happens. Like many of my colleagues, when faced with personal stories like this one, I wish I could find immediate and concrete solutions to alleviate the difficulties in my patients' lives. Of course, sometimes I am only able to observe these difficult situations as they emerge from the everyday lives of the people who search for my help, not finding an actual practical and instant solution.

After a mental digression about this issue, I regained my role as a therapist, abandoning sympathy for my patient in favor of empathy. I invited her to mentally go back to her last vacation and talk about that.

She saw herself sitting on a pier in a Croatian village as she was admiring a wonderful sunset with her husband. She recalled some sweet words they shared in the twilight. Then, almost awakening from that description, she said she was once told that "reality starts with a dream" and that she now felt ready to dream again of an experience like that with her husband, which allowed her to look to the future and be positive again.

At the end of the session, the tensions she had been feeling had diminished. We planned one more session. On that occasion, she told me that she spoke to her husband about what emerged during the treatment. They decided to commit to a future together in which they would again live magic moments like the ones they had already experienced together.

CHAPTER 9

Processing Emotions
Using CST and SER for Integration and Release

There can be no transforming of darkness into light and of apathy into movement without emotion.

CARL GUSTAV JUNG,
"PSYCHOLOGICAL ASPECTS OF THE MOTHER ARCHETYPE"

When exploring the potential of CST and SER in scenarios involving separation, loss, abandonment, and bereavement, the role of the Facilitator in the practice and implementation of these therapies is outlined by specific protocols and principles. Although every single interaction between Facilitator and patient is unequivocally unique, just like everyone is unique as an individual, there are specific criteria that Facilitators cannot disregard:

- The voice of the patient's non-conscious must be perceived through the Significance Detector.
- The Facilitator must try to foster dialogue between the patient's conscious and non-conscious.
- The Facilitator must encourage the positive resources that emerge in scenarios of separation, loss, abandonment, and/or bereavement, transforming destructive scenarios into constructive potentials for the benefit of the patient's present and future.

CST and SER work with the emotionality of ongoing situations and past experiences. As Dr. Upledger advised, the Facilitator must follow the instructions of the patient's Inner Physician—the Higher Self—in facilitating the intrinsic self-correcting mechanisms of the organism.

Patients often complain of physical symptoms that do not seem to have any connection with situations involving separation, abandonment, or loss and consequently grief. Even more often, they are not even aware of the real causes of the physical symptoms that prompted them to turn to a therapist.

In such cases, Facilitators must focus on themselves and on assuming the correct attitude (correct approach) with their patients. Facilitators must transform all attitudes that are potentially shallow, self-centered, and self-referential into a positive/constructive approach, which will allow them to manage any context their patients want to address. Above all, Facilitators must be absolutely aware that they will have to deal with the delicate and crucial domain of their patients' individual emotions and experiences.

To better understand the approach Facilitators must assume, it is essential to first understand the energy of emotions. To begin, the energy held back or expressed through destructive emotions, such as rage, fear, hate, and possessiveness, is exactly the same energy that also constitutes constructive emotions, such as calm, relaxation, joy, serenity, and safety. To preserve the energetic potential of individuals and facilitate the improvement of their self-confidence, it is essential not to use avoidance techniques or to force the analysis of emotions on the patients. On the contrary, the objective is to convert/transform the emotion that has a destructive connotation into its opposite, the constructive energetic potential of that same emotion.

Facilitators must not define their patients' emotions as *positive* and *negative* but rather as *constructive* and *destructive*. Similarly, it is crucial to debunk the erroneous equations *positive = favorable* and *negative = unfavorable*. Describing the positive potential of a "negative" emotion with destructive energy, Dr. Upledger himself noted:

> Anger might give you the superhuman strength to cripple Hulk Hogan were he to attack you. But when this anger continues, it becomes destructive. Anger is a spender. It demands of your heart, your lungs, your liver, your stomach, your colon, your entire physiology. It works just like the sympathetic nervous system. It will save your life in an emergency and keep you going under stress, but it will also hasten your demise. It is destructive when the emergency is over and your life has been spared. Hate, anger, jealousy, fear, and guilt will consume and destroy their owner if they maintain an ongoing residence.[1]

Patients may be facilitated in their attempt at expressing their emotions by being supported as the emotional energy outflows rather than by being led or vehemently encouraged to let said emotions out.

As soon as the emotion-related destructive energetic component (entropic energy) emerges, Facilitators can neutralize it with their intention and then convert it into syntropic energy with the cooperation of their patient's non-conscious. That energy thus remains available and can later be employed constructively.

Sometimes patients are not aware of the retained emotions connected with their symptoms. It is the Facilitator's aim to let a patient's non-conscious express those emotions. Through it, patients can acquire awareness of the primary and secondary causes for their symptoms. It goes without saying that there is no need for intervention when the emotions involved are constructive (for example, happiness, joy, serenity, and the like).

Traditional Chinese medicine holds that emotions gather in specific organs of the body. Dr. Upledger used the term *visceroemotional* to define these correspondences between internal organs and emotions. We will analyze them later in more depth (see chapter 13). Before addressing such a complex subject, however, we should first define what *emotion* actually means.

DEFINING EMOTION

Neuroscience has recently described the functioning of the emotional process, outlining a specific systemic context of organized components connected to emotional processes of perception, monitoring, and adaptation. In practice, this context involves specific cerebral areas and neural circuits as well as sensory mechanisms. Therefore, neuroscience regards emotions as biological functions that play a key role in the evolution of living beings and contribute to guarantee both their survival and reproduction. Research in this field also has drawn attention to the centrality of simple positive emotions as useful evolutionary tools for individuals and, more generally, for the species.

When providing a definition of emotions, it is essential to distinguish between emotions and feelings, the latter being a product of consciousness, a subjective classification made by the individual on unconscious emotions.

Before further analyzing the distinction between emotions and feelings and examining the organs and systems involved in the functioning of the emotional process, let us take a step back and see how emotions were considered in different historical periods, before neuroscience took them into account and defined them on a structural and organic level.

Emotions in History

We are going to analyze how different scientists, thinkers, and philosophers regarded emotions, starting from a relatively recent period. The first intellectual we want to mention is French philosopher and mathematician René Descartes (1596–1650), who claimed that body and mind are clearly divided. He attributed a nonmaterial foundation to the mind, identifying it in the human organism with the brain. In fact, Descartes considered the brain to be the repository of all superior functions as well as the organ responsible for all intellectual processes (e.g., reasoning, language, morality). On the contrary, he connected emotions with a much humbler area of the body, the lower abdomen, which he regarded as the seat of the most animal-like instincts of human beings.

From Descartes through the past century, emotions have been seen as "transient states and reactions that are able to interrupt the flow of mental activity between the reception of a stimulus and the response from the individual."[2] This type of conviction actually has roots in far more ancient history, dating back to the age of classical Greece, when man was believed to be a dualistic being divided between logos (thought/word) and pathos (emotion/passion). This particular dualism was passed on over time as a model that could guarantee the implementation and consolidation of logical thinking, intellect, and objectivity. The latter were considered the characteristics of the rational individual who does not deviate from critical thinking for any instinct or emotion.

In the time of ancient Greece, the philosopher, logician, and scientist Aristotle (384–322 BCE) added on to the dualism of logos and pathos, proposing instead a tripartite system of ethos, logos, and pathos (character, thinking, and emotion). Nowadays, these are still considered the three main components that, along with their variables, constitute what we could call the "art of communication" (*ars retorica*) and allow us to analyze the structure and content of a message as well as the type of communication that is necessary in order for it to be received and/or divulged.[3]

Much more recently (more precisely, in 1990), this concept was expanded and surpassed by psychologists Peter Salovey and John D. Mayer. They described the new notion of "emotional intelligence," creating the basis for a new science of communication: "Emotional intelligence involves the ability to access and/or appraise and express emotion; the ability to access and/or generate feelings when they generate thought; the ability to understand emotion and emotional knowledge; and the ability to regulate emotions to promote emotional intellectual growth."[4]

The concept of emotional intelligence was then further actualized by well-known psychologist and science journalist Daniel Goleman, who published in 1995 a book titled *Emotional Intelligence: Why It Can Matter More Than IQ*. In this book, he built the structure for a veritable school of communication with motivational purposes and the objective of acquiring "personal and social emotional competence," including leadership competence and the speculative management of others' emotionality and one's own.

The new current of communication based on emotional intelligence was quickly noticed and awakened the interest of several psychologists, psychotherapists, and scientists, including biologists and neuroscientists, who all tried to examine in depth what we could define as the "organic structure of the emotional system."

Organs, Systems, Emotions, and Neuroscience

We are now moving on to some of the most significant conclusions made by neuroscientists and psychotherapists in relation to their clinical studies and scientific research on the organic structures involved in the emotional process.

Neuropsychologists Mark Solms and Oliver Turnbull note, "The structures that form the core of the emotion-generating systems of the brain are identical to those that generate the background state of consciousness. . . . These phylogenetically ancient structures lie in deep regions of the brain, in the middle and upper zones of the brainstem."[5]

Joseph LeDoux, an American neuroscientist who manages the Center for the Neuroscience of Fear and Anxiety at New York University, studied the functioning of the limbic system and its interactions with emotional states as well as its correlation with the modes of expression of human personality. In 1996, LeDoux theorized the existence of a dual route in the transmission and processing of information, going from sensory organs to the brain and mainly involving two cerebral nuclei: the amygdalae (with one nucleus in each cerebral hemisphere).

The first pathway of the dual route, also called the low, short, or direct route, is activated through the sensory organs that receive external stimuli, which are translated into sensations, perceptions, and electrical impulses and then sent in the form of information to the thalami (cerebral nuclei of the center of the brain), where the first processing takes place. Subsequently, the thalami send other electrical impulses to the amygdalae, which further process the information, producing new and different electrical impulses meant to send orders and tasks to the effectors (lungs, heart, muscles, etc.) according to the information the amygdalae received. The effector organs, in turn, produce an immediate behavioral response to express the emotion.

The second pathway, also called the high, long, or indirect route, also involves the thalami and their processing of the impulses coming from the sensory organs. In this case, however, the thalami send the new electrical impulses to the cerebral cortex, not to the amygdalae. Only after the new impulses arrive in the cortex are they processed and sent to the amygdalae, which process them again. The amygdalae produce other impulses and send them to the effector organs to stimulate the response of the organism.[6]

In short, the direct route from the thalami to the amygdalae makes it possible to immediately assess external stimuli as they occur, allowing a quick response to fight-or-flight situations. On the contrary, the longer pathway from the thalami to

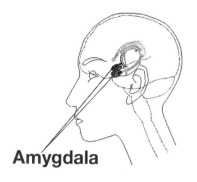

Fig. 9.1. Amygdala. There is one amygdala for each cerebral hemisphere. On a cellular level, they hold the memories of occurrences connected with experiences of survival. They also play a crucial role in emotional contexts involving aggressiveness.

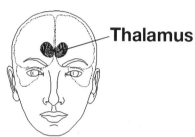

Fig. 9.2. Thalamus. It selects the sensory impulses directed to the brain, especially the emotional ones. If the impulses are too many, it can become dysfunctional.

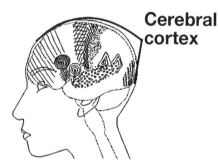

Fig. 9.3. Cerebral cortex. Its main purpose is communication. It influences cognitive choices to solve issues through specific strategies, from the simplest to the most complex.

the neocortex and then to the amygdalae allows the superior cognitive systems of the brain to make a more detailed assessment of a single stimulus and how it relates to other stimuli, representations, and experiences, thus bringing a person to an emotional response that is more complete, articulated, and aware. Responding through conscious feelings means involving more superior cognitive systems, which offer the opportunity to regulate emotional response.[7]

According to LeDoux, the quality of cognitive regulation of emotions seems to be determined both by the quality of the representation of the cognitive system and by the strength of neural pathways going from the prefrontal cortex to the amygdala.[8]

When LeDoux wrote about his observations, neuroscientist Paul MacLean reacted vehemently. MacLean, whom we mentioned in chapter 6 as the father of the triune brain model, accused LeDoux of overlooking some aspects of emotions because MacLean did not recognize a distinction between emotions and feelings and connected them both only to the cerebral structures and neural circuits of the cerebellum that are linked with the limbic lobe.

On the contrary, LeDoux clearly distinguished emotions (derived from a primary stimulus) and feelings (derived from the conscious processing of unconscious emotions), always considering them in relation to the limbic system but regarding feelings as being further processed and then transmitted as information to the neocortex.

It was Richard D. Lane, professor of neuroscience, psychiatry, and psychology at the University of Arizona, and his colleagues who, in 1998, provided scientific evidence proving that the neural correlates of emotional awareness include the activity of the anterior cingulated cortex.

In 1990, Lane had started his research on cerebral functions involved in the emotional process, employing psychology and neurobiology to outline the nature of emotional awareness and the mechanisms through which emotions contribute to physical and mental health. His research allowed him to delineate a protocol that can be used as a model to study, assess, and address emotions. It is a cognitive-developmental model that focuses on individual differences in the emotional experience and expression. To devise it, Lane evaluated the neural foundation of emotions and emotional awareness by using positron emission tomography (PET) and functional magnetic resonance imaging (fMRI), which locates the areas of the brain that are activated during a certain activity, in interaction with peripheral physiology, vagal tone, and neurovisceral integration, even examining the mechanisms through which emotions can initiate a sudden cardiac arrest.

In order to enhance the clinical application of this model, in 2000 Lane and his collaborators developed an assessment scale of emotional response, known as Levels of Emotional Awareness Scale (LEAS), studying behavioral, neuroanatomical, and clinical correlates of emotional awareness. It is described as follows:

The LEAS divides emotional awareness into five primary levels:

1. physical sensations;
2. action tendencies;
3. single emotions;
4. blends of emotions;
5. blends of blends of emotions.

It poses evocative interpersonal situations and elicits open-ended descriptions of the emotional responses of self and others, which are scored using specific structural criteria applied to the emotion words used in the responses.[9]

Marie T. Banich, executive director and professor of psychology at the Institute of Cognitive Science of the University of Colorado at Boulder, further developed

LeDoux's studies in order to examine them from the point of view of cognitive and behavioral neuroscience. More precisely, she conducted her research through neuroimaging techniques (medical imaging of neuroradiology). Professor Banich's work focused on the comprehension of the neural systems that allows us to manage our attention and actions in order to set priorities, organize, and direct our behavior toward specific objectives, thus delineating the abilities that are usually defined as "executive functions." Her comparative studies examine both healthy individuals and individuals with ADHD or behavioral issues, especially of ages typically considered by neurodevelopmental studies.

Modern neuroscience (or neurobiology) applied to cognitive and behavioral science embraces an extremely wide scientific, sociological, and psychological field, including emotional learning as the global process of learning through positive and negative emotions. For our purposes, it is enough to just summarize some of the conclusions of the various research on emotions conducted in the neuroscientific field:

- Amygdalae are essential for processing the impulses sent by sensory organs through a direct pathway connecting the thalami and the amygdalae and through an indirect pathway connecting the thalami, the cortex, and the amygdalae. Neurotransmitters are involved in both pathways (high route and low route).
- Among the main neurotransmitters that manage our emotions are dopamine (connected with pleasure and gratification), serotonin (associated with memory, learning, and relaxation), and norepinephrine (which keeps stress and anxiety levels low).
- Emotions and cognition are activated in different cerebral areas, but they are bound to meet in the prefrontal cortex.
- Acquiring awareness about one's own emotions is fundamental in order to be able to address, process, and overcome emotional traumas and/or the destructive emotional elements in physical traumas.
- The processing and transformation of trauma starts when negative and/or positive emotions transform into constructive (syntropic) energy.

Another useful source is the work of social psychologist Barbara Fredrickson, professor at the University of North Carolina:

According to the broaden-and-build theory of positive emotions developed by Barbara Fredrickson (in 1998), positive emotions, as well as negative ones, have an adaptive function, motivating individuals to carry out activities that are adaptational on an evolutionary level. Not only do positive emotions increase physical, intellectual, and social resources, but they are also involved in the improvement of the individual's state of health. For instance, positive emotional experiences broaden the scopes of the cognitive system and foster a more creative and flexible thinking pattern, while at the same time also facilitating the ability to face stressful situations and everyday adversities.[10]

EMOTIONS VS. FEELINGS

We are going to mention yet another neuroscientist, Portuguese neurologist, psychologist, and essayist Antonio Damasio, director of the Brain and Creativity Institute of the University of Southern California and professor at the Salk Institute for Biological Studies, one of the most prestigious scientific research institutes in the biomedical field. He brought to the academic world and the public the appreciation of emotions and their current scientific evaluation through his book *Descartes' Error: Emotion, Reason and the Human Brain*.

Descartes's error, as the book calls it, was failing to understand that "nature appears to have built the apparatus of rationality not just on top of the apparatus of biological regulation but also from it and with it."[11]

Damasio himself clearly differentiates between emotions and feelings, dividing them into three fundamental "states":

- emotion, which is provoked and takes place unconsciously
- feeling, which can be represented unconsciously
- feeling of feeling, which means that the feeling is consciously perceived and the organism is aware of both emotion and feeling[12]

The difference between emotions and feelings was excellently summarized by psychologist, music therapist, and neuropsychoanalyst Pietro Aquino:

Keeping a clear-cut separation between emotions and feelings, the latter being the private, mental experience of an emotion, there are some conclusions to be drawn:

- It is not possible to observe a feeling in anyone else, but it is possible to observe a feeling in ourselves when, as conscious beings, we perceive our own emotional states.
- Some aspects of the emotions that originate feelings are clearly observable.
- Basic mechanisms behind emotions do not require consciousness since the occurrence of a feeling in a limited window of time is by itself conceivable without the organisms actually noticing it.

- We are not necessarily aware of what induces an emotion and cannot control emotions with our will, which means that they can manifest below the level of consciousness and still provoke emotional responses.
- It is possible to acquire the ability to conceal some of the external manifestations of emotions but not to block the spontaneous changes occurring in our bowels and inner environment.
- Emotions are triggered on a completely unconscious level and are therefore hard to elicit consciously since they depend on deep cerebral structures, which cannot be controlled with our will.

Therefore, we know we are experiencing a feeling when in our mind we perceive a "feeling self," whereas we acknowledge an emotion when we feel it occur in our organism.

Experiencing an emotion is simple since it consists of mental images arising from the neural schemes that represent the variations occurring in the body and brain and constituting the emotion itself.

Nonetheless, we know we are experiencing a certain feeling only after building the second-order representations that are necessary for the "core consciousness."

Experiences play a crucial role in all of that since each of them leaves behind a conscious or unconscious trace that generates emotions and feelings with positive or negative connotations.[13]

THE IMPORTANCE OF BEING CONSCIOUS OF EMOTIONS

In CST, it is essential to know emotions and, above all, to distinguish them from feelings. Emotions are connected with specific organs and systems of the human organism, the limbic system in particular, and they can actually be responsible for emotional and physical dysfunctions. Moreover, in order to focus on the Therapeutic Imagery and Dialogue of SER and act on the possible dysfunctions caused by emotional trauma, it is important bring the individual to the conscious awareness of the emotions that could be provoking the issue. We must therefore move their attention from the feeling, which is deceiving and speculative and hides the true nature of the emotion itself. Once more, we must remember: "Any kind of stimulus, whether it causes fear or happiness and whether it is activated consciously or unconsciously, initiates a chain of responses that alters the initial state of the organism."[14]

Clinical Observations

A patient once came to my office with a common physical symptom: chronic migraines.

On a fascial level, her superior trapeziuses were contracted and their connection with the base of the occipit was causing a strong tension in the system of the vertical intracranial membranes.

I started the treatment focusing on the Significance Detector, and we almost immediately initiated the Therapeutic Imagery and Dialogue.

During the first part of the session, when the craniosacral rhythm stopped, I asked the patient what she was thinking about. She started talking about a very precise and painful moment of her life, the end of the Second World War, when the borders between the former Yugoslavia and Italy were redefined.

While my hands were placed on the patient's thoracic inlet, she perceived a huge weight in that area. As she was expressing that sense of uneasiness, I felt drawn toward the pericardium.

The patient told me she was born in a village in the region of Istria, which had been part of the Italian territory just before the war, and where she had lived with her parents all her childhood and part of her adolescence. When the national borders were redefined just after the conflict, her parents did not want to live in a territory that was under the new regime of Yugoslavia, so they took part in the exodus as refugees and moved to Italy.

At that time, she still depended on her parents. Therefore, even if her friends, her school, and her habits were in Yugoslavia, she had to follow her parents in the exodus. She found herself changing every aspect of her life and was forced to get used to a completely different environment, which sometimes was hostile to her.

After a while she started complaining of strong migraines, but no clinical exam could detect a specific physical cause.

During the Therapeutic Imagery and Dialogue, as she was telling me about her memories, she was reliving the emotions she had experienced during the period following the war. She confessed that she had never talked about that subject in such personal terms. She had always thought it was not appropriate since so many other refugees had to face the same situation at that time. What the Therapeutic Imagery and Dialogue made extremely clear was that she had never been aware of the importance of her experience and of its connotation from the perspective of abandonment and loss.

By treating her pericardium and lung meridians, I proposed the facilitating action her non-conscious suggested to me and supported the patient during the dialogue. That is how her story emerged as I have just described it. Her extracranial and intracranial fascial tension was already fading even during the treatment.

Through self-realization (the contact with her Inner Physician), my patient became aware of the destructive emotional charge that she was holding back as a vestige of her experience.

The treatment sessions continued, and we set four other appointments. Each time her migraines faded a little more. During the fifth session she declared that she wanted to visit the places of her childhood, which before then she could barely stand to think about, let alone consider seeing again.

After some time, the patient called to tell me that she was now aware of the trauma and the subsequent loss the separation from her homeland had caused.

She is currently living where she used to live as a child and is now able to think about her oldest memories. Most importantly, her migraines did not come back.

❧ A CST-CENTERED VISION ❧

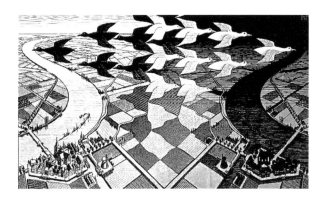

Fig. 9.4. *Photo of Day and Night*, by Maurits Cornelis Escher

M. C. Escher's works are particularly appreciated by scientists, logicians, mathematicians, and physicians for the rationality of his geometrical distortions and his original interpretations of scientific concepts, which allowed him to create paradoxical effects.

In his work *Day and Night* (fig. 9.4), two specular sides of the same landscape suggest that one single situation can take on different connotations according to circumstances. Similarly, CST facilitates the transformation of a situation that is energetically destructive into a constructive potential. Its transformative power is in line with this image, in which the black-and-white transformation shows two opposing and opposite aspects of the same landscape (which we could associate with the patient's emotional scenario).

CHAPTER 10
Constructive and Destructive Energy
Harnessing Polarity for Transformation

*When THE WHOLE starts its creations with the principle of polarity,
the paradox of the universe manifests itself.*

THREE INITIATES, *THE KYBALION*

In discussing the Holmes and Rahe Stress Scale (chapter 8), our focus was directed to specific situations that could be considered negative and could feed a kind of energy that is potentially destructive for the individual's Life Cycle. In CST and SER, the Facilitator works to draw from the constructive resources that reside inside each person in order to bring any traumatic negative situation to a positive/constructive epilogue and dissipate the potential destructive energy.

It is crucial to note that the integrative functionality determined by positive-negative polarity is the most natural of phenomena. One need only think of the magnetic polarity of our planet or of our very cells to find natural examples of polarity with a functional interaction.

The principle of polarity is the basis for theory and experimentation in various fields, such as science and philosophy. As an example, one of the best-known philosophical principles based on the assumption that there is no life without polarity is the concept of yin and yang in ancient Chinese philosophy.

In psychotherapy, the concept of polarity has been widely employed and developed by Franz Perls's Gestalt psychology. Assagioli, too, was inspired by studies on polarity (concerning the polarity axis of the egg in particular) when he invented the Egg Diagram (fig. 10.4, page 114) that represents the process of psychosynthesis.

In accordance with the ideas developed in Gestalt therapy and psychosynthesis, Dr. Upledger further extended the concept of polarity, adopting it as one of the foundations for the transformation and dissipation of destructive energy associated with a trauma.

In order to better understand his work, we will reiterate the concept of trauma as cause of an Energy Cyst. In the experience of Dr. Upledger, trauma can be kinetic, pharmacotoxicological, emotional, spiritual, environmental (caused by earthquakes or other natural disasters), social, et cetera.

As described earlier, the most common situation leading to the formation of an Energy Cyst is the presence of destructive emotions, such as fear, manifesting when trauma occurs. Such destructive emotional experiences are not always caused by a single traumatic event. In fact, they usually are constituted by a series of negative/destructive emotions resulting in an accumulation. The presence of a series of positive/constructive emotions weakens the effects of trauma and fosters the disappearance of the Energy Cysts. Through this phenomenon, we see an important principle: Extreme fear and extreme love represent the two opposite poles of human polarity.

In practice, we see the following:

- Past experiences with destructive emotions (e.g., fear, anger) and the negative feelings connected with them (e.g., sense of guilt) promote the formation of Energy Cysts.
- Past experiences with constructive emotions (e.g., joy, happiness) encourage positive feelings (e.g., love) and promote the disappearance of extrinsic destructive energies.

As soon as the patient relives the trauma and becomes aware of the destructive charge of the emotion connected to it, the last effects of the Energy Cyst disappear. This emotional release seems to be particularly effective in achieving a complete therapeutic effect.

CONTEMPORARY PERSPECTIVES ON POLARITY

Isabella M. Treacy, a student who graduated in Natural Science at the University of Padua, wrote an essay that examines in simple and understandable terms the notion of polarity and its use in disciplines such as chemistry, biology, philosophy, and literature. In the conclusion, she regards polarity as an intelligible reality of life, humankind, and the universe: "In its different acceptations, polarity is an essential and indelible characteristic of reality in general and human condition in particular. The tension between opposites that is typical of polarity is definitely not a negative feature. It must be kept and valorized, at least within certain limits."[1]

In 1925, Italian theologian, writer, and naturalized German Romano Guardini (1885–1968) wrote "Der Gegensatz," an essay in which he recognized in polar opposition the unity of body and spirit. About polarity, he wrote:

It is no mere exclusion, since that would mean contradiction, and not even pure inclusion, which would mean sameness. From this perspective, what we actually call opposition is a peculiar kind of relation, made of mutual exclusion and inclusion at the same time. The concrete-living manifests as unity, but it is a kind of unity that is possible only in an oppositional way. The passage between one side and the other does not occur with a slide or a gradual increase, but rather with a "leap" from a field of quality and meaning to another. We must then underline with similar decisiveness that one side can exist only in relation to the other and with the other. Both are life, but life is more than the single sides and more than their sum.[2]

In 2004, psychotherapist, mathematician, philosopher, and theologian Giuseppe Vadalà worked with psychotherapist Sandra Pierpaoli to write "Il benessere come equilibrio tra le polarità psicocorporee." Discussing the polarity between the mind and instinct, the two authors note that as the human species developed, the achievement of the upright position brought with it the connection of rationality and thought with the upper body, while the lower body, recalling the animal-like posture on all fours, was connected to animal-like instinct. Indeed, in the Western world in particular, there is a tendency to give more importance to the brain over the rest of the body, creating an imbalance that causes both physical and psychoemotional unity to be dysfunctional and can even jeopardize the life force of the individual. The imbalance also can occur for the opposite reason: If the instinctive part is given too much importance in relation to the psychoemotional one, the unnatural division between mind and instinct may lead to the inability to channel the instinct in a constructive way. This can make it impossible for the individual to develop a life with a balanced emotional state. Whatever the dominant side is, the imbalance creates conflict, generating a destructive process. Conversely, the integration of the parts produces a uniform flow of life energy that influences the entire organism. In fact, it is detectable through the individual's posture, maturity, harmony, relations, and ability to think and act constructively.[3]

In 2018, clinical psychologist, psychotherapist, and writer Carmen Di Muro published an article about quantum physics. Here is a part of it:

The phenomenon of polarity can be found everywhere, from the simplest matter to the most complex cosmic phenomena. Today, fringe science helps us more and more to clarify its subtle laws. Let us consider the atom, the smallest unit composing what surrounds us: its nucleus is made of two poles, the proton with a positive charge and the electron with a negative charge. The principle of polarity itself can be found on a biological level in both animal and vegetal cells in which the nucleus is positively charged and the cytoplasm—the substance located between the plasmatic membrane and the nuclear membrane—has a negative charge. This difference in the electric potential determines the vitality of cells.[4]

These examples comprise only a fraction of recent affirmations made by academics and therapists in relation to their observations, research, and clinical studies on human polarity. The volume of material explored in studies and interdisciplinary experimentations in this respect is certainly much wider and much more articulated. In fact, polarity plays a large role in human knowledge since it derives from the very properties and relations, such as symmetry, antithesis, orientation, conditions, positions, and movements, of all organic and inorganic elements, both in themselves and in relation to other elements.

We are now moving on to explore other definitions of polarity in order to allow us to focus even more clearly on the role of Facilitators and their understanding of the implementation of their technical competence when they assess and treat the polar energetic framework of the human body.

ASPECTS OF POLARITY

We should note that polarity is relevant to the following:

- physics (of a body, an electrical device, a magnetic field)
- quantum mechanics (polar coordinates, wave function)
- organic and inorganic chemistry (molecules, electronegativity, covalent bonds of atoms)
- Earth science (sedimentology, geotectonics, geophysics, crystallography)
- biology (physiology, morphology, embryology)
- statistics (C. E. Osgood's and P. R. Hofstätter's semantic differential scales)
- medicine (epithelial polarity, genetic polarity of the "operons," physiological polarity in homeopathy, physiopathological polarity in anthroposophic medicine)
- psychology (behavioral characteristics)
- philosophy (mutual dependence of opposite and complementary elements)
- grammar (positive or negative value of a sentence)
- art and literature (e.g., G. W. Goethe's essay "Theory of Colors," Robert Louis Stevenson's novella *Strange Case of Dr. Jekyll and Mr. Hyde*)

Let's look at the concept of polarity through the lens of some of these perspectives and fields of study.

Philosophy

In philosophy, similar to simple dualism, polarity assumes a constructive foundation thanks to the undividable complementarity of the two poles, which makes the existence of one essential to the existence of the other.

Eastern Philosophy

In East Asian cultures, the highest expression of the concept of polarity is the Tao. Translated from Chinese, this word can mean "path" or "way," but it represents the matrix of the universe. At the beginning of time, the Tao was in its nonbeing state, the state of *wu ji* (pure energy, lack of polarity, and lack of differentiation). It then gave birth to the *being*, and the being had two poles that represent the fundamental principles of the universe in all natural elements:

Yin: female, cold, negative, lunar, passive, cloudy, hidden, mutable, wet, black

Yang: male, hot, positive, solar, active, limpid, clear, constant, dry, white

According to Laozi, the philosopher and writer of ancient China who is reputed to be the author of the classic text known as the Tao Te Ching, opposite poles are inevitably connected in a single unit and are mutually dependent, which means that one cannot be understood without the other.

The concept of polarity characterizes all East Asian philosophies and healing techniques, such as those of Indian and Chinese traditional medicine, in which it has always been natural for philosophy, religion, spirituality, and science to merge.

For instance, we find the concept of polarity in Indian chakras, which in an overly simplified manner could be defined as energetic centers of the human body. There are seven major chakras and twenty-one minor chakras. The seven major

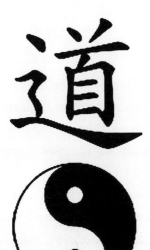

Fig. 10.1. The symbols for Tao and for yin and yang

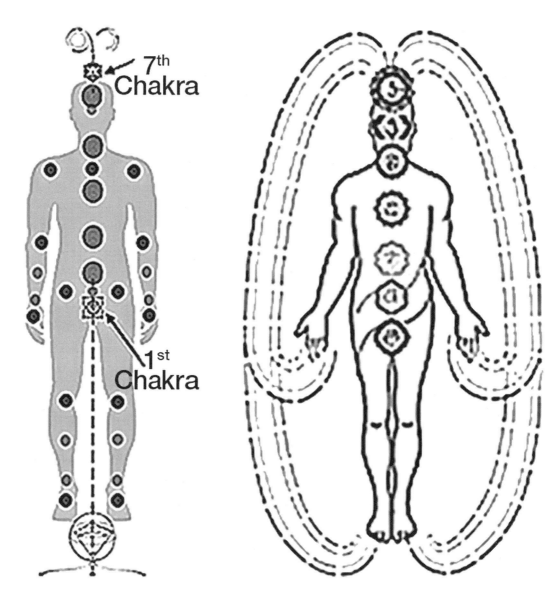

Fig. 10.2. The major and minor chakras and their energy field

chakras trace an energetic path of the human being, from the top of the head to the pelvis (more precisely, from the fornix to the sacral-coccygeal plexus) and then to the toes, creating a polarity that establishes a constant channeling of energy exchange between the energy of the cosmos (seventh chakra, on the crown) and the energy of the Earth (first chakra, the pelvic area).

Each of the major chakras is connected to one or more organs of the human body, and the energetic channels traced by the minor chakras are ideally analogous to the energy channels, or meridians, in traditional Chinese medicine. Since the macrocosm reflects the microcosm and vice versa, the polarity of the structural organization of the major chakras can also be found in all the other chakras.

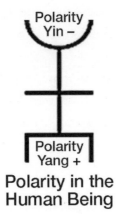

Polarity in the Human Being

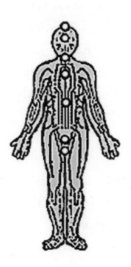

Fig. 10.3. Energy meridians—their polarity and a map of their channels

The direction of the polar structure of chakras is opposite to the energy flow, from male to female (yang and yin). Like meridians, chakras may become blocked, meaning they become overloaded with energy or voided of it, consequently not allowing the constant and harmonious flow of energy in the body.

Just like chakras, meridians embody polarity in their flow and connection to yin and yang principles. They also are associated with the organs of the human body and pass through them longitudinally, from either the front or the back side.

The imbalance between the forces of yin and yang manifests the illness in one of the twelve organs that are known to Chinese medicine: lungs, large intestine, spleen, pancreas, heart, small intestine, bladder, kidneys, gallbladder, liver, pericardium or heart minister, and triple burner or sanjiao (*sam-se'u,* meaning "regenerated organs" in traditional Tibetan medicine). . . . Each body part has its own polarity: the frontal part of the head is yang, whereas the occipital part is yin;

the palm of the right hand is positive, whereas the back is negative; the palm of the left hand is yin, whereas the back is yang. The same goes for fingers and toes.[5]

We will cover the subject of chakras and meridians more in depth later (see chapter 16). In particular, we will look at the energetic framework arising from the chakras and the emotions linked to the different organs and systems of the human body. For now, we'll close our discussion with the list of the polarities of the main meridians, according to the principle of yin and yang.

Yin Meridians	Yang Meridians
conception vessel	gallbladder
heart	governing vessel
kidney	large intestine
liver	sanjiao
lung	small intestine
pericardium	stomach meridian
spleen	urinary bladder

Western Philosophy

In the West, philosophy addresses the subject of polarity mostly in relation to dialectics, unlike Eastern philosophy, which embraces universal aspects that can be applied to nature, medicine, spirituality, and the human dimension.

The concept of logos (thought/word) in contraposition to pathos (emotion/passion) is attributed to Heraclitus (535–475 BCE), the pre-Socratic Greek philosopher. Logos and pathos by themselves may be seen as a dual opposition between rational and irrational, but Heraclitus brought this concept even further in his theory, called the Doctrine of Flux and the Unity of Opposites, which identifyies logos with the principle of nature. According to such doctrine, every law that regulates nature (and human beings) is subordinate to the polarity of opposites. In Heraclitus's view, the balance of the universe is dynamic and based on the constant succession of conflicting opposites.

> The opposites do not exclude one another, but they act simultaneously, thus creating harmony. "Intellect" as logos, as intended by Heraclitus, allows us to acknowledge the mutual dependency of the opposites, which cannot live without each other and thus are one single unit. Our senses perceive the world as an incessant series of opposites, as Heraclitus explained through his famous aphorism "Panta rhei," meaning "everything flows." Each opposite seems to exclude the other, but logos allows us to see everything clearer and harmoniously organized; everything implies its opposite and the world is therefore the reign of the unity of opposites.[6]

Polarity dominated much of the philosophical reflection in ancient Greece, but Plato (428–348 BCE) made polarity explicitly evident through the theories of his Unwritten Doctrines, especially in the Supreme Principle of the One and the Indefinite Dyad, in which he laid out his thoughts on order and harmony.

> All perceivable things can be explained only by tracing them back to the unity of the corresponding Ideas. According to Plato, multiplicity cannot be explained if not through unity. All levels of reality have a bipolar structure, which means that two principles, the One and the Dyad, merge in a reasonable balance. In *Philebus,* the Socratic dialogue written by Plato, the One is presented as limited and the Dyad as limitless, and the being is a mixture of limited and limitless.[7]

In ancient Egypt, polarity was considered one of seven "universal laws" or "natural laws of truth," which are listed in *The Kybalion,* the text attributed to Hermes Trismegistus that was made available to the general public only in 1908. Hermes Trismegistus is a mythical figure commonly situated in the Hellenistic period (323–30 BCE). He was a king, philosopher, minister, and prophet who was frequently associated with the god Thoth by ancient Egyptians. He is believed to have founded Hermetic technical and philosophical thought and Hermetic literature, which provided the foundation of the alchemy of the Middle Ages and Renaissance. According to the law of polarity, as explained in *The Kybalion,* "Everything is Dual; everything has poles; everything has its pair of opposites; like and unlike are the same; opposites are identical in nature, but different in degree; extremes meet; all truths are but half-truths; all paradoxes may be reconciled."[8]

Plotinus (204–270 CE), a philosopher native to Lycopolis in ancient Egypt, further examined Plato's concept of polarity, serving as a junction between Eastern and Western thought. Thanks to the versatility of his reasoning, Plotinus inspired for centuries to come theologians and mystics, metaphysicists and gnostics, esotericists and alchemists, and pagan, Christian, Jewish, and Muslim thinkers and philosophers. According to Plotinus, the One is neither the Intellect nor the Good but comes even before. The polarity of the world comes from the structure of the One, which is an opposition of elements and constitutes their synthesis. That occurs in all different dimensions of reality, which are progressively inferior, creating the universe, but the One always remains transcendent from them. According to Plotinus, the One can exclusively be defined through "what it is not," analogously to the Eastern concept of Tao. Thanks to Plotinus, Neoplatonists embraced this thought and maintained it from the third century until the beginning of the sixth century.

Later on in history, the Neoplatonic principle of polarity was developed by Christian theologians, the most famous probably being Nicholas of Cusa (1401–1464), also referred to as Nicholas of Kues or Nicolaus Cusanus, a German cardinal, theologian, philosopher, humanist, jurist, mathematician, and astronomer. He applied the concept of polarity to the relationship between God and the world, seen as having an "enfolding/unfolding" nature in which God is an "implicit universe" and unfolds in the universe we know. To Cusanus, God is not immobile in his perfection but is characterized by motion and action with an infinite and eternal spiritual energy. This energy has the constant creating power of the One, which contains all parts. Therefore, God reveals himself in the universe as a macrocosm with its respective human microcosm.

German idealism, a philosophical current derived from Neoplatonism and developed in the eighteenth century, retrieved the vision of a being (One) existing above the subject/object dualism. Two of its most well-known exponents, Friedrich Schelling (1775–1854) and Georg Wilhelm Friedrich Hegel (1770–1831), recovered Plato's concept of polarity. Schelling introduced Soul and Nature as the two opposite poles that coincide and are in relation with the unknowable "Absolute." Hegel criticized Schelling's concept of the Absolute, deeming it a mistake to conceive it as imperturbable and static and therefore "indifferent." He thus proposed the concept of the "Whole" instead of the Absolute. In the Whole, "differences are not annihilated and are not static Substances, but rather dynamic Subjects developing through a progressive realization. According to Hegel, the being 'is' and 'is not,' which means it is contradictory and divided into dialectic polarities contradicting and synthesizing each other. Everything refers to its opposite and is at the same time itself and its opposite and the synthesis of both."[9]

Coming from a perspective that focused not on philosophy and theology but rather on politics, history, and society, German philosopher, economist, historian, sociologist, political analyst, and journalist Karl Marx (1818–1883) created his own theory about polarity, stressing its negative meaning. In his view of polarity in the "theory of historical development," the concentration of wealth promotes the process of polarization between social classes, which then progressively brings an intensification of conflicts, overcoming old forms of economical organization.

Psychology and Psychotherapy

In light of his clinical experience with SomatoEmotional Release, Dr. Upledger believed Jung's analytical psychology, Gestalt psychology, and Assagioli's psychosynthesis to be the most adequate approaches in the field of psychology and psychotherapy to address the individual's psychological and emotional side. Therefore, we are going to consider the concept of polarity only in these three schools of thought. Once again, our discussion will be a schematic summary taken from the general context to address the subjects we are interested in, but the reader is certainly encouraged to further research any of these subjects.

To address the field of analytical psychology, developed by Swiss psychiatrist, psychoanalyst, anthropologist, philosopher, and academic Carl Gustav Jung (1875–1961), we are going to examine the analysis of modern-day psychologist and psychotherapist Chiara Miranda. In the context of Jung's perspective on the sense and functioning of the principle of compensation of the opposites, she writes about his recognition of Freud and Adler's merits:

> Freud was focused on the analysis of the past, whereas Adler on the subject as tending to the development of individual potentials in the future, so Jung clearly had to find a synthesis of these opposites, which do not exclude one another but rather integrate each other. From here, he started to elaborate the concept of psychological types, recognizing that individuals have within themselves two conflicting polarities that constitute the foundation of individual personalities—introversion and extroversion. . . . Individual personality mainly manifests one of these polarities, while the other remains in the background. These two tendencies may be imagined as the two extreme opposite points of an imaginary line going from absolute introversion to absolute extroversion. In Jung's theory, a mechanism called "compensation" has the task to balance introversion and extroversion. Such mechanism acts both on a conscious and on an unconscious level, allowing a self-regulation between them.[10]

In Gestalt psychology, in particular in the vision of its greatest exponent, German psychotherapist and naturalized American Friedrich "Fritz" Salomon Perls (1893–1935), the focus on polarity is directed toward the "dialectics of the opposites." In Perls's book *Ego, Hunger, and Aggression,* "the differentiation into opposites is described as a 'characteristic' that does not only belong to human mind, but also to life in general and all its expressions. . . . In fact, Perls believed that any form of evolution is connected to the process of polar differentiation. . . . In his view, the more the Ego is able to expand in the wide range of polar differentiations that it can reach, the more it develops different functions and thus progress."[11]

Moreover, in Gestalt theory, "the psychoanalytical concept of unconscious is replaced by the concept of consciousness, more precisely by the polarity of consciousness/unconsciousness. . . . Experience is actually nothing more than a figure in relation to a background: the relationship between the figure and the background can be described in polar terms, so that existence is seen as a field dominated by polarity."[12]

Roberto Assagioli (1888–1974), psychiatrist, theosophist, and founder of psychosynthesis, decided to use the shape of the egg to represent a series of concepts, including polarity. Taking an interest in the single biological characteristics of eggs, and especially in the polar distribution and orientation of their internal materials,

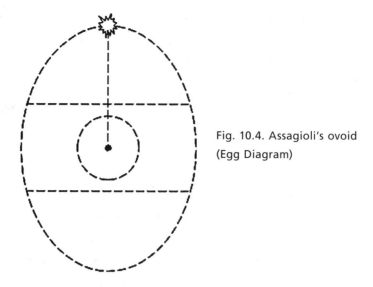

Fig. 10.4. Assagioli's ovoid (Egg Diagram)

Assagioli conceived the Egg Diagram (fig. 10.4, above) to graphically represent the psychosynthetic process. In the following chapters we will have the chance to examine several other aspects of psychosynthesis, but for now we are just going to summarize polarity in Assagioli's Egg Diagram. Italian writer Vittorio Viglienghi, who teaches at the Istituto di Psicosintesi of Ancona, an institute founded by Roberto Assagioli himself, analyzed the axiality of the Egg Diagram in relation to its polarity:

> Since the circle is symmetrical in relation to one center, but the ellipse is symmetrical in relation to two focal points, the introduction of this latter kind of axiality implies duality, or polarity, and therefore choice.... Assagioli had to choose as a geometric symbol of the structure of psyche a figure that is intrinsically characterized by duality. To incarnate or to manifest oneself means to enter the world of duality, of polarity, in which the One/Whole (the circle) "splits" into spirit and matter, in up and down, right and left, front and back, past and future, in order to express and evolve. Evolution and transformation require necessarily the condition of duality and polarization, an environment that is geometrically represented by the ellipse, not by the circle.[13]

Embryology

We have just seen how Assagioli took inspiration from the structure of the egg for his diagram. We are now going to see the biological characteristics of the egg through the specific discipline that studies this subject, embryology. Let us then analyze the polarity of the primary oocyte, the female germ cell that divides by meiosis, producing the polar globule.

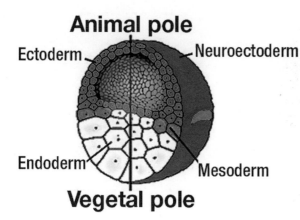

Fig. 10.5. Gastrulation—from vegetal pole to animal pole

The Egg

The polarity of the egg is found in the specific distribution of the materials constituting the ooplasm (the cytoplasm of an egg), which change their orientation according to the polar axis of the egg.

> An embryo is divided in two hemispheres. Its so-called animal pole is generally where polocytes or polar bodies are emanated, and it reveals the eccentric location of the nucleus or germinal vesicle; its antipode, at the opposite side of the axis, is called the "vegetal pole." The two poles of the egg are defined as superior and inferior when the egg is rich in yolk, which gathers in the vegetal hemisphere, causing it to be the lower part thanks to gravity. This polarity is a characteristic of all eggs and is connected to the organization of the future embryo.[14]

Therefore, even though its shape is generally spherical, the most important characteristic of the egg is polarity. In a mature egg cell, polarity consists in the stratification of the yolk (or vitellus), a reserve material that contains molecules of various kinds, including RNA. Polarity between the animal pole in the upper part and the vegetal pole in the lower part increases constantly and progressively during the earlier stages of development, when it is visible through the shades of color that show the increased density of the yolk. The color blending is vertical, going from the animal pole to the vegetal pole.

The Oocyte

The female germ cell (oogonium) is the main element of oogenesis, which starts in the fifth month of embryonic life. It derives from primordial germ cells and is the precursor of primary and secondary oocytes and polar globules. The oocyte derives from the oogonium and produces polar bodies and the primary oocyte through meiosis, the process of separation and reorganization of chromosomes in the cell. The

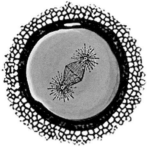

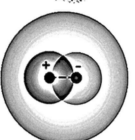

Fig. 10.6. The oocyte—polarity in the female germ cell

first meiotic division of the primary oocyte produces the secondary oocyte and the first polar globule. The second meiotic division generates the second polar globule, a mature gamete ready to be fecundated. The organization of the egg predetermines the structural and functional characteristics of the adult.

Biology

Polarity is an essential property for the development of plants and animals, both in their evolution and in their individual complexity. Animals, plants, single cells, and unicellular organisms are all composed of different parts that are constantly organized in a specific direction.

Polarity can take on different meanings depending on the context. Let us compare two definitions. First:

> In biology, polarity is defined as a persistent and asymmetrical structural distribution along an axis. The axis of alignment indicates not the polar direction but only the relation between the axes and some external points of reference. The direction of the asymmetrical and organized distribution of the structures is called the orientation of the axis.[15]

And then:

> In biology, polarity manifests itself in morphological and functional differentiations, differences of intensity in the metabolic activity (respiratory exchanges, sensitivity to toxic agents), and differences of chemical composition and electrical

charge or potential. Even cellular structures often display a complete polarity, which means that the different functions correspond to the morphologic differentiations. Sometimes polarity regards solely behavioral factors (physiological or functional polarity).[16]

Cell Polarity

Cell vibrations play a crucial role in the release of the entropic energy held by an Energy Cyst within an organism. Each vibration has its own polarity.

Each cell of the body emits its own electromagnetic vibration, defined by American biologist Bruce Lipton as "cellular consciousness," a kind of energetic signature varying according to the health conditions of the cell. If the state of the cell deteriorates, the change of vibration entails as its consequence a pathology, more or less severe. Everything is connected to the phenomenon of cell polarization, in which the cell membrane is the boundary line between the intracellular fluid, which has a negative charge (K+ ions), and the interstitial extracellular fluid, which has a positive charge (NA+ and Cl– ions).[17]

Let us further investigate cell polarity by extrapolating only some of its multiple characteristics described by Dr. Diana Oliveri, researcher in neurochemistry and developmental neurobiology:

Cell polarity and its conservation are based on an asymmetrical distribution of the cytoskeleton and the activity of proteins in the cell. The concentration of specific proteins in a specific cellular region is an essential part of the process. . . .

The cell membrane of mature epithelial cells is divided in two; an apical part is in contact with the external environment, whereas the basement part is in contact with the internal environment and the vascularized area.

Within mature epithelial tissues, polarity regulates cell morphology, intracellular signals, asymmetrical cell division, cell migration, cellular physiology, and histological physiology, as well as organogenesis.

The polarity of each single cell is essential in the development of complex multicellular organisms since the division of a polar cell generates daughter cells that are not equivalent, allowing a differentiated development.

In most cases, the development of the polar axis requires an input coming from a biological signal or from the physical environment, such as a gravity stimulus or slight gradient.

Although polarity characterizes all multicellular organisms, since it is essential for the differentiation of cellular functions and for the formation of the organs, the requirements that allow polarity to be generated depend on the mobility of the organism.[18]

Chemistry

In chemistry, polarity is a property of a particular group of molecules called polar molecules; all the others are called nonpolar. A polar molecule has a partial positive charge (+) and an opposite partial negative charge (−).

A molecule's polarity is connected with its type of bonding (ionic bonds involve electrostatic attraction, while nonpolar and pure covalent bonds involve the sharing of electron pairs between atoms) and with its geometry, meaning the three-dimensional arrangement of the atoms constituting the molecule.

Even atoms have their own polarity since they are made of subatomic components, which are protons (with a positive charge +), neutrons (without any charge), and electrons (with a negative charge −). The atoms of the same element are all alike. Between atoms of different elements, however, there are differences in how they combine with each other through chemical reactions to form molecules.

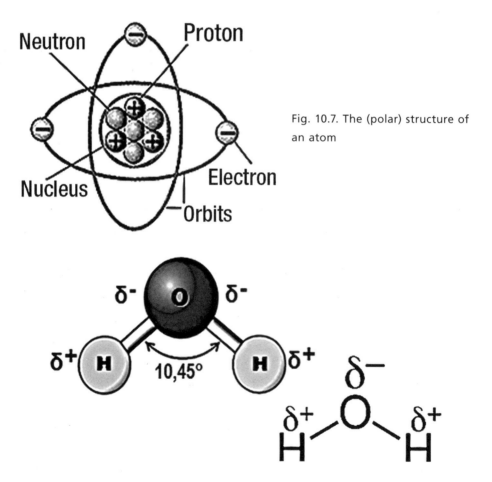

Fig. 10.7. The (polar) structure of an atom

Fig. 10.8. The (polar) structure of a water molecules

As a general rule, we could say that all symmetrical molecules are nonpolar, while asymmetric molecules are polar. The polarity of molecules also depends on their molecular geometry. An example of polarity can be found in the molecule of water (H_2O). An example of nonpolarity can be found in molecules composed of two equal elements, such as O_2 or H_2, and symmetric molecules, such as CH_4 or CCl_4.

Physics

In physics, polarity is the property that makes certain physical entities gather at the opposite poles (generally north and south) of a body, such as a magnet or polarized light.

> Polarity also refers to a property of the bodies that have electrical or magnetic poles, or are subjected to electrical current, and whose magnetization or electricity is indicated by a vector with a clear direction. For instance, an electric or magnetic dipole has a polarity because the vectors (indicating the electric or magnetic induction) have a precise direction. A battery has a polarity because the electromotive force that it generates has a precise sign, which means that the positive and the negative poles are clearly determined.[19]

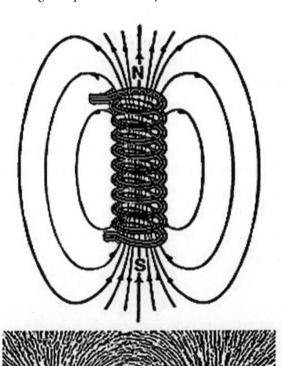

Fig. 10.9. Magnetic field lines created by the poles of a solenoid

Geometry

In geometry, polarity can be seen in the particular homography (bijection between dimensional figures) between the points and the lines on a plane in which, under certain circumstances, for each point (pole) there is one and only one line, called polar.[20]

Geophysics

Geophysics considers geomagnetic polarity, which is the direction of the primary magnetization of the minerals in a rock in accordance with the dipole of Earth's magnetic field at the moment of a rock's formation. Since there are periodic inversions of Earth's magnetic field throughout geological periods, geomagnetic polarity can be normal (when the field points north) or inverse (when it points south) in relation to the current magnetic field.

Geology

Geological studies include many disciplines that evaluate polarity on various levels, starting from Earth's magnetic field, also known as the geomagnetic field, generated by a magnetic dipole located at the center of Earth. Many other planetary bodies share the same phenomenon.

Sedimentology is the specific study of the overall characteristics of sediment. Its purpose is to determine the original source of that sediment, as well as its size, structure, composition, layering, fossil content, and so on. The layer that can help in identifying the original source of the sediment is magnetic polarity; otherwise it is called homogeneous.

Orogeny assesses the characteristics (amplitude and direction) of the orogenic waves that produce a corrugation in the layers of Earth's crust. The deformation of an orogen (an extensive belt of rocks) depends on various phenomena (magmatic, tectonic, metamorphic, sedimentary, etc.). It displays a decreasing intensity when an initial corrugation of the orogen moves away from the axis of alignment, either with a polar direction from the inside out or toward both directions.

Earth's Polarity

In order to talk about Earth's polarity, we return to geomagnetism, the series of magnetic phenomena analyzed by geophysics. Geomagnetism is a wide subject, subdivided in many different sectors. We are going to list only some of its aspects, in particular those that are useful in confirming the analogies between different energetic fields generated by polarity (Earth, atom, cell, human being).

Magnetic fields are connected to the law of conservation of energy, one of the fundamental physical principles that can be observed in nature. This law states that,

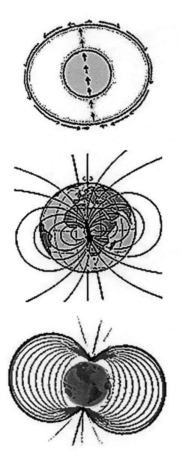

Fig. 10.10. Magnetic field lines—the vector field created by the Earth's poles

although energy can be transformed and converted from one form to another, the total energy of an isolated system remains constant. This principle is inclusive of all possible forms of energy, among which are mass and momentum (after Einstein).

The magnetic field around Earth (geomagnetic field) is a natural physical phenomenon of planet Earth. It is comparable to the magnetic field generated by a magnetic dipole whose poles are not static, do not coincide with the geographical poles, and have an axis that is inclined in respect to Earth's axis of rotation. Its field lines (vector fields) enter the Northern Hemisphere (Boreal Hemisphere) and come out from the Southern Hemisphere (Austral Hemisphere).

Earth's magnetism is essential for all life forms on the planet. It extends for several tens of thousands of kilometers into space, creating an area called the magnetosphere, which generates a sort of electromagnetic shield able to deviate cosmic rays and all charged particles, diminishing the number of those that reach the ground.

The geomagnetic pole and the geographic pole do not coincide. Moreover, the two magnetic poles of Earth periodically reverse their positions, which means that polar inversions occur in Earth's magnetic fields.

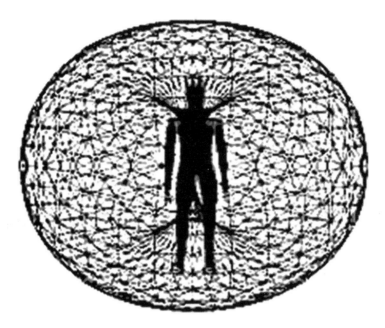

Fig. 10.11. Toroidal magnetic field of the human body

Toroid

A toroid is an algebraic plane curve consisting of the contour of the projection of a torus (a geometrical surface produced by the rotation of two circumferences, such as a meridian and a parallel).

The toroid has an elliptical shape with a hole in the middle (like a doughnut), a central axis, vortices, and a surrounding coherent field. In cosmometry, it is the fundamental form of balanced energy flow in sustainable systems on all scales (e.g., cells, human beings, Earth, cosmos). It is the primary component of the fractal embedding of energy flows (toroidal flows), going from the microcosm to the macrocosm, in which every individual entity keeps its own unique identity while still remaining in contact with the whole (fig. 10.11).

POLARITY IN CST AND SER

As we have seen, duality and, more specifically, polarity are crucial in natural and behavioral phenomena and in human thinking. They affect even the human organism and its functioning. If the macrocosm is reflected by the microcosm (and vice versa), this is only a part of what the Facilitator can perceive during a treatment session.

As an example, let us stop for a minute to analyze the orientation of the fascia to understand how Energy Cysts can modify its original structure.

The fascia originates in the mesoderm, the intermediate in a series of three embryonic layers, during the third week of life for a fetus. It wraps around all organic

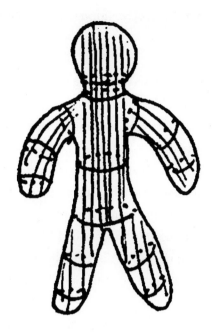

Fig. 10.12. Direction of the fascia in the human body

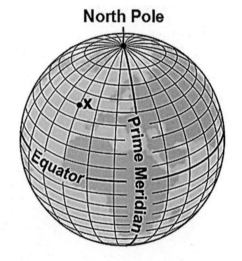

Fig. 10.13. Earth's meridians and parallels

structures, generally following a longitudinal direction (from the head to the feet) within the body. However, in some areas of the body its direction is horizontal (for example, next to diaphragms or joints). The horizontal structure of the fascia creates barriers to defend the brain from information overloads caused by traumas or dysfunctions that produce impulses and stimuli in the organism, even including the response of the central and peripheral nervous systems.

We could imagine a graphic stylization of the direction of the fascia in the human body (fig. 10.12) as a diagram of Earth's meridians and parallels (fig. 10.13). Like a geological orogen provoking an orogenic wave in Earth's crust, an internal dysfunction can cause a wave in the structure of the tissue, provoking a change in the fascia.

Physiotherapist Giacomo Leone, a Visceral Manipulation (VM) therapist and student of osteopath and VM developer Jean-Pierre Barral, described the fascia as follows in a seminar:

> Anatomically speaking, the term "Fascia" designates a membrane of connective tissue with a protective and nutritional function. The tissue constituting the Fascia is all connected and continuous, allowing the different anatomical elements to be considered as mechanically supporting each other.
>
> The connective tissue is the base for all the Fascia and actually constitutes 65 to 70 percent of all tissues of the human body. Even though different parts of it can take different names, it has the same embryonic anatomical structure.
>
> We could use the metaphor of tubes sliding into other tubes, like in a telescope. When the tubes are oiled, everything works fine; but an alteration could provoke the movements to stop being fluid and cause a dysfunction. The functions of the Fascia are several and very complex. The connective tissue provides support to structures that are highly organized. Since it contains embryonic mesenchymal cells, connective tissue provides a specific type of tissue that is able to originate more specialized elements under particular circumstances.
>
> The Fascia is divided into Superficial and Deep Fascia. The Superficial Fascia is a continuous layer of tissue attached to the dermis of the skin and to the Deep Fascia. The Deep Fascia surrounds the muscles and is attached to the periosteum of the bones, to ligaments, and to tendons.
>
> Fascial layers provide passageways for nerves and lymphatic vessels. Fascia is

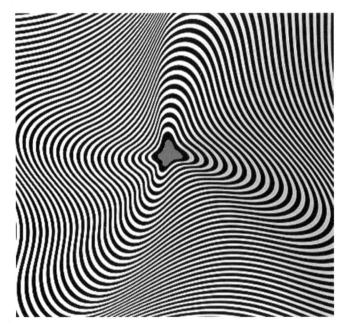

Fig. 10.14. Graphical representation of restrictions in the fascia caused by an Energy Cyst

composed of elastin, collagen, and ground substance. To sum up, we can say that the fascia is the only tissue made of collagen that connects, supports, surrounds, and nourishes. Almost our entire body is Fascia; if we took it out, we would only have bones, muscles, and few other structures. On the contrary, if we were to take out the structures it contains, the fascia would not lose its shape and our body would keep its overall appearance.

When Energy Cysts form in the tissues, they reshape the fascia and create restrictions or expansions. They also alter its functionality and change the orientation of its movement. Though the fascia is still able to keep its longitudinal arrangement, its deviation from its correct path inhibits its ability to move fluidly.

CONCLUSIONS ON POLARITY

We will later see the critical role of polarity in the development of various techniques that Facilitators can implement (e.g., the realignment of the vector/axis system in the energetic framework of the human body) as well as the importance of the toroidal model in the visualization of the energetic field and the space of communication between Higher Selves.

In the meantime, remember that the adjectives *constructive* and *destructive*, which we use in this text to define advanced emotional processes, are the consequence of the positive or negative impression left by a primary emotion. Whether the emotion is considered negative or positive, it may have a destructive outcome or, equally likely, evolve in a constructive way for the individual.

By considering negative-positive polarity to orient the path of management and processing of emotions that brings us toward a constructive result, we could refer to multiple effective schools of thought and disciplines. However, in this text we are going to use Assagioli's psychosynthesis as our preferential reference.

Polarity and Transformation Exercise

The objective of this simple exercise is to identify in any context (e.g., finances, social life, work, etc.) an objective or subjective event involving loss that is commonly considered negative, such as the stressful events suggested in the Holmes and Rahe Stress Scale, and then find a positive consequence, a favorable outcome connected to a possible transformation of the problem that the event has caused. In order to do that, let us ask ourselves the following question:

How can I take concrete action right now to transform the feeling, sensation, or emotion of loss caused by the situation I am experiencing?

A sample table and the instructions below will help you complete the exercise.

1. In each cell of the first column, *SITUATION*, write a few words to describe a current or past situation that is causing a problem in your everyday life right now.
2. In each cell of the second column, *NEGATIVE*, write a few words to describe the dysfunctional aspects of the objective and/or subjective loss connected with the situations in the first column.
3. In each cell of the third column, *POSITIVE*, write a few words to describe/represent a positive aspect of each problem (the negative aspect in the second column) you have associated with the situations in the first column.

SAMPLE TABLE

Situation	Negative	Positive
overwork	no free time	financial gain
not enough work	lack of money	free time (self-management)
breakup	loneliness	new opportunities (friendships, traveling)
new relationship	change of habits	support and complicity

SELF-ASSESSMENT

Situation	Negative	Positive

MEMORANDUM

I was teaching a class to first-level students of CST. In order to introduce the topic of the cerebral hemispheres, I started to explain how the impulses that reach the brain through the central nervous system are organized.

It probably is clear by now that even the two hemispheres of the brain ideally represent two polarities connected to each other through a hypothetical axis, which in this case is the corpus callosum.

To stimulate the students' interest, I usually trace a vertical line in the middle of the whiteboard. Each of the columns thus created represents one of the hemispheres, the right hemisphere (intuitive/creative) and the left hemisphere (analytical/rational). After that, I proceed to write two lists of professional categories, one for each column, sorting the categories according to their specific competence and how much they stimulate one or the other hemisphere. I also ask the students to suggest professions, which I then add to the lists. In the column corresponding to the right hemisphere (intuitive), I normally write professions such as writer, artist, inventor, or musician; in the column of the left hemisphere (rational), I list professions such as accountant, mechanic, engineer, chemist, and so forth. At a certain point that day, I wrote "surgeon" in the list of the left hemisphere since I believed it to be an extremely analytical profession that requires precision—one need only think of the incisions surgeons have to perform on their patients' bodies.

As soon as I wrote that word in the column, one of the students raised his hand. That student was Giovanni Giuricin, a medical doctor and surgeon with a specialization in orthopedics, who at that time worked in the operating room of the hospital Ospedale Maggiore of Trieste and now works as an orthopedist, craniosacral therapist, and instructor of naturopathy in Austria. When I encouraged him to speak, I thought that Gianni (as I call him now that we are good friends) just wanted to suggest other professions to add to the list. Instead he told me, "I have an objection, sir. You put my profession in the column of the left hemisphere, in which rationality prevails. Even if I need to attentively analyze every gesture I make and every part of the body that is involved in the surgery, every time I make an incision I actually open a window on the unique universe of the patient's body. On that occasion I have the privilege to observe that universe and interact with it."

Since I did not have anything to say to object to that, I turned again to the whiteboard and also wrote "surgeon" in the right column.

DR. UPLEDGER'S HERITAGE

It is evident that no one is solely rational/analytical or solely creative/intuitive. As we have seen, the macrocosm reflects the microcosm, and vice versa.

When Facilitators employ CST and SER, they are connected with *THE WHOLE* in a space—the Third Space—where the contact between their own Higher Self and the Higher Self of the person they are treating takes place. Two different realities, divided and distinct, unite in a space that is one, unique, and transcendent.

It is through this kind of knowledge that Dr. Upledger left his spiritual heritage to all Facilitators, reminding us that with the aptonomy of the touch we implement to improve other people's health, we *make the world a touch better.*

Clinical Observations

In the case I am about to illustrate, a negative traumatic event initiated a destructive process in a person who, later, once she was able to face her issue, was able to make a constructive, radical change in her life.

It might sound incredible, but this case could appear among the articles of a newspaper, with a dramatic headline that would state, more or less, "Trauma caused her to give up lucrative job and risk unemployment—she turns her life around."

Everything started when a middle-aged woman who worked as a bank teller came to my office. The bank she worked in had been robbed, and she had been directly involved in dealing with the robbers. After the occurrence, the bank had organized therapeutic sessions for all the staff who had been involved and had reported post-traumatic stress symptoms. In addition to receiving sessions with the psychologist who was available to all employees, she had decided also to come to my office.

After I let her in and made her sit, I started to write down her general information and asked her the reason she had chosen CranioSacral Therapy. Her answer was "I didn't come here because I needed to; I came here because the bank I work in pays for these treatments. I want to retaliate against them and make them pay as much as I can."

I raised my eyes from the paper and looked at her, not knowing whether to feel surprised or discomforted. At that point, she felt she needed to explain the situation further and added, "I can't stand to work at the bank anymore. It is an awful job, and I feel exploited and underrated."

Normally I would ask such a patient to leave my office, since I find it unethical to start a treatment with that sort of motivation. Nonetheless, something was holding me back, so I invited the woman to lie down on the therapy table anyway.

While listening to her craniosacral rhythm, I asked her whether she wanted to tell me about the bank heist. She must have been eager to vent, because she started to speak and went on and on without ever taking a pause. What she said helped me understand why she had decided to say those things to me, a complete stranger, rather than to the psychologist hired by the bank.

She told me her story more or less as follows:

When the robbers came in, my colleagues got scared, but what I saw was an opportunity to inflict a loss to the bank. Under my desk I had a drawer with not much cash and in a small door underneath a bag with a substantial amount of banknotes. As soon as they entered, one of the robbers walked toward me. His face was covered and I could only see his eyes. In that moment, I saw him as a modern-age Robin

Hood. My hands were already under the desk to open the small door and give him the contents of the bag. When he arrived in front of me, I noticed his hand underneath the jacket and understood that he was probably armed. Looking at me, he said, "Open the drawer, you big dummy, and give me all the money!"

That gratuitous insult made me feel like the world had been pulled out from under my feet. I thought that the robber had the same lack of consideration as those who shared everyday life with me at work. So I decided to do exactly as I was told and gave him the small amount of money inside the drawer, not what was in the bag. By insulting me bluntly while I was already feeling threatened and stressed, he missed the opportunity of going home with ten times more money.

Upon hearing her story, I felt even more astonished than before. However, I was perceiving her tensions relaxing on a myofascial level, and her craniosacral rhythm, which had been slower than average, became normal.

After that session, I worked with her again and learned that at the beginning of her career she expected great things from her job, but she had soon realized that her workplace was filled with various discriminations. Decisions were based not on merit but on mere aesthetic factors. She was short and not very attractive by aesthetic standards of that time. Therefore, even with great skills and competence, she found herself cast aside, something that did not happen to her female colleagues who were less capable but more eye-catching. Over time, this had caused her to feel a grudge against her coworkers and bosses, and even toward the whole institution for allowing the discrimination to take place. That grudge was trapped inside her, creating a nonlocalized discomfort that manifested itself through various physical issues, always different and hard to diagnose. She had started to call in sick to work more and more often, which had contributed to the lack of consideration she had already noticed in the management.

Being called "big dummy" by the robber, though he did not even know her, was only the tip of the iceberg. It was what had made her realize the destructive component of her grudge.

We worked together on that emotion, and after various sessions in which I energetically treated her liver meridian in particular, her trauma changed and became a stimulus to transform her future, prompting her to quit her job at the bank and become a freelance financial advisor. She was very competent, and her success as a financial advisor actually proved it.

For a period she continued to come to my office to receive CST treatments even though she had to pay for them herself, since neither the insurance nor the bank would cover that cost anymore.

☙ A CST-CENTERED VISION ☙

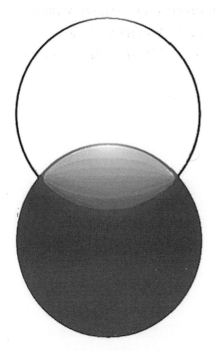

Fig. 10.15. Color is produced by the meeting of light and darkness.

British physicist, mathematician, philosopher, astronomer, historian, theologian, and alchemist Isaac Newton (1642–1727) claimed that darkness is the absence of light. A century later, in his book *Theory of Colors,* German writer, poet, and playwright Johann Wolfgang von Goethe (1749–1832) opposed that theory. According to Goethe, who studied science, theology, philosophy, humanism, painting, music, and other arts, darkness exists as a polarity interacting with light. Colors are not contained in light but originate from the interaction of light and darkness, manifesting themselves through the phenomenon of polarity.

Austrian esotericist and theosophist Rudolf Steiner (1861–1925), who founded anthroposophy, took inspiration from Goethe. He, too, believed that colors originate from light and darkness, and he developed a spiritual theory about the administration of color in various forms, anticipating current chromotherapy.

❧ ❧

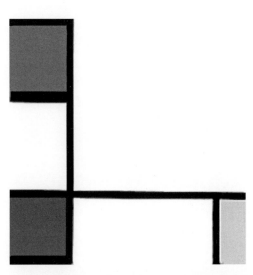

Fig. 10.16. *Composition No. IV with Red, Blue, and Yellow*, by Piet Mondrian
(In color, red is the top left rectangle, blue the bottom left, and yellow the bottom right.)

Dutch painter Pieter Cornelis Mondrian (1872–1944) used Steiner's works as a reference. Mondrian searched for formal and chromatic balance in the relations between primary colors (yellow, red, and blue), arranged between uniform white fields and vertical black lines. In his purely abstract art, the formal and chromatic balance is connected with a precise spiritual symbolism. Yellow is associated with the energy of the sun, red with the union of light and space, and blue with spirituality.

That is the universal balance that, according to theosophy, sees only the three primary colors between light (white) and darkness (black). Or as paraphrased from Goethe's *Theory of Colours*, color is produced by the meeting of light and dark.

Between white and black: colors. Between constructive and destructive: the multiple shades through which an individual appears to the Facilitator. In the magic of primary colors, which create all the other colors, using CST and SER with patients supports them in their path toward self-healing.

CHAPTER 11
The Cerebral Hemispheres
Connection and Harmonization

There are two brains in the head, one which gives understanding, and another which provides sense perception.
DIOCLES OF CARYSTUS (GREEK PHYSICIAN, FOURTH CENTURY BCE)

In previous chapters we examined some aspects of emotions and learned how they were considered in opposition to logic. Starting from this contraposition, we analyzed polarity to better understand the function of opposites and their natural and necessary interaction and integration.

Different stimuli, notions, and concepts that at first glance seem to be a mere digression from the main path of this text are actually the tiles of a theoretical and experiential mosaic gradually forming a complete picture. Among intuitive sceneries and logical passages, we will see in this picture the involvement of all the structures and their connection with CST and SER treatments.

How can our brain give a constructive structure to what it is presented with, especially in such a heterogeneous context as the discourse on separation, bereavement, and loss? First, let us proceed with a brief review of anatomical/physiological and functional concepts in order to comprehend what later will be our priority focus when addressing topics, situations, and scenarios involving loss, separation, death, and bereavement on a biological level.

THE TWO HEMISPHERES

The brain is the main organ of the central nervous system. It is at least partly responsible for the regulation of vital functions and is the seat of homeostatic regulation.

In human beings, cerebral activity gives birth to the mind, its superior cognitive functions, and, more generally, psychic and emotional functions.

The brain is divided into two hemispheres, right and left, which are completely separated and communicate between each other via about 300 million axonal fibers

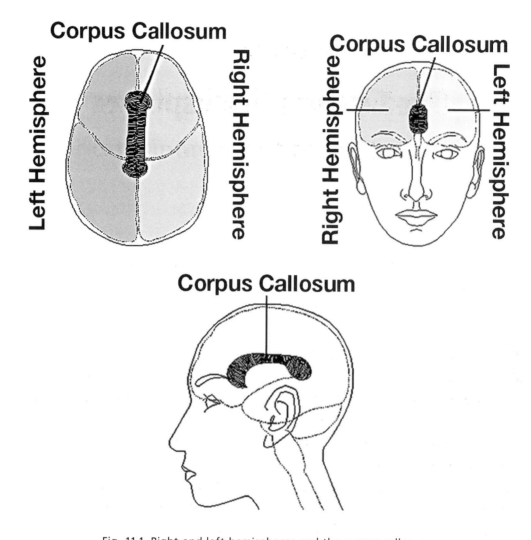

Fig. 11.1. Right and left hemispheres and the corpus callosum

(bundles of axons) of the corpus callosum. Axons are nerve fibers conducting electrical impulses in a centrifugal direction, away from the nerve cell body.

The cerebral hemispheres are symmetrical but not identical. The left hemisphere is analytical, practical, organized, logical, and rational. It manages the past and the future. It functions in a linear and methodical way. Its task is to gather details in the present, catalog them, and organize them. The left hemisphere connects us and our inner world with the outside world and separates the inner world of the individual from the rest of the world.

The right hemisphere is synthetic, artistic, creative, spatial, nonverbal, global, and perceptive. It is focused on the present, on the here and now. It reasons through images and learns through the movements of the body. The information arrives in this area in the form of energy and, at the same time, flows through the sensory system in order to produce a representation of the present moment (smells, tastes, sensations, sounds, and visual perceptions). Through the awareness of the right hemisphere, it is possible to perceive a connection with the energy that surrounds us.

The differences between the two hemispheres also concern many other cognitive activities, such as memory. The left hemisphere is connected with procedural, semantic, and autobiographical memory. The right hemisphere mostly manages visual, spatial, temporal, and emotional memory.

The two hemispheres can carry out their functions either symmetrically or asymmetrically. In left-handed people, the functions of the two hemispheres often are reversed.

The symmetries between the two hemispheres involve the control of the movements of the two halves of the body (left and right):

- The muscles of the left half of the body are controlled by the motor cortex of the right hemisphere.
- The muscles of the right half of the body are controlled by the motor cortex of the left hemisphere.

The asymmetries between the two hemispheres involve several functions, such as language and expression:

- Language centers are located exclusively in the left hemisphere, which is slightly larger, as are functions that govern the formulation and expression of concepts.
- The right hemisphere manages some aspects of musical functions and visual perception and is involved in the expression of emotions and in artistic sensitivity.

Although they have specific peculiarities that differentiate them, the two hemispheres work synergistically. Even when one tends to predominate over the other, the brain always works using both hemispheres.

It is important to highlight that a single cognitive function can be managed by either the left or the right hemisphere according to its specific purpose. For instance, musicians perceive music in two different ways: If they just want to relax and acknowledge the harmony, they listen to it almost unconsciously with the right hemisphere; on the contrary, if they want to analyze the melody on a technical level, the left hemisphere automatically comes into the picture.[1]

Since specific areas of the brain control specific functions, the characteristics of a certain dysfunction are determined by the location of the cerebral damage that caused it.

THE CORPUS CALLOSUM

The two cerebral hemispheres are connected to each other by a bridge of nerve fibers, the corpus callosum, which allows them and the central nervous system to exchange any information in real time. We previously defined the corpus callosum as the axis connecting the two poles of the right and left hemispheres. We also could define it as the layer that connects logic to emotions.

The corpus callosum is a cerebral commissure. In neurology, the term *commissure* indicates a formation of gray or white matter that is similar in appearance to a flat bundle and connects two quite homologous areas of the central nervous system. This connection is made along the cerebrospinal axis through specific nerve fibers called commissural fibers.

As noted earlier in this chapter, the corpus callosum is made of almost 300 million bundles of myelin fibers that connect corresponding areas of the two hemispheres, joining them in the central-lower portion of their medial side. It is the most important commissure of the brain since it connects the four lobes (frontal, temporal, parietal, and occipital). It ensures the transmission of information and coordination between the two hemispheres.

The upper surface of the corpus callosum is covered by a thin layer of gray matter that constitutes part of the dorsal hippocampus and extends almost to the membranous portion of dura mater that separates the two hemispheres. On the lower surface of the corpus callosum is the insertion of the septum pellucidum; its posterior part makes contact with the crura of the fornix.

Fibers of the corpus callosum enter and leave all regions of the neocortex, constituting the callosal connections. The fibers link cortical areas connected with peripheral motor and sensory functions. Physiology shows that the corpus callosum allows the processing of visual, auditory, and tactile information and that it intervenes in the coordination of movement and language. It also helps us monitor fear and calm an overexcited RAS, fostering the passage from one phase of our Life Cycle to the next. (As discussed in chapter 6, the RAS affects almost every other system in the body and is activated by stress, according to the fight-or-flight principle.)

THE CENTRAL NERVOUS SYSTEM

Not even the most sophisticated computer can boast a complexity of circuits, correlations, processing units, and information channels as remarkable as the human nervous system. All the expressions of our personality, such as thoughts, hopes, dreams, wishes, and emotions, are functions of our nervous system. It is the seat of the

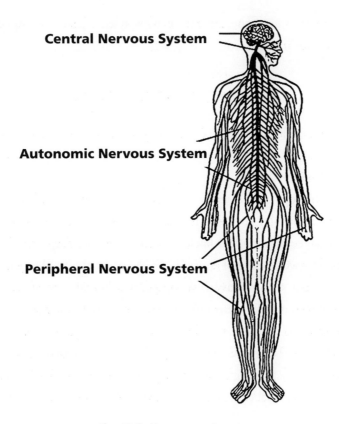

Fig. 11.2. Nervous system

reception, processing, and transmission of data concerning the whole human body. In fact, it is the system of regulation of bodily functions.

The nervous system includes all the nerve tissues of the human organism. These tissues transport information and instructions from one region of the body to another. The main functions of the nervous system include:

- providing sensations about both the internal and the external environment
- integrating sensory information
- coordinating voluntary and involuntary body processes
- regulating and monitoring peripheral structures and apparatuses

Nerve tissues include two different types of cell: nerve cells, or neurons, which are responsible for the transmission and processing of information in the nervous system, and glial cells, or neuroglia, which isolate neurons and provide a support network. Glial cells are more numerous than the neurons and represent about half the volume of the entire nervous system.

In neurology, the central nervous system is referred to as *white matter*. It is made of neurons whose axons are wrapped in what is called the myelin sheath. *Gray matter,* in contrast, is the tissue of the central nervous system that is composed of neurons whose axons are not myelinated.

QUANTUM PERSPECTIVES

The fundamental evolutionary discoveries of quantum physics have opened the door to a new approach to observing reality, not only in the field of physics but also of biology and medicine.

As regards biology, we already have seen how new branches of this science (epigenetics, for example) consider the energetic component involved in the reactions that take place on a molecular level and their transformative action on RNA expression and the well-being of individuals. Now, in the field of quantum biology, as it's known, recent studies have investigated the possibility of transferring information to the nervous fibers through the production of biophotons (quanta of an electromagnetic field in quantum biology) and electromagnetic waves.[2] Meanwhile, the study of quantum electrodynamics (QED) is now bringing a new perspective on living matter, considering it not merely as a series of biochemical, anatomical, and physiological reactions in an organism but also as a single Open-System Human Being.

According to the principle of complementarity of quantum physics, a quantum—an elementary particle associated with a given force field—can be both corpuscular and wavelike (wave-particle duality). These two aspects exclude each other depending on the type of experiment (intentional observation), which determines the behavior of the particles involved.

Just as a quantum can be described both as a corpuscle and as an electromagnetic wave, a CST and SER Facilitator's touch also can have both a physical nature and the function of a directional energy wave. In CST, the technique known as Direction of Energy sets up the conditions that allow the Facilitator to send syntropic energy through intention and touch toward an energetic blockage (entropic energy), creating a constructive reaction in the organism of the individual. We will later see how the technique of the Direction of Energy can be implemented to harmonize the cerebral hemispheres.

Note that Dr. Upledger substantiated this technique after thorough studies on quantum mechanics, in particular on quantum superimposition as illustrated in the paradox of Schrödinger's cat.

Quantum Biology

To analyze some of the aspects of quantum biology that are relevant to our path, we are now going to propose them through a synthesis of the words of Paolo Manzelli, professor of physical chemistry at the University of Florence and president of the NGO EGOCREANET, from some of his articles on the subject.

> The cells of all living systems produce in the UVA and visible frequency range faint light quanta—the Biophotons—which derive from the metabolism of several molecules able to "structure" the electromagnetic energy in the frequencies of their double bonds.... We know that the brain is the seat of an electromagnetic field and its channels are the "bioelectrical synapses" of the dendrites (gap junctions), which produce sparks of quantized light caused by the asymmetrical distribution of ions between the two sections of the synaptic fissures. This emission of Biophotons allows the interactive communication between various areas of the brain and, in the "Higher Areas of the Cerebral Hemispheres," the production of the endorphins that are necessary for the processes of the biochemical synapses. ... The emission of Biophotons as bioelectrical twinkling can activate our system of perception.... As light quanta, Biophotons then allow the brain to process the epigenetic information, acting as a "quantum computer" to create images, sounds, colors, and other sensations, which we actually perceive.[3]

> All that was said above can change radically the approach to health, disease, and healing, highlighting the "Energetic" contribution of the communication of Biophotons as light quanta and of Biophonons as sound quanta. That gets us closer to the intuitions and practices belonging to ancient conceptions and representations of Vital Energies and Subtle Bodies.[4]

Quantum Interdisciplines

Thanks to the concepts of quantum mechanics and physics, more and more scientists are finding connections between different scientific disciplines. As pointed out by Aldo Sacchetti, hygienist, professor, scientist, and one of the fathers of Italian ecology:

> Only quantum electrodynamics can account for the instantaneous wide-range processes governing biology. In fact, they are supported by coherent oscillations with high and low frequencies involving at the same time water molecules and message macromolecules carrying bioinformation—such as DNA, RNA, or proteins. That underscores the limits of the current biomedical approach, while also giving a higher scientific dignity to alternative medicine such as homeopathy.... The sensitivity of life at the level of quanta is widely documented nowadays, also in the context of photons, the particles composed of the minimum indivisible quantity of electromagnetic energy.... Our body is the constant and coordinated pulsing modification of interatomic and intermolecular bonds that are more than the

number of stars in the universe. This indivisible and coherent dynamic composition between energy, matter, and shape is the main manifestation of life.... In my opinion, quantum electrodynamics could allow us to overcome [the] seventeenth century's harmful fracture between physics and metaphysics.... In fact, biological structures can, inside themselves, convert mechanical vibrations into electromagnetic oscillations and vice versa.[5]

Quantum Electrodynamics (QED)

Consistent with the general laws of physics and the evidence of an interrelation between physical elements (field-particle), QED has brought a new holistic vision on living matter. Not only biological organisms—from the particle to the cell, from every single biological system to the entire human organism—but all of reality constitute a single unit made of an almost infinite number of field-particles that the coherence of QED actualizes on the physical level.

Giuliano Preparata (1942–2000), researcher at the CERN of Geneva and professor at the universities of Princeton, Harvard, Rockefeller, and Milan, wrote the following words:

The Oneness (Unity): the Universe as a unified quantum field.

The Oneness emerges from a deep understanding of the concept of the quantum field. The Universe is a single field. The field is the Oneness of the Universe.

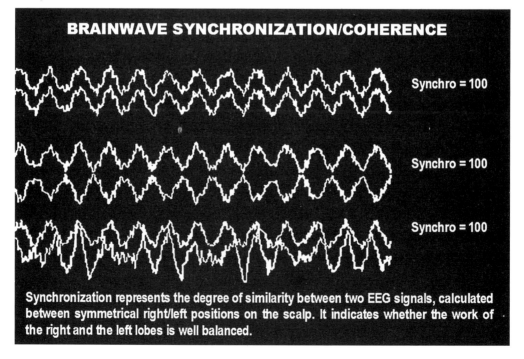

Fig. 11.3. EEG showing brainwave synchronization/coherence

. . . The particles and every phenomenon are an aspect of this Oneness. . . . Coherence springs from the same conceptual structure of these fields, [and] then it is miraculously realized as a real fact of nature and then as a generator of observed phenomena.

The theory of quantum electrodynamics coherence has to do with the interaction between the matter fields and electromagnetic fields in unison, on certain particular carrier frequencies, with certain phase relationships. The theory of quantum electrodynamics coherence is a particular aspect of coherent realization of quantum field theory to which we had originally given the name of "super radiance," a term coined by Robert H. Dicke, physicist of Princeton, who was the first to conceive of this coherent behavior, of oscillations in phase, between atomic systems and electromagnetic fields. . . . Life is therefore a delicate balance between coherence and incoherence.[6]

Emilio del Giudice (1940–2014), physicist at the Italian National Institute for Nuclear Physics, researcher, and science communicator, wrote about the universal quantum field as well:

Quantum field theory is the deepest response so far historically proposed to the problem of "one" and "many." The Universe is described by a set of quantum fields, each of which extends indefinitely in space and time. . . . The quantum field has in fact double characteristics; it is a set of quanta, of granules that provide the "intensity" of the field, but it is also governed by a "phase" (which roughly defines the way the field swings) that emerges spontaneously from the global dynamics of the set of quanta. . . . The local point of view and the global one are therefore complementary aspects in the context of quantum field theory. The Universe, which is deeply one, can also be seen, to a limit, as a set of separate individual realities. . . . The physical states closest to the existence of Oneness are coherent states in which an undefined set of "particles" is described by a well-defined phase in space and time, which ensures a related and cooperative behavior (hence the name coherency) of all the components that, in the process, lose their nature of separate individuals. . . . The trapped electromagnetic field has with it a constant companion, the "vector potential," a totally immeasurable quantity in classical physics, but that, in quantum field theory, influences the phase of a coherent system. The potential vector, unlike the field, is not trapped; it extends to a wide surrounding area, transporting not energy, but only information, and exerting its "subtle influence," we could say, like in computing science, by changing the phase of the coherent present systems. Among the various coherent systems it is therefore open to the possibility of a "subtle dialogue," a communication without exchange of energy, which involves only the phases, which therefore escape to each type of parcel measure and can be perceived only by those who put themselves in a wave ambit. . . . The "subtle influence" of the potential vector is then undertaken to correlate all these coherent structures in the unity of the living. . . . It seems the archetype of life: from a collection of unattached individual objects to an object that is "everything." This may be one of the ways to understand the emergence of consciousness from matter.[7]

DIRECTION OF ENERGY

We have dwelled on the theoretical explanations of eminent scientists to reiterate a concept that will be useful to illustrate the practical aspects of the technique of Direction of Energy.

By implementing the Direction of Energy, the Facilitator stimulates communication between symmetrical and asymmetrical areas of the cerebral hemispheres and, through the corpus callosum, simultaneously encourages communication between the right and the left hemispheres, allowing an optimal recovery of the energy flow in the organism. The directional energy the Facilitator employs through intention is syntropic energy that dissipates any residual entropic energy in the hemispheres and corpus callosum, which can cause communication to be inefficient and problematic.

The Facilitator then has the chance to work with the patient to:

- interact with energetic structure to optimize anatomical, physiological, biological, and cognitive functions
- develop the ability to interact with stimuli and information coming from the senses
- enhance all the stimuli and information coming from the organism to the brain

Objectives

For treatment of the cerebral hemispheres and their connection with the corpus callosum and nervous system through the Direction of Energy, a CST Facilitator will have to work extensively with intention, remembering that the body is a unit, and structure and function are interconnected. The Facilitator's objectives are:

- to restore the functionality of the corpus callosum and encourage optimal communication between the two hemispheres (right and left) of the brain
- to develop the ability of intention to restore optimal energy flow in the organism through treatment
- to develop the ability to visualize the anatomical and physiological structures involved in the treatment

Technique

Through application of the Direction of Energy technique, a Facilitator will:

1. connect with the two cerebral hemispheres
2. connect with the central nervous system
3. support the path chosen by the Open-System Human Being, helping individuals in their delicate passage from one phase of their Life Cycle to the next

Hand Placement

Choose one of the three cranial vault holds. If you are not able to touch the patient, use the same technique as described below, but keep your hands in proximity to the two hemispheres.

Direction of Energy Exercise

1. Place your hands on the patient's head using one of the three cranial vault holds pictured below (fig. 11.4) and connect with the two hemispheres.
2. Through the intention, start to send energy from one hand to the other. Listen.

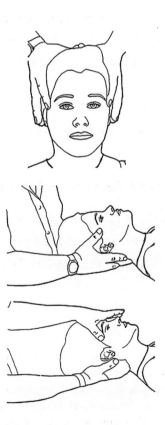

Fig. 11.4. The three cranial vault holds

3. As soon as you perceive any modification, or physical or energetic change, ask each hemisphere to express itself, using Therapeutic Imagery and Dialogue with the patient's non-conscious.*

   Ask the left hemisphere (rational):
   - What are you experiencing right now?
   - What would you like to experience instead?

   Ask the right hemisphere (creative):
   - What are you experiencing right now?
   - What would you like to experience instead?

   Ask the corpus callosum:
   - How can you facilitate the communication between hemispheres?
   - Can you find balance and an acceptable solution for both parts?
   - If you can, what is it?

4. Ask the patient's Higher Self or Inner Physician to bring to the patient's consciousness the answer of the corpus callosum in order to find a balance between the polarities of the rational and the creative hemispheres.
5. Thank all the structures involved in the treatment for contributing to the patient's well-being and the transformation of destructive energy into constructive energy so that the individual can experience in the best way possible the present stage of their life, whatever it is.
6. At this point, you can resume the Therapeutic Imagery and Dialogue as needed.

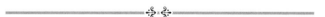

Self-Listening Direction of Energy Exercise

If you like, you can try to practice Direction of Energy on yourself—obviously without the part of the Therapeutic Imagery and Dialogue—by placing one hand on each hemisphere (fig. 11.5) and following these steps, without rushing:

---

*The modification is a change in state (from the current state to a new different state) and can be felt both in tactile perception (change in position or volume, always talking about quantum movements), and in listening to the craniosacral rhythm, both in energetic perception and in the acquisition of a message from the Inner Doctor, or a Significant Detector, etc. Basically any type of change that the facilitator can perceive while listening to the two hemispheres. So when we talk about modification we are talking about the sensation/perception that reveals a modification.

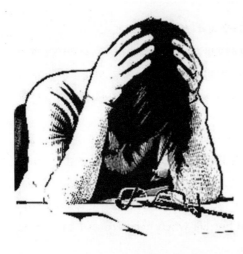

Fig. 11.5. Self-listening exercise—the connection of the two cerebral hemispheres

1. Let thoughts give way to the sensation of an intimate listening to your own internal rhythm.
2. Start asking questions of the hemispheres and the corpus callosum, as detailed above.
   Those who have never before tried to perceive the craniosacral rhythm will need to use their intention (the confidence in their own ability to perceive):
   - in this situation
   - in this moment
   - with this purpose

3. At the same time, in complete tranquility, you can listen to your own primary breathing and your own Inner Physician's voice.
   It is possible!

It is crucial to focus on the fact that, as we concentrate on this exercise, we also are connecting with what we have learned so far and widening our ability to understand. Essentially, we are giving ourselves the chance to connect with our Inner Physician (our Higher Self) and open up to a new perception of what we still need to learn.

This exercise improves both our perception and our concentration and will later be useful in helping us understand the mechanisms regulating our connection with our entire physiological, energetic, emotional, and spiritual system.

Clinical Observations

A woman once came to my office complaining of a sense of physical discomfort in all of her body. She was feeling a small, nonlocalized pain that increased every time she was in a relationship. That situation had been going on for years, never stopping regardless of who her partner was.

I started to treat her, and we almost immediately directed the session toward SomatoEmotional Release, during which I visualized the image of the sun. I asked the patient what meaning the sun could have for her. She answered that she associated it with summer, a season she did not like because it reminded her of a particularly unhappy moment of her life when her parents had started to fight almost every day.

She also remembered that, since they had a house with a tree-lined garden, every time a fight broke out she had to go out in the sun and stay on her own in the garden, where there was also a small inflatable pool. At the end of the summer, her parents had definitively decided to separate. From that moment on, summer stopped being her favorite season.

After her parents' separation, she had grown up blaming herself for their fights. She believed that she was somehow the cause, even if she could not remember why.

Eventually she had started to have romantic relationships, but they never lasted long. Her constant physical discomfort increased and became a subtle pain right in the moments when she should have relaxed, preventing her from feeling content or satisfied with the person she was with.

The temporal development of her story, together with what had emerged from her non-conscious during the treatment and what I had perceived from the Significance Detector when she told me she had suppressed the reason why she felt guilty about her parents' fights, made me understand that I had to analyze with her the emotional aspect connected with their separation.

That analytical aspect was completely lacking. Her connection with the left hemisphere was probably blocked.

The session ended. I asked her how she was doing, and when she told me she felt a little confused but relaxed, I encouraged her to come back.

In the following session, I started to treat her with the Direction of Energy between the hemispheres in order to connect the emotional aspect with the analytical aspect and allow her memories to come back to her consciousness. I felt that the situation of responsibility she could not remember concerned exclusively the relationship between her parents, not her.

I perceived that the right hemisphere did not accept communication from the left, whereas the left hemisphere was trying to communicate with the right to send information that could rebalance and channel her emotions constructively. Even her corpus callosum was blocked in a sort of impasse. It could not transmit any signal or message because the right hemisphere was blocking any impulse coming from the left hemisphere.

In a nonverbal context, I located an Energy Cyst in the right hemisphere. I started to send syntropic energy to dissipate it, and then I continued the Therapeutic Imagery and Dialogue by inviting the patient to verbalize.

What emerged was that the patient thought she could not allow herself to be happy or to have any long-lasting relationship since she had not allowed her parents to do so. This sense of guilt was fed by her right hemisphere, which gave stability to the constant scenario of punishment and atonement related to what had happened to her parents.

In fact, she had never analyzed coherently what had happened during her childhood. Children often blame themselves for events that are completely independent of any responsibility of their own. She had accepted her own guilt, even though she did not know what it was, and resigned herself to the unhappiness it implied.

In the end, the patient realized she needed to ask her parents for an explanation about their separation. She had never done that, as she had never even considered the possibility that there could be another plausible reason for the end of her parents' relationship apart from her own responsibility.

When she came back to my office, she told me she had asked her mother why her relationship with her father had ended. More surprised than relieved, she found out that her parents had separated because their characters were not compatible and they had contrasting ideas about the future of their relationship and family. Moreover, her mother had told her that they had always sent her away from where the fights were taking place, sending her to the garden in the sun, only because they wanted to protect her from the vehemence of those fights.

The patient needed more sessions to process the loss of that sense of guilt, which had become an omnipresent companion in her life to the extent of not letting her have relationships with other real-life companions. She finally succeeded in setting herself free from the Energy Cyst, the blockage of the right hemisphere that inhibited the role of the corpus callosum and caused the inability of her hemispheres to communicate, the sense of guilt, and the physical discomfort that prevented her from having any relationship.

❖ A CST-CENTERED VISION ❖

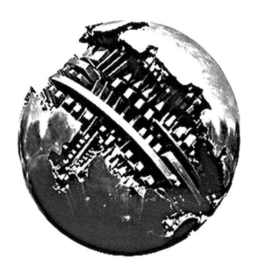

Fig. 11.6. *Big Sphere*, by Arnaldo Pomodoro

Arnaldo Pomodoro is one of the greatest Italian sculptors, goldsmiths, and engravers of international fame. The spherical shape in his art represents, and can be the realization of, one's own space within the larger space in which one lives and moves. In 2008, he wrote, "I believe my sculptures to be crystals, or nuclei, or eyes, or fires, for the frontier and the journey, for the complexity, for the imagery."[8]

Pomodoro's *Big Sphere* (fig. 11.6), divided in two parts, is sectioned to let the observer glimpse the parts composing each hemisphere. It is an interesting analogy to our brain: divided in two hemispheres, each constituted by several parts, from the bigger to the infinitesimal—atoms and electrons. Each part interacts with the other and, if it is functional, keeps the entire sphere in balance within the surrounding environment (homeostasis).

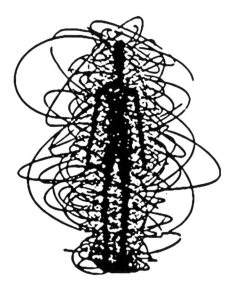

Fig. 11.7. Reproduction of a piece from the *Feeling Material* series, by Antony Gormley

Antony Gormley is a sculptor, architect, and archaeologist from London who dedicates most of his work to anthropomorphic sculptures. He invented a new artistic language that explores the envelope of the body both as architecture and as seat of the mind, positioning each artwork in wide architectural or natural spaces in relation with its surroundings. He uses the cast of his own body as matrix and measure for the works, thus becoming the subject, the tool, and the material of his research.

Gormley's *Feeling Material* (fig. 11.7) is a series of sculptures the artist used to represent the human figure, with a spiral orbiting next to the body and then continuing its movement in the space around it.

As Dr. Upledger once said, "One of the characteristics of consciousness is intelligence; therefore a particle of energy can certainly decide when and where it will go."⁹ The title of the sculpture series, *Feeling Material,* fits perfectly in this concept, with the term *feeling* meaning to be conscious of the energetic potential that we can transmit into matter.

CHAPTER 12

Transformation

The Concepts of Psychosynthesis

Diego Maggio, BSc (hons), DO, CST-D and Euro Piuca, MD

Every space of certainty is a dead space, since it abolishes any possibility of transformation.

CARLOS BUBY, "CATIMBÓ"

This chapter was written in collaboration with Dr. Euro Piuca, a surgeon; the former director of the dialysis and nephrology department at the Ospedale Maggiore of Trieste; a therapist in the fields of psychosomatic medicine, medical hypnosis, and unicist homeopathy; an Instructor at Upledger Italia, the Osteopathic College, the Centro Organizzazione Interventi Medicina Attiva S.R.L a Tavernola Bergamasca (Bergamo) (Intervention Organization Center of Active Medicine S.R.L in Tavernola Bergamasca), and the Accademia di Maestria of Trieste center for holistic research; and the developer of the seminar "CST & SER, Jung, Assagioli and Psychosynthesis."

Psychosynthesis introduces the same work of transformation that we are proposing with the purpose of overcoming traumas caused by separation, loss, small deaths, and bereavement. In the experiential interpretation we are applying, pairing psychosynthesis with the approach we propose in this text can be useful in the process of integration and transformation to:

- foster personal transformation
- identify the best way to start the energetic transformation from destructive to constructive and maintain its results
- use the non-conscious and the cooperation of mind and body to achieve this change

- get the maximum results with minimum efforts, using what Assagioli called "wise will"

Before delving into the core of this approach, however, we are first going to touch upon the main contact points between some of the figures involved in this field who also inspired Dr. Upledger in his research on SomatoEmotional Release: Carl Gustav Jung, Fritz Perls, and Roberto Assagioli, who is also the father of psychosynthesis. In particular, Jung's analytical psychology, Perls's Gestalt, and Assagioli's psychosynthesis share some affinities of fundamental thoughts that influenced Dr. Upledger in his work:

- Human beings are essentially healthy organisms in which temporary dysfunctions may occur.
- Symptoms do not necessarily imply a pathology; they are only the superficial manifestation of a problem.
- In the organism, nature always tends to make harmony prevail over dysfunction.
- The human psyche always tends to reconcile opposites.
- During therapy, individuals must be helped to become aware of their own personality and enabled to transform it by integrating the contradictions that cause the dysfunction.
- An individual's spiritual/transpersonal aspect plays a key role in the development of their higher psychic functions.
- Introversion and extroversion indicate the interests of the individual in life.

TRANSFORMATION: BETWEEN BEING AND BECOMING

We have seen Heraclitus's concept of *panta rhei* (everything flows), which holds that reality is constantly changing in a process of perpetual transformation, and all things are born, grow, die, and transform.

Psychologist and psychotherapist Pasquale Angelo Montalto detailed a helpful comparative synthesis of Heraclitus's concepts and those of Parmenides, a Greek philosopher of the fifth century BCE:

> In Heraclitus's vision, our Being fights for Life in the process of transmutation. Life is conceived as a dynamic unit, containing multiple moving elements that tend to realize the harmonic multiplicity of opposites through transformation processes, in a sort of "concordant discord" produced by the tension of achieving the path of truth. . . . On the contrary, Parmenides sees the idea of Being as something univocal, unitary . . . immutable, eternal, and necessary. . . . It exists and cannot but

exist, since the world of pure reality is uncreated, indestructible, . . . perfect, and out of time, in a perpetual present. Unlike reality, which lies somewhere else in the pure Being, our existence is immersed in a constant flow . . . and consists of a fabric of appearance.

We tend to hold on to a useless and wearying self-centeredness. In order to continue Being and "stay in the race" with life, we often completely forget to transform our actions in accordance with the life flow of the universe we live in. At this point, conscious reflection interweaves with the urgency of taking action, maintaining Being and Becoming separate but not opposed, in the joy of living and continuing to rely on experience as a scientific datum to help us build reality.[1]

POLIVERSION: POLARITY AND INTERACTIONS IN PSYCHOSYNTHESIS

The psychosynthetic goal is to acquire the ability to direct energies at will—that is, through the directing function of the will—in any direction and fashion, according to specific purposes, intentions, needs, and demands. This can be called poliversion.

ROBERTO ASSAGIOLI, *THE ACT OF WILL*

One of the objectives of psychosynthesis is to enable contrasting or opposite elements of the human psyche to converge (synthesize). In order to do so, it is essential to become aware of the inner polarities of the individual and consider the different ways to deal with them. Assagioli proposed an analytical approach to get closer to this synthesis of polarities. For instance, extroversion and introversion can coexist in one individual when their relationship is mutually exclusive; if the first polarity represents the usual conscious attitude, like an extremely strict behavior, the other acts unconsciously to compensate it and break one-sidedness. In fact, these are the two poles of the oscillation of the normal thinking process, and in this oscillation the role of the unconscious is to constantly correct conscious processes.

When dealing with separation, bereavement, loss, and small deaths, it is essential for the Facilitator to never judge the patient's emotional reactions. It could be useful to consider that any emotional excess often hides exactly the opposite aspect, which is repressed.

In fact, it is sometimes hard to see the polarity of some individuals because they seem to display only one side of their emotional life to its full extent. If that were the case, they would meet stagnation. Contrast and dialectic are necessary for continued growth, and a lack of interaction can bring stasis, close-mindedness, and energy blockages.

Another emotional tendency—perhaps the most common—common in patients who are processing any kind of loss is the oscillation between opposite poles. Oscillations can be brief or go on for years. They are often the cause or result of some type of emotional repression that arises during the processing of trauma and grief.

Conflict and Synthesis of Opposite Poles

Inner conflict is an inevitable consequence of the total and unaware identification with one aspect of ourselves, often displayed during the grieving process, causing anxiety, incoherence, and loss of energy.

The Facilitator's task is to help the patient go back to a state of creative tension based on the clear recognition and acceptance of the emotional extremes (poles) that generated the conflict. In order to do so, the Facilitator can use the non-conscious to connect with the patient's Inner Physician to find the space of balance and healing where the Higher Self resides.

In inner life, a balanced tension between two poles produces exchange and mutual enrichment and therefore growth. To achieve this result, we must bring to patients' awareness the fact that one part of themselves, which they probably have rejected, actually has an essential contribution to offer to the rest of the personality. When we can observe the two poles objectively, the tension between them fades so that they can converge and merge into their synthesis, bringing new constructive energy.

A synthesis is created when two elements merge and give birth to a new entity (e.g., hydrogen and oxygen + spark = water), potentially starting a transformation. In a scenario of loss in which conflicting emotions emerge (introversion and extroversion in the expression of pain, in actions, and in the contemplation of the consequences of loss), the release of destructive energy that follows the perception of the loss causes the appearance of a new quality that includes both opposites and the sensation that none of the original poles was really lost.

The Whole Is Greater Than the Sum of Its Parts

Aristotle's maxim "The whole is greater than the sum of its parts" is simple and essential. It can be observed in any circumstance, both in the natural world and in strictly human contexts; a melody is more than the single notes constituting it, just like an organism is superior to the single cells that form it.

This Aristotelian maxim became one of the bases of Fritz Perls's Gestalt psychology, but it also was adopted by numerous schools of thought for the universal quality of its message.

Assagioli observed that the human psyche is constituted by various elements—sensations, impulses, desires, ideas, intuitions, et cetera. Some of these elements are connected; some are in conflict; others exist side by side even if they are alien to each other. It is rare for the human psyche to have the unity, organic harmony, and synergy that we can find in the human physical organism.

Through psychosynthesis, Assagioli created a psychological method that helps to achieve that synthesis. It is practical, open to any contribution, and applicable in many fields, such as CranioSacral Therapy and SomatoEmotional Release.

ACCESSING LATENT ENERGIES

The main objective of psychosynthesis is to lead individuals to wholeness and facilitate their access to a higher level of integration using a comprehensive approach to deal with the most essential aspects of human existence. At the same time, psychosynthesis employs an essentially practical method in order to help individuals:

- identify the unconscious forces controlling them
- discover their own will with techniques that sharpen their minds and awaken their intuition
- use imagination to create new tools to enrich their individual inner realities (individual = undivided)

By using psychosynthesis, we stimulate forces that are already inside us, latent energies that we are sometimes able to actually see in action. These latent forces operate when:

- an emotional wound slowly heals, creating an Energy Cyst
- we discover an unexpected courage in ourselves in a moment of crisis
- we suddenly find the solution to solve a problem that has haunted us, after searching for it in vain for a long time
- a spontaneous transformation takes place inside us

The effectiveness of psychosynthesis, just like the effectiveness of CST and SER, actually comes from the activation of these positive latent forces. In fact, psychosynthesis, just like CST and SER, does not promise to remove all obstacles, but it gives great importance to their transformation in each step of the growth process. It prioritizes creativity over the deceitful certainty of standard answers, recognizes the great variability of human beings, and thus does not guarantee the same result for everyone.

The psychosynthetic process develops through three interconnected steps:

1. Know yourself.
2. Own yourself.
3. Transform yourself.

To achieve our objective in our work with CST and SER, we are going to briefly explore some of the aspects of the psychosynthetic process, especially developing Assagioli's third point (transform yourself), with the following goals.

- We must learn to accept the parts of ourselves that are connected with inabilities and limitations. (It is of great importance to overcome fear, depression, denial, etc., in any situation of loss, including the loss of losses.)
- We must allow all sides of our personality to exist, since those we ignore can hide talents and abilities that we have never used. (It is crucial to use all of our resources to advance in all phases of our Life Cycle and address any blockages in the vital energy continuum.)
- We must nurture the aspects of ourselves that allow new creative talents to emerge in order for our personality to fully express. (This is essential for the process of interaction that brings us to our Higher Selves.)

WILL TO MEET THE HIGHER SELF

Will enables the individual to grasp wider existential meanings and reach self-realization. We experience it through its potential, which is developed in everyday life. In the psychosynthetic process, the human being goes from a chaotic mixture of conflicting tendencies to the harmonization of different elements around a center, the Higher Self.

In an integrated individual, the Higher Self is able to coordinate all the different functions of the psychophysical organism through the action of will.

To outline how various psychological functions interact with each other and trace the path toward a perfect integration and self-realization of the individual, Assagioli listed ten laws:

1. Images or mental pictures and ideas tend to produce the physical conditions and external events that correspond to them. Every image has in itself a motor element.
2. Attitudes, movements, and actions tend to evoke corresponding images and ideas; these, in turn, evoke or intensify corresponding emotions and feelings.
3. Ideas and images tend to awaken emotions and feelings that correspond to them.
4. Emotions and impressions tend to awaken and intensify ideas and images that correspond to or are associated with them.
5. Needs, urges, drives, and desires tend to arouse corresponding images, ideas, and emotions.

6. Attention, interest, affirmation, and repetitions reinforce the ideas, images, and psychological formations on which they are centered.
7. Repetition of actions intensifies the urge for further reiteration and renders their execution easier and better until they come to be performed unconsciously.
8. All the various functions and their manifold combinations in complexes and subpersonalities adopt means of achieving their aims without awareness and independently of (and even against) our conscious will.
9. Urges, drives, desires, and emotions tend to and demand to be expressed.
10. The psychological energies can find expression directly, through discharge and catharsis; indirectly, through symbolic action; or through a process of transmutation.

These ten laws are the keys to the activation of the personal transformational process. They highlight the best modalities to initiate the change and maintain its results, taking advantage of what the mind-body relationship can offer. In this way, we can achieve the maximum results with minimum efforts, using what Assagioli called "wise will."

WISE WILL

In psychosynthesis, as opposed to the traditional Freudian psychoanalytical conception of will, at the center of the inquiry are not only the unconscious but also the existence of an autonomous and conscious will of the Self, or Personal Self. In order to conceive the conscious will, we need to become aware of the essential difference between the Self, or Personal Self, and the Higher Self, or Transpersonal Self.

In fact, will is the function that is structurally most strictly connected with the conscious Self or Personal Self.

Assiagioli's Egg Diagram (fig. 12.1) can help us trace a synthetic map of our inner reality. Though it has the limitation of being a static description of a fluid concept (just like every other diagram), it is useful because it allows us to consider the different dimensions we can encounter in our CST and SER work.

The Egg Diagram represents the following elements:

1. lower unconscious
2. middle unconscious
3. higher unconscious or superconscious
4. awareness field

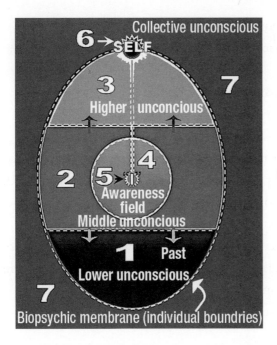

Fig. 12.1. Assagioli's Egg Diagram

5. conscious Self or "I"
6. Higher or Transpersonal Self
7. collective unconscious

Note that the distinction between lower and higher unconscious does not concern a moral judgment but rather a development: The lower unconscious is simply a more primitive part of ourselves, and it is not bad, only more ancient. On the other hand, the superconscious is everything we can achieve during our evolutionary path.

Lower Unconscious

The lower unconscious is the most primitive and childish part of ourselves. It often dominates us *(I don't know why I did it; I don't know what got into me; I lost it; I was out of my mind),* taking over and making us act in ways we normally would disapprove of.

Our task is to acquire a certain degree of knowledge and mastery of this part of ourselves—to contact this dimension, become familiar with its energy, and become able to guide it and channel it.

This level includes and originates:

- the basic psychological activity presiding over biological life
- the clever coordination of physiological functions
- primitive tendencies and impulses
- many psychological complexes with a strong emotional tone

- dreams and elementary imaginative activities
- various morbid manifestations, such as phobias, obsessive ideas and impulses, and paranoid delusions
- certain uncontrolled, spontaneous parapsychological faculties

Middle Unconscious

This level of consciousness is similar to the psychoanalytical concept of the preconscious. It represents everything we are not aware of in all given moments but that we can retrieve when we need to. For example, when we are asked for our phone number, even if a minute ago we were thinking of something completely different, we immediately remember it because it is available to us as if it were part of an internal archive. The middle unconscious is also the site of a form of psychological gestation, where ideas take shape before their emergence into awareness.

At the level of the middle unconscious, the following processes occur:

- processing of experiences
- preparation for future activities
- most theoretical and practical intellectual work, imaginative processes, and artistic creations of medium degree and value

Higher Unconscious or Superconscious

This is the highest level of the unconscious, the origin of all of our happiest states. When we have a bright idea or an ecstatic experience, when we feel a deep feeling of peace or disinterested love, when time seems to stop or we feel in a state of grace, elements of the superconscious have entered our awareness field.

It generates:

- higher artistic, philosophical, and scientific intuitions
- brilliant creations
- ethical and altruistic imperatives
- states of enlightenment, contemplation, and ecstasy

It includes, in a latent and potential form, the higher energy of the Spirit and elevated supernormal faculties and abilities. Therefore, the superconscious represents the source of human potential, artistic creativity, enlightenment, ecstasy, altruism, and everything that inspires great geniuses, artists, and mystics.

Like the lower unconscious, the superconscious is essentially different from our usual way of feeling and thinking. Therefore, it cannot be directly assimilated in the awareness field. Defense mechanisms filter and censor it, excluding it from consciousness.

Why?

It happens because the contents of the superconscious are so much more intense, bright, and wide than our usual awareness. If they emerge copiously and too fast, they could upset our personality. Though it may seem strange, we want not only to avoid the perception of the most primitive and pitiful aspects of ourselves, such as aggression and triggers arising from childhood traumas, but to defend ourselves from the sublime, desperately trying to maintain the current structure of our psyche, as limited and unstable as this balance may be.

Awareness Field

The term *awareness field* is not completely exact, but it is clear and convenient to use to define the part of our personality that we are directly aware of at all times: the constant succession of psychological elements and emotions of all kinds (e.g., sensations, images, thoughts, feelings, desires, impulses, etc.) that we can observe, analyze, and judge.

Conscious Self or "I"

The "I" is often confused with the aware personality (awareness field), but they do not actually coincide. The contents of consciousness (thoughts, feelings, etc.) are one thing, but the "I" is the center of consciousness that contains them and perceives them. The human beings who go with the flow, not lingering on self-analysis or wanting to know themselves, do not make this distinction. They identify themselves with the changing contents of their consciousness, confusing a moment of depression with *I am depressed* and a moment of anxiety with *I am anxious*.

Nonetheless, we can disidentify from this flow of contents and find our "I"—what we are, or the conscious Self behind our awareness field. This is a fundamental experience in the process of the psychological maturation of an individual. To find one's own "I" means to stop being controlled by ideas and emotions, reaching a sort of psychological distance. According to psychosynthesis, we can be dominated by everything we identify ourselves with and master and guide everything we disidentify from.

Therefore, the "I" is not an emotion but rather a pure center of consciousness.

Higher or Transpersonal Self

The conscious "I" often seems to fade and disappear (for example, during sleep, fainting, or hypnosis), only to come back and suddenly be found again, without us knowing how. This fact brings us to consider that behind or above the conscious there must be a permanent center, the true "I" or Higher Self.

The position and mutual relationship of the Self and the Higher Self are displayed in the Egg Diagram through the dotted line going from the middle of the awareness field (conscious "I") to the star at the top of the whole conscious and unconscious personality (Higher or Transpersonal Self).

The Transpersonal Self is the central part of the superconscious, the truest essence of our being. At this level there are no blockages or anxiety, dualism, or sense of separation. Becoming conscious of the Self is an extraordinary experience that makes us feel as ourselves and, at the same time, connected with everyone else and the universe as a whole. The Self is what we truly are.

Collective Unconscious

Human beings are not isolated. In the diagram, the external border of the egg is dotted to indicate that it delimits but does not separate completely from the outside. Consider it to be similar to the semipermeable membrane surrounding cells, which allows the existence of a constant and active exchange of fluids with the biological environment of the body. In the same way, there are constant processes of psychic osmosis, both between human beings and between each individual and the general psychological environment.

This level of consciousness corresponds to Jung's concept of the collective unconscious, but Jung did not give a clear definition of what it is and included in it very different and contrasting elements, putting together primitive and ancestral structures, higher archetypes, and superconscious activities.

It is constituted of the psychological life of mankind as it developed over the centuries. We all take part in this life, more or less consciously; we are all immersed in an ocean of thoughts and emotions that do not belong to us only but also to all of humanity; and we all participate in a common heritage of experiences that perpetuates in us, making other individuals our peers, not alien creatures.

The Indivisible "I"

Assagioli's Egg Diagram helps reconcile two facts that could seem mutually contradictory:

The apparent duality of "I"s: There seem to be two "I"s because the ordinary "I" theoretically and practically ignores the other—which is latent and does not reveal itself directly to the consciousness—to the extent of denying its existence.

The actual unity and indivisibility of the "I": In fact, there are not two "I"s, or two entities that are completely different and separated. The "I" is one; it simply has different degrees of manifestation, actualization, and awareness. One might say that the Personal Self or "I" is what we can perceive in a given moment about the Transpersonal Self; it is an emanation, a projection of the Self in the conscious personality. We could say it is like a reflection of light, which is distinct from the light source but does not have its own autonomy since it is not another separated light.

Let us be clear: The "I" must not be disregarded; it is the culmination of individuality, a conquest, something we achieved in an evolution of millions of years. The Self keeps this sense of individuality, but it transcends its limits and possesses the ability to perceive universality.

TRANSPERSONAL WILL

In addition to the will of the Personal Self, there is also the will of the Transpersonal Self to consider, a will that tends to attract the Personal Self upward, manifest through it, and guide the entire personality. One of the objectives of spiritual or transpersonal psychosynthesis is to make the will of the superconscious, or Higher Self, a conscious experience. Essentially, according to psychotherapist Piero Ferrucci, who trained with Roberto Assagioli, "the will is the ability of an organism to function freely in accordance with its intrinsic nature instead of following the influence of external forces."[2]

Assagioli was convinced that when will is lacking, and therefore the individual is not able to choose or is afraid of taking the responsibility for a certain choice, suffering, depression, and anxiety are inevitable. What can help us heal and grow is understanding that in some measure we are responsible for our lives.

Our will is expressed through our choices. When we realize that we are the ones who make choices for ourselves, we get rid of situations in which we feel we are the victims, and we become free because we know the ability to choose is ours again.

This is what happens when we realize that injustice occurs because we do nothing to prevent it. We get sick because we do not take care of our health. We are alone because we are afraid of contact with other people. Misfortune haunts us because we see only negativity. Prevarications take place because we always expect them, and so on.

When we are aware that our will to choose can give us freedom, our psychic and spiritual voltage increases and we start to discover our own identity, which can be an effective weapon to overcome several negative/destructive emotions, such as anxiety, fear, anger, depression, the sense of powerlessness, et cetera, and all the other emotions/scenarios that are connected to situations of separation, small deaths, loss, bereavement, or death.

TRANSFORMATION OF ENERGIES

The first illusion we need to discourage is the conviction of being an immutable monolithic entity (being) in order to realize that we are a mixture of conflicting and changing elements (becoming). Each one of us reveals a different personality depending on the relationship we have with others.

Our attitudes influence our perception of the world and our way of being. For each of them, we can develop a corresponding image of ourselves and a series of physical tensions, gestures, emotional states, behaviors, and opinions. This constellation of elements constitutes by itself a sort of micropersonality, more or less complete, that Assagioli's psychosynthesis defines as a subpersonality. Each subpersonality has a definition and a peculiar energy of its own.

The more we accept our subpersonalities, even those that seem the most unpleasant and neurotic, the more we feel whole. This is because we cannot erase any part of ourselves; we can only transform it. In order to do so, we must do the opposite of what we normally would do—we must accept it.

We should avoid judging our energies in any way, because it makes transformation impossible. This is the first essential step on the path of transformation; if we refuse it and fight any part of ourselves and its energy, we cannot move a single step ahead. Moreover, as usual, our reality reflects on the reality that surrounds us.

Humankind is like a single being with a single fate and a single evolution; on this planet floating in the immense space, we are a single entity. Our energy blends with the energy that surrounds us.

USE OF ENERGIES

In physics, especially in regard to the second law of thermodynamics, and in the field of information theory, entropy is a key concept. The tendency toward disorder that exists in nature on a molecular level is undeniable, and there is evidence to prove it. While specific scientific claims on entropy are irrefutable, philosophical deductions generally are extreme and unilateral. Over the past years, many studies have been carried out on the spontaneous tendency toward order and organization in nature. As Belgian scientist and Nobel Prize winner Ilya Prigogine stated, in any chaotic system there are "fluctuations" bringing that system toward greater order.

In similar fashion, whenever entropic energy triggers a destructive process in a patient, the Facilitator's job is to help the organism transform that entropic energy into syntropic energy.

Energies, tendencies, and latent potentials are plastic and mutable forces. Working with them on different levels often requires encouraging their transformation—the same sort of transformation that constantly occurs within us spontaneously. Just like heat becomes movement or electric energy, and movement becomes heat and electricity, our emotions and impulses transform into actions or imaginative and intellectual work (sensations become images, ideas become resolutions or actions).

From this perspective, we can see that any kind of energy—even the energy we consider extremely negative/destructive (e.g., anger and aggression)—is a natural energy and, as such, is neutral, just like the energy of the wind, sun, atoms, rivers, et cetera, which can cause catastrophes as well as prove to be incredibly useful.

Therefore, when treating patients and initiating a transformative process, Facilitators ask the destructive (entropic) energy to transform into constructive (syntropic) energy, supporting a natural phenomenon and changing its objective without changing its intensity.

Energy can become destructive when it is not regulated or conveyed correctly, but in its most advanced form it has a regenerative power. If we direct it creatively, it provides the correct impulse to act positively/constructively.

DIRECTION OF ENERGY THROUGH ATTENTION

Assagioli always stressed the importance of avoiding one particular common mistake: "Many people believe that we must follow our emotions, whereas it is our emotions that must follow us."[3]

It certainly is not possible to come up with an emotion or a brilliant idea exactly when we would like to. Even though our will cannot act directly on emotions or intuition, we should choose and chase the emotions that promote life, such as joy and interest, because they moderate and transform the emotions connected with crises.

Our will can help us seek and pursue constructive emotions. In fact, it is a fundamental function of our psyche that is able to move our attention as it likes, preventing it from being at the mercy of chance and our own obsessions.

Attention gives energy. Giving attention means feeding and nurturing. Our will can make this choice; we choose what we give attention to. Taking attention away from something means letting it die. More specifically, the absence of attention weakens emotions.

By following this simple principle, we can discover our ability to recreate our entire internal world and, little by little, learn to use our will to accentuate positive/constructive values, attitudes, and behaviors and allow them to be more influential than negative/destructive emotions.

It is dangerous to follow our emotions as if they were oracles, but we cannot deny them, for this would mean repressing valuable parts of ourselves. On the contrary, we must be aware of them, not let them overwhelm us, and learn how to manage them with our will.

It is through the center, the Higher Self, that we can truly see an emotion as it really is, understand the truthfulness of an emotion or feeling, and decide how to respond to it accordingly. Therefore, Piero Ferrucci reminds us, "we need the attentive 'listening' of feelings, even the feeblest ones, a clear vision, and an active attitude!"[4]

This means choosing which feelings deserve our attention and which feelings we must ignore (i.e., not feed). When negative emotions, such as depression, resentment, envy, fear, or anxiety, emerge, we can choose from among our options:

- We can give them full attention, understand them, and express them.
- We can ignore them.
- We can do both things alternately, which is often the wisest choice.

IDENTIFICATION WITH THE HIGHER SELF

Up until now we have seen that we should not always deal with depression, anxiety, and other negative/destructive emotions by merely acting as if they were not there. If we act as if a particular negative emotion does not exist without acknowledging its presence and understanding its nature, we only repress it; we do not weaken its force. As it turns out, understanding the nature of our emotions is key, since we can afford to ignore only what we have already understood.

Therefore, it is clear how essential the acknowledgment of the Higher Self is on a theoretical, practical, spiritual, therapeutic, and educative level, and how crucial the methods to become aware of its nature consequently are.

It is hard to understand what we are—our real nature. As we will see, situations of separation and loss are often very effective incentives in the search for this understanding. In fact, they take us at first to scenarios in which we feel unhappy and dissatisfied with our lives, but this is exactly the reason why they then encourage us to change and transform.

In order for us to change, improve, and grow, it is necessary first and foremost to know what we are—to acquire awareness about ourselves in the present moment and express it. If we identify with our personality or our Ego, which are both unresolved remnants of childhood, we are not able to know our limits, to be completely aware of our own individuality as opposed to that of others, and at the same time to feel part of a whole.

It is those who succeed in identifying with the Higher Self (Transpersonal Self) that identify with their very essence and observe every part of themselves, without ever coinciding with any of them completely, whether they are physical parts, emotions, desires, or thoughts. If the observation is made through the perspective of the Higher Self, even form loses its limiting aspect because each form includes all forms. We can see the whole universe even in a grain of sand.

The Higher Self is the space of healing. During CST and SER treatments, Facilitators may encounter a mysterious internal barrier that allows them to immediately acknowledge something they have just perceived or never even guessed was there.

In that moment, they can receive an extraordinary flow of intense intuitions, images, feelings, and physical sensations. It means that they are in contact with the most elevated part of their being, the Higher Self, which blends with the patient's Higher Self and with the whole universe (melding, as Dr. Upledger called this phenomenon).

Sharing is a spontaneous impulse of the Higher Self. If all barriers fade between two individuals—the Facilitator and the patient, in our case—and both of them perceive themselves as part of an organic and harmonious whole, they perceive a sense of liberation because control in the Higher Self is replaced by the need for releasing oneself to the gifts of life. In other words, the Higher Self manages and uses personal will in a constructive (transpersonal) way, setting it free from subjugation to desires and dominant impulses.

In the Higher Self, the energy of will, the energy of love, and the energy of the mind meld. Therefore, we could define the actions taken in accordance with the Higher Self as the consequences of a caring will in action.

CREATIVE THINKING: IMAGINATION

The human mind is a creative tool that can connect us with our highest potentials. Thinking is a type of energy we can use to develop constructive qualities, attitudes, and conditions that we think should prevail. By using our reasoning consciously and creatively, we can change ourselves, our lives, and the external environment.

No image is neutral. Every image has a motor power—that is, the tendency that stimulates the organism to transform that image into reality.

Without imagination, we could not make choices because we would be incapable of picturing the consequences of our choices; we would be prisoners of reality and incapable of understanding what is possible and even what is not or does not seem to be, which is what enables us to have great intuitions.

Allowing images to emerge yields precious information, since every image is a living reality that pulses, transforms, has its own intelligence, and is able to interact with us. We can dialogue with images, ask them questions, and listen to their answers.

Evoking images, sounds, tactile sensations, gestures, smells, and flavors helps us train and use creative imagination, which is simply the connection with a part of ourselves that is much wiser than our ordinary conscious levels. It is the superconscious (Higher Self) that generates our intuitions, creative inspirations, epiphanies, ethical impulses, ecstasy, and unconditional love and is the freest, wisest, sanest, and most creative part of ourselves.

Imagination also has an actual influence on the organism. Several parts of our brain are activated in the same way, whether we do something or we just imagine doing it. In some research experiments, people connected to electroencephalograms were asked first to move one finger and then only to imagine doing it; in both cases the EEG showed exactly the same cerebral activity.

We can therefore assume that it is possible to train our imagination to prepare for a certain activity.

We all can find a guiding image inside ourselves or create an ideal model to use in the work on ourselves. This is how a Facilitator can treat patients when the external conditions pose an objective obstacle to the treatment (e.g., when a patient is intubated, tracheotomized, intravenously fed, forced to bed, in a difficult position, etc.).

How can we learn to let creative imagination express itself?

Through the connection between our two hemispheres, we can bring to our own awareness anything emerging from the non-conscious and connect the rational/analytical/critical part with the imaginative/artistic/intuitive one. By doing so, we allow ourselves to listen to ourselves as we tell ourselves a story made of the intuitions our non-conscious allows to emerge.

Similarly, Facilitators need to listen to what their patient's non-conscious brings to their attention. In fact, Facilitators are trained to dialogue with the organs and systems of the human body following Dr. Upledger's recommendations, which means without judgment and by letting themselves be free to listen and use their intention in what other people may deem to be just the fruits of fantasy.

In practice, the Facilitator asks the non-conscious to *feel free to tell me a fairy tale and fill it with many different characters, sounds, smells, and tastes. And don't worry, I will pay attention and stay here in awe as I listen, understand, and accomplish for your sake.*

COOPERATING WITH THE INEVITABLE

People who use phrases without wisdom sometimes talk of suffering as a mystery. It is really a revelation.

OSCAR WILDE, *DE PROFUNDIS*

Psychosynthesis is meant to cooperate with the inevitable, considering especially negative situations as if they were some sort of school, some sort of boot camp useful for understanding, learning, and developing new skills.

We will see later that the creative transformation of negative/destructive emotions and feelings, such as anger, pain, depression, sense of failure, et cetera, is the cornerstone of CST and SER work, especially when the focus is on loss (all kinds of losses, from the smallest to the ultimate loss, the loss of losses, the last passage of the Life Cycle).

It is quite likely that we all know in some way or another that suffering is an inevitable part of human life and that it is possible to experience it as a step ahead in our growth, instead of as an awful prison. If suffering cannot be removed, it at least can be dealt with cleverly. Even though it often is ignored, one of the most crucial human abilities is the ability to change perspectives when observing a situation.

Will can influence but rarely change the reality of the external world. However, we have the ability to search for an internal change—that is, to effect cognitive reframing. Anyone can potentially transform suffering into a lesson, evoking resources that were previously repressed and therefore could not be used. When pain cannot be avoided, we must learn how to suffer in a smarter way.

Unfortunately, what often happens is the opposite. In the face of suffering, the human organism employs a wide range of reactions that tend to freeze in an Energy Cyst and constantly reoccur. That is exactly why a Facilitator's intervention is so important. By itself or in combination with other therapeutic methods, it can help the organism use its own resources even through suffering and disease and support the individual's resilience—meant in particular as the ability to overcome trauma—in retrieving homeostasis, thereby guiding the individual on their path to well-being.

Psychosynthesis takes pain, suffering, and failure and transforms them into creative situations that can help individuals understand themselves better and discover new resources. CST and SER also make use of the resources that are available to every person to transform the negative/destructive energy connected to painful and stressful traumas caused by separation and loss and process the consequent grief, releasing all its residues from the organism.

By doing so, we can accelerate the process of change and the restoration of the vital energy continuum, fostering an optimal passage from one phase of the patient's Life Cycle to the next.

Clinical Observations

I had recently come back to Italy and was trying to implement Dr. Upledger's courses, proposing some international seminars that had not been organized in Italy previously. I decided to suggest the Intensive Program, which I had already attended both as a student and as Dr. Upledger's assistant at the Upledger Institute Clinic in Florida.

When I received Dr. Upledger's approval to adapt the program to meet the requirements of the Italian Ministry of Health's continuing medical education guidelines for therapists, I carefully created the protocol of the intensive treatment for Italian students and patients. The Intensive Program takes place over the course of five days, during which time doctors, therapists, and health care professionals with solid experience in CST and SER give their contribution. The peculiarity of this course is that it is one of the few in which patients play a crucial group role.

Five patients are treated in the same room at the same time. Each patient has three Facilitators working on them, using CST and SER, for a total of five hours a day. There are three breaks each day and short intervals for coming together to discuss the experience. The dialogue is supervised by the conductor and a doctor, who has the chance to assess the medical history of all patients at the beginning of the course and is supposed to make an evaluation at the end.

When I organized this particular event, I invited some of the best therapists and professionals in Italy, as well as some fellow Instructors from the United States to take part in the first edition.

I was introduced to one of the five patients by a therapist who was also one of my students. She proposed him for the program because she had never worked on a similar case in her entire experience as a Facilitator, which was not short.

This is the story of that patient, as told by my student and then confirmed by the patient himself during the intensive treatment:

The patient was a young graduate in economics and corporate law. His field of study had been decided by his family, which owned a big Italian company. He had gone to Florida to get a master's degree. One day as he was sitting in a rented convertible and waiting for the green light at an intersection, he was brutally robbed by a group of criminals. They shot him repeatedly and escaped, leaving him severely wounded in the vehicle.

One of the bullets pierced his abdomen and got stuck in his sacrum. When an ambulance finally came to bring him to the hospital, he was already in a coma. He miraculously woke up after six months and came back to Italy, but at that point he was paralyzed from the waist down.

His life fell apart. Life before trauma and paralysis was just a memory full of potential and unattainable projects. Now he was bitter, angry, resentful, and frustrated, and he alternated these feelings and emotions with periods of intense depression.

His parents kept supporting him and never stopped devoting all their efforts to get him the best care available, even though they knew he would never walk again. He was aware of his parents' efforts and agreed to take part in the intensive treatment only because he did not want to offend them—exactly as he had done before with all the other therapies they had provided him with. He was not expecting any beneficial effect from the treatment. Moreover, he did not trust the integrity of anyone who had treated him before or was now going to treat him, since he believed they were all people who only wanted to take advantage of his parents' money.

What is more, he did not have any desire to go on living a life he was not recognizing as his own anymore, and this is exactly what he said when he introduced himself to the other patients of the intensive treatment at the beginning of the first day.

I will not list all the techniques we employed during the treatments of those five days, but what I want to note is that on the last day he was sad because the experience was about to end.

I and some other Facilitators who had participated in the program continued to treat him for a long time afterward, at his request.

Life as he had known it before the incident would never return, but after some years he was able to use his potential and find some value in his disability and his academic studies, founding a company that produces equipment for disabled people. Not only that, he designed a catamaran equipped for the disabled and had it constructed. He even crossed the ocean on it, reached America, went back to the place where he had been assaulted, and had the personal gratification of being treated by Dr. Upledger himself.

This was the story of a patient who did not want to live anymore but was helped through CST and SER to take his chance at cooperating with the inevitable in the spirit of psychosynthesis.

❧ A CST-CENTERED VISION ❧

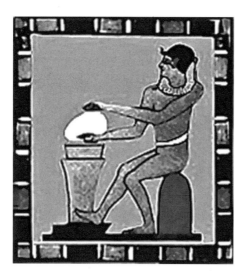

Fig. 12.2. The cosmic egg shaped by the god Ptah

From the cosmic egg to the philosopher's stone to Bosch . . . and beyond.

Over the centuries, the egg has stood as a symbol and archetype of birth, life, and transformation for civilizations, cultures, and philosophies all over the world. We have evidence dating back to 2000 BCE to prove that. Its sacred cosmogony can be found in the ancient peoples of Mesopotamia, India, Egypt, Greece, Africa, and China and in Celtic culture.

In the art of ancient Egypt, we find the representations of the "Egg of Life" shaped by the god Ptah (fig. 12.2) and in the myth of the birth of the god Ra, deity of the sun born from a cosmic egg.[5]

In sacred interpretations, the egg is also considered one and triune; one in the form, three in the physical substance (shell, yolk, albumen) and holy essence (birth, death, resurrection). It represents life as a mystery in the symbolism of birth and life after death, just like the phoenix, the mythological bird that arises from its own ashes.

In Piero della Francesca's painting *Brera Madonna,* sometimes called *The Holy Conversation* (fig. 12.3), the egg suspended over the Virgin Mary alludes to her maternity.

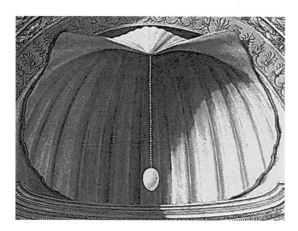 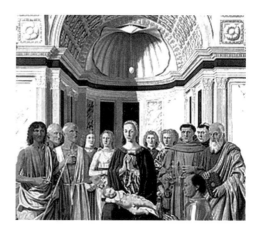

Fig. 12.3. Details of *Brera Madonna,* by Piero della Francesca

In *La via dell'alchimia cristiana,* Severin Batfroi wrote: "As a symbol of the primordial origin of the world, the egg was considered an archetype able to bring all elements back to their original purity. For this reason, the 'Philosopher's Stone' . . . for its ability to transmute poor metals into gold was compared to an egg."[6]

The egg became the object/subject of many surrealist works by Salvador Dalí, René Magritte, and Man Ray. It shows secrets, reveals the pure form, represents the primordial womb, and tells the story of the becoming.

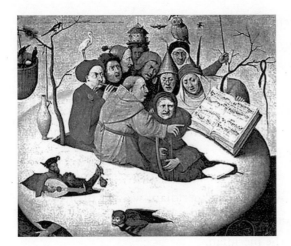

Fig. 12.4. *Concert in the Egg,* by Hieronymus Bosch (or a follower)

Hieronymus Bosch chose to represent the egg for its allegoric and symbolic value. In his painting *Concert in the Egg* (fig. 12.4 sometimes attributed not to Bosch but to one of his followers), the choir emerges from the philosopher's egg used by the alchemists for transmutations.

The symbol of the egg in the history of art, representing the entire Life Cycle and transformation, does not stop here. It seems incredible! Did Assagioli know when he chose this symbol for his psychosynthesis? We believe he did.

CHAPTER 13

Seats of Emotions
The Viscera and Meridians

As you get up in the morning, smile to your heart, stomach, lungs, and liver. After all, there is a lot going on thanks to them.
                    THICH NHAT HANH, *ANGER: WISDOM FOR COOLING THE FRAMES*

Our viscera are the seats of emotional energy. According to Dr. Upledger, in CST and even more so in SER, we can use six major meridians to balance the energy that is typical of the various organs.

Each organ is the seat of a specific energy connected to a specific emotion, and each organ is crossed by a meridian. By treating a meridian, we can dissipate any destructive energy accumulated in the organ it is connected with or any Energy Cyst blocking or altering the energy flow of the meridian.

Bear in mind that emotions are a normal physiological response to the stimuli of the external environment. There are no negative emotions; each of them has its own function and exists to ensure and support life. It is emotions that are excessive or excessively restrained, along with the obsessive feelings connected with them, that can become destructive for the organs that contain them and for the entire physiological system.

Here are some examples:

- Reflection is necessary to give form to thoughts, but excessive reflection can cause excessive worry and foster dysfunction in the spleen.
- Sadness sometimes encourages an internalization and perceptive sensitivity, but excessive sadness or an unwillingness to release it (through crying or laughing, for example) causes dysfunction in the respiratory tract and lungs.
- Fear prompts us to act carefully and save energy, but when it is disproportionate and unreasonable, it provokes a loss of fluid and energy that are essential for the kidneys and the entire organism.
- Anger sometimes can be a release valve to preserve the integrity of the liver, but excessive anger damages it.

In this chapter, we are going to discuss the major meridians that correspond to the organs and the main emotions, as Dr. Upledger considered them, with a particular attention to the emotions and feelings that are connected with situations of separation, loss, and bereavement.

We will also examine the emotional level of death (that is, the fear of death) and small deaths (that is, objective and subjective loss), and we will observe how CST and SER offer us the chance to express our constructive energetic/emotional potential to oppose the destructive emotional/energetic charge.

ENERGY CYSTS AND MERIDIANS

As we have seen, Energy Cysts are spots where the energy flow is blocked; they also can be generated in the organism in response to the emotions arising after a trauma. Energy Cysts inhibit the flow of vital energy, substantially modifying the craniosacral rhythm and its ideal symmetry, quality, amplitude, and rate, thus affecting the entire craniosacral system.

Palpation of the meridians is yet another method of assessment that can help locate an Energy Cyst, in this case one that blocks the flow of energy in the meridian it is located in. However, as Dr. Upledger observed, an Energy Cyst can obstruct the energy flow anywhere on an acupuncture meridian, and pain might then occur either in the connected organ or in any other part of the meridian. Therefore, we cannot count on the location of pain to find the Energy Cyst.

A change or blockage of the energy flow in a specific point of a meridian might be the residue of a problem that is no longer active or the effect of a lesion that is still active—that is, an Energy Cyst.

When they are dysfunctional, meridians can be either empty (obstructed, blocked, deprived of energy) or overloaded (containing an excessive amount of energy). When

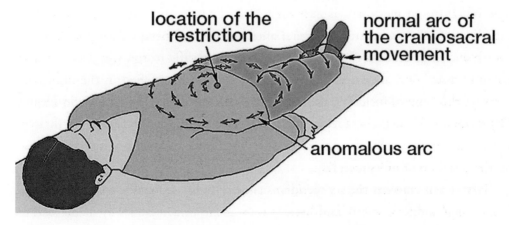

Fig. 13.1. Arc of movement of Energy Cysts and craniosacral movement

Facilitators perceive an empty or extremely full meridian, they can trace it with their hands to detect the presence of an Energy Cyst altering its usual flow. If an Energy Cyst is located along the meridian, Facilitators can feel its peculiar vibrations as they get closer to it, like we have seen with the Arcing technique. It also is possible to perceive various qualitative alterations in the organism, such as warmth or other sensations connected with the increase of energy.

With their destructive energy, Energy Cysts indicate that negative emotions are trapped in the organs. They can affect the entire physical and emotional balance of the individual, sometimes even altering the person's entire personality. For example, the anger trapped in an Energy Cyst might give an angry connotation to the manifestations of the individual's character.

In order to dissipate an Energy Cyst, the Facilitator does not follow the acupuncture method of traditional Chinese medicine or the acupressure of shiatsu but considers only six meridians:

Pericardium–Heart–Lungs–Kidneys–Spleen–Liver

During the treatment, these six meridians are considered merely as access and exit channels, used respectively for the inlet and the release of syntropic energy.

Once the meridian where the Energy Cyst is located has been found, the Facilitator must use intention to dissipate the destructive energy that is trapped and fed by the Energy Cyst and impregnates the energy of the meridian. Once the Energy Cyst disappears, its energy is released and constructive energy enters, though never surpassing the energetic potential that the organism is able to accept.

Thanks to the meridians, which reach various organs as energy channels, we have another reference in CST and SER to assess the organs involved in the individual's dysfunctions and discomfort.

THE SIX MERIDIANS OF CST

The literature on meridians is extremely vast. That is only fair, considering that meridians are the foundation of several ancient forms of therapy dating back to the fourth and third centuries BCE. Clearly there is a specific reason why Dr. Upledger chose to assess only six meridians among all of those mentioned in the numerous texts on this subject, including the twenty that are recognized by the World Health Organization. There is also a reason why Dr. Upledger himself instructed Facilitators to treat the meridians by placing one hand on the organ involved, and the other hand on the distal point of its meridian.

First, let us consider the six meridians chosen by Dr. Upledger: the pericardium, heart, lungs, kidneys, spleen, and liver. If we want to understand why he decided to choose these six, we must take into account the electromagnetic parameters ascribed to two subjects we have already mentioned: quantum electrodynamics and traditional Chinese medicine.

> In the world of quantum physics, the "field" consists of quantities that do not always have well-defined values. . . . We cannot count the quanta, but the particles have perfectly synchronized oscillations in phase and give us matter. . . . These two conditions of the same reality (energetic and material) exchange information by means of electromagnetic emissions. The exchange takes place in all possible directions, between homogeneous elements, whether they are cell clusters or organs, thus able to receive and decode the signal transmitted. . . . However, we are dealing with an open system kept stable by multiple regulation processes that generate a continuous stream of EM signals related to all cellular activities, from the flow of nutrients to the antioxidant-oxidant balance, from the production of ATP to pH regulation, etc.[1]

When sending syntropic energy into the organism through the energy channels and simultaneously releasing the entropic energy they detain, a Facilitator is taking advantage of the electromagnetic (EM) signal transport channels—that is, the meridians. The Facilitator essentially serves as an external agent whose electromagnetic emissions result in the general adjustment of the organism's homeostatic values. As it turns out, cell resonance with variations in the electromagnetic spectrum in the six meridians chosen by Dr. Upledger is extremely specific, especially on a cerebral or spinal level, and involves the entire craniosacral system.

Traditional Chinese medicine (TCM) recognizes seven emotional states, each of them with a specific location in specific vital organs. The number seven in TCM correlates to the six spatial directions plus the center (qi) in which human beings are oriented through the choices their emotions lead them to.

When considering the seven emotions, we see that in some cases the same organ is involved in more than one emotion:

1. Anger affects the liver.
2. Joy affects the heart.
3. Pensiveness affects the spleen.
4. Worry affects the spleen and the lungs.
5. Sadness affects the lungs.
6. Fear affects the kidneys.
7. Shock affects the kidneys and the heart.

In sum, as you can see, the seven emotions involve only five organs.

Ultimately, Dr. Upledger's chose to work with the meridians that are associated with the main organs, not all the viscera. By doing so, he found himself addressing once again the concept of polarity, in this case the balance between the two poles of TCM, yin and yang. Within this balance, he acknowledged the key role of a membranous organ that is not included in the seven emotions: the pericardium, which serves as the energetic center of will.

> For traditional Chinese medicine, in the human body the vital organs with yang active elements are the liver (wood), the heart (fire), the spleen and pancreas (earth), the lungs (metal), and the kidneys (water).
>
> The functions of these organs are carried out by the yin passive elements that correspond to the gallbladder, the small intestine, the stomach, the large intestine, and the urinary bladder.
>
> In addition to these five yin-yang pairs that determine the psychic and spiritual state, there is another pair that is mainly responsible for the spiritual dimension of human beings, the pericardium (energetic center of will) and the triple burner.[2]

The six yin-yang couples form six main elements affecting the entire balance of the vital energy (qi).

This structure substantiates the choice made by Dr. Upledger, which consists of proposing a CST treatment that employs the most distal point of each meridian and the respective organ crossed by the meridian.

We now return once again to quantum electrodynamics, in particular through a reference to the studies of Giuliano Preparata and Emilio Del Giudice.

> The millenary experience of the Chinese in the study of singular points of the human body and the related network of interconnections (meridians) solves the problem [of how to transport EM signals that bring neurons into coherence]. . . . It identified the meridians, the energy channels that mostly extend longitudinally in the body, carrying the field emitted by the external standard to the part of the organ involved. Meridians allow us to approach the considered source from closer to the terminal point of the path of magnetic transport, which is normally a finger or a toe, rather than directly on the area involved, thus making the test much more practical and faster. . . . It is now known that in the human body there are great numbers of singular points of the skin—400 according to the World Health Organization (WHO)—which are the spots of superficial emergence of the 20 major meridians. . . . These points are characterized by a low resistivity compared to the rest of the dermis . . . because of a high density of gap junctions, hexagonal complexes of proteins that form channels between adjacent cells. . . . The value of the short circuit current available at any examined point varies proportionally with

the level of the homeostatic regulation in the organ or the part of the organ that is located along the meridian. The interaction with the external standard provokes a variation in the current, which can therefore be used as a variable parameter measurable with proper techniques.

The correlation of the abovementioned singular points with well-defined areas of the body was . . . validated . . . with imaging techniques . . . or through the injection of radioisotopes in anomalous points to follow their path. . . . This interconnecting network of points is constituted of an independent system connected with the cerebral cortex through the nervous system. . . . A new organizational model for the correlation between these points has been recently set forth . . . proposing a direct connection between single points and the cerebral cortex, followed by a return to the organ that is controlled by primary and secondary messengers—hormones, neuropeptides, cytokines, and more. . . . This and similar works . . . make use of fMRI (functional magnetic resonance imaging) to correlate the measuring point with the corresponding cerebral area.[3]

MOLECULES OF EMOTION

We have already mentioned Candace Pert, and we will return to her again later. She was a neuroscientist with a degree in biology and a doctorate in pharmacology from Johns Hopkins University School of Medicine. She conducted research at the National Institute of Mental Health (NIMH), wrote more than 200 scientific publications, and worked in collaboration with neuroscientist Solomon H. Snyder and with Dr. Upledger.

In an interview, she said that her 1997 book *Molecules of Emotion* offers "a systematization of our research in the field of neuroscience." She explained:

As I went more and more in depth in the research on emotions, I understood how powerful they are for the individuals, even for their healing. At first, my guess was that emotions are situated in the head or brain, but I later concluded that they also express in the body and are a part of it. They are energy and information, but we can map them as molecules in the body.

My most recent studies focused on the general concept of well-being and what is actually needed for an individual to feel good. They showed that emotions are part of the informational energy of the organism, but they also transcend the single individual's health and spread in the surrounding environment. In other words, emotions seem to "jump" from one person to another, from one body to another, from one culture to another. They are planetary, and this nature of transition from microcosm to macrocosm is an extremely interesting aspect. In my opinion, to know emotions, to control them, to let them flow is the key to start the "global shift" that is necessary today for our future. . . .

The healing process always implies a process of spiritual transformation, and it is extremely complex, so it cannot be considered exclusively as the mere removal of tumors, bacteria, and pathogens. When we are searching for the cause of a disease, we need also to look elsewhere. At the origin of the pathologic process there is an essential flaw, an obstacle in the communication network, so the healing must involve the entire body-brain system in order to be effective. I believe we need to establish a new paradigm of healing in which emotions play a key role, Eastern and the Western perspective on the body are connected, and we make use of guided meditation, psychology, and other techniques—music, work on the body, massage—that accept the role of emotions in human health.[4]

ORGANS AS SEATS OF EMOTIONS AND CONNECTED FEELINGS

Nowadays, many scientists find strong correlations between the recent discoveries of neuroscience and the influence of emotions on the organism, as described by Eastern medicine and philosophy, especially traditional Chinese medicine, Ayurveda, traditional Tibetan medicine, and yoga. With this in mind, Dr. Upledger proposed a connection between organs and emotions.

Pericardium

This organ covers and protects the heart, providing it with a defense mechanism. However, if its defensive action is excessive, it prevents any work or interaction with the heart.

Destructive Emotionality	Constructive Emotionality
Excessive protection	Protection
Sense of persecution	Security
Oppression	Preservation
Hostility	Defense

Pericardium and Heart

The pericardium is the fascia that covers and protects the heart. If the pericardium is dysfunctional, it becomes atrophic and inhibits the rhythmic movement of the heart. The heart is vulnerable to the emotions of shock caused by sudden and unexpected events and suffers when dealing with turbulent emotions or emotions connected with fear. Chronic dysfunctions of the heart also can involve the kidneys, which are connected with fear as well.

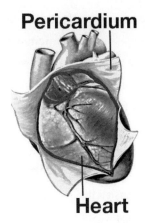

Fig. 13.2. Pericardium and heart (cross-sectional view)

Heart

The heart is the seat, filter, and supply of the fear of getting hurt in affective relationships. It may compromise our ability to love, or even the possibility of love, because of the fear of losing love itself.

Destructive Emotionality	Constructive Emotionality
Excessive euphoria	Joy
Withheld emotions arising from shock	Love
Fright	Contentment
Inability to express emotions	Enjoyment

Lungs

These paired organs are the seats of unresolved pain and deep or durable sadness as well as anxiety, preoccupation, melancholy, and grief. They filter, seat, and supply spiritual pain as well. The lungs work in close contact with the heart. Any unresolved pain, deep sadness, or sense of negation of one's physical and vital space due to the interruption of the vital energy continuum may cause respiratory problems, dysfunctions, and diseases.

Emotions following bereavement, such as sadness and pain, reduce the will to live and pose a significant threat to the lungs.

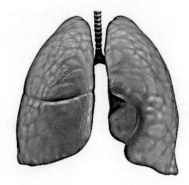

Fig. 13.3. Lungs (cross-sectional view)

The anxiety connected with excessive preoccupation affects the lungs as well as the large intestine (see the meridians of traditional Chinese medicine) and the spleen. Anxiety prevents a person from using their energy well and can provoke shortness of breath, asthma, colitis, ulcers, and inflammation of the large intestine. Anxious preoccupation also is associated with the stomach and, sometimes, with gastrointestinal problems.

Destructive Emotionality	Constructive Emotionality
Emotional pain	Sensitivity
Sadness	Responsiveness
Sorrow	Openness
Anguish	Lucidity

Kidneys

These paired organs are the seats of the fear of death or the interruption of the life continuum. They filter, seat, and supply fears connected with the negation or end of biological existence and/or chromosomal immortality (the inability to reproduce and preserve the species). In TCM, the kidneys, along with the brain and heart, are known as the "imperial organs." They maintain the correct water:salt balance in the organism (75 percent of our body is water) and take care of the depuration of blood.

Fear and shock are the most dangerous emotions for the kidneys and can undermine their functionality in retention and evacuation, sometimes even causing them to lose control of their functions. The emotions of shock can undermine a person's emotional strength and confidence.

Destructive Emotionality	Constructive Emotionality
Fear	Willpower
Indecisiveness	Confidence
Panic and fright	Readiness

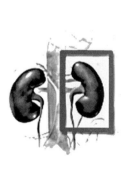
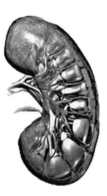

Fig. 13.4. Kidneys (cross-sectional view)

Spleen

This organ is the seat of disillusionment and disappointment (about oneself and about humankind in general), melancholy, overthinking, and excessive preoccupation (leading to anxiety), which can affect the spleen itself as well as cause fatigue, lethargy, and difficulties in concentrating. Melancholy in particular can also affect the digestive tract and stomach, causing the buildup of gas and swelling. This organ filters and holds the disappointment arising from issues such as human cruelty against peers or those who are in a position of difficulty, weakness, inferiority, or discomfort.

Destructive Emotionality	Constructive Emotionality
Melancholy	Thoughtfulness
Excessive preoccupation	Concentration
Excessive mental/intellectual effort	Reflection
Anxiety	Gratification
Closure/isolation	Open-mindedness

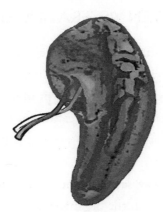

Fig. 13.5. Spleen

Liver

This organ collects and holds anger and depression. It can absorb and detain strong depressive shocks caused by the powerlessness felt due to events involving loss (such as the objective loss represented by an unexpected death), which subsequently can develop into rage and/or desperation, sometimes even causing depression.

The liver produces the bile that gathers in the gallbladder. The issues occurring over time in reaction to anger may be expressed through digestive disturbances, abdominal cramping and swelling, nausea, lack of appetite, ulcers, and gastritis..

The throat and the intestines are also part of the digestive tract. The throat is involved in swallowing and in verbal expression, and explosions of anger can affect it as much as suppressed words. Rage and anger also can cause strong migraines, neck and shoulder tensions, high blood pressure, and dizziness.

Destructive Emotionality	Constructive Emotionality
Anger	Courage
Resentment/grudge	Serenity
Irritability	Inner calm
Rage	Proactive attitude
Self-doubt	Decisiveness
Frustration	Moderation
Depression	Trust

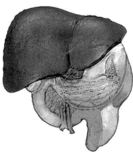

Fig. 13.6. Liver

COMMUNICATION BETWEEN VISCERA AND EMOTIONS

Let us try to understand how the communication between organs and emotions occurs in the organism. As Candace Pert once explained, neuropeptides are chemical substances—small chains of amino acids—that are produced by neurons, and they seem to function as a form of internal communication for the body. Like other compounds in the body, such as neurotransmitters, specific neuropeptides "dock" only at specific specialized receptor sites, much like a lock (the receptor) and key (the neuropeptide) mechanism. In this way, said Pert, neuropeptides "hold the key to understanding the chemistry of emotions in the organism. . . ."

She continued:

> I believe that neuropeptides and their receptors are a key to understanding how mind and body are interconnected and how emotions can be manifested throughout the body. Indeed, the more we know about neuropeptides, the harder it is to think in the traditional terms of a mind and a body. It makes more and more sense to speak of a single integrated entity, a "body mind."[5]

For those who have a deeper knowledge of Dr. Upledger's therapeutic work, the affinity connecting these neuroscientific studies to the contents of his books *A Brain Is Born* and *Cell Talk* should be clear. In fact, these texts describe a method of treatment with the dialogue of SomatoEmotional Release to listen to and communicate with the cells of the various organs and the brain for an individual who has experienced emotional trauma. Does not everything vibrate energetically in syntony with the universe? And is not human voice—meant as the emission of biophonons—a vibration too?

AN ENERGETIC TECHNIQUE TO TREAT EMOTIONS HELD IN THE VISCERA

To treat the viscera and the emotions they hold, we must employ the technique of emptying the destructive energy from the meridian connected with the organ and filling it with constructive energy. To do this, we might act both through intention (nonverbally) and through Therapeutic Imagery and Dialogue, following the instructions of the patient's non-conscious.

In both cases, we are working to release destructive energy connected with a traumatic emotion that generated one or more Energy Cysts and compromised the optimal energy flow of the entire meridian. Let us see how.

Objectives

For a Facilitator, the technique of emptying and filling the meridians is another method of assessment and treatment. It requires that one become familiar with the meridians considered in CST, learning the path of each and their respective organs. The goal is to assess the flow in a meridian, with the following objectives:

- To establish whether it is functional
- To establish whether it is energetically empty or energetically overloaded
- To establish whether it is interrrupted (Energy Cyst), and if so, where that interruption is located along the path
- To release the emotional charge connected to destructive energy held in the associated viscera

Hand Placements for the Six Meridians

Pericardium Meridian

To treat the pericardium, place one hand on the organ and the other on the distal point of its meridian, which is the middle finger of the left hand (or the left inner wrist).

Then, with one hand still on the pericardium, move the other hand to the middle finger of the right hand (or the right inner wrist)

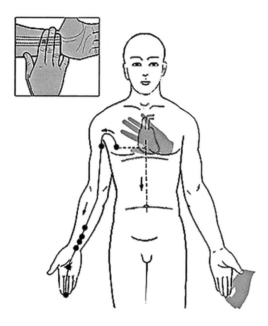

Fig. 13.7. Hand placement for the pericardium meridian

Heart Meridian

To treat the heart, place one hand on the organ and the other on the distal point of its meridian, which is the little finger of the left hand.

Then, with one hand still on the heart, move the other hand to the little finger of the right hand.

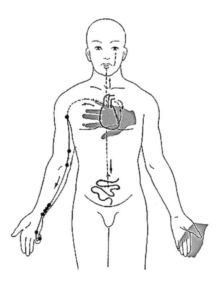

Fig. 13.8. Hand placement for the heart meridian

Lungs Meridian

To treat the lungs, place one hand alternately on each of the two lungs, and at the same time, place the other hand alternately on the respective distal points of the organ's meridian—the thumb of the right hand for the right lung and the thumb of the left hand for the left lung.

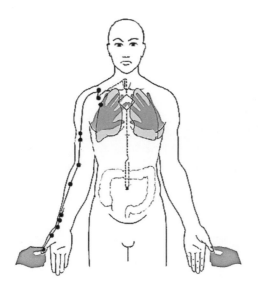

Fig. 13.9. Hand placement for the lungs meridian

Kidneys Meridian

To treat the kidneys, place one hand alternately on each of the two kidneys, and at the same time, place the other hand alternately on the respective distal points of the organ's meridian—the beginning of the metatarsi on the middle part of the right foot for the right kidney, and the same point on the middle part of the left foot for the left kidney.

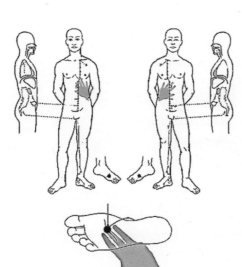

Fig. 13.10. Hand placement for the kidneys meridian

Spleen Meridian

To treat the spleen, place one hand on the organ and the other on the distal point of its meridian, the hallux of the left foot.

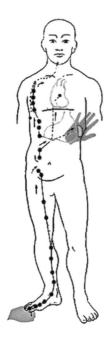

Fig. 13.11. Hand placement for the spleen meridian

Liver Meridian

To treat the liver, place one hand on the organ and the other on the distal point of its meridian, the hallux of the right foot.

Then, with one hand still on the liver, move the other to the hallux of the left foot.

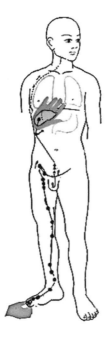

Fig. 13.12. Hand placement for the liver meridian

Meridian emptying and filling technique

- In order to dissipate energy cysts, Dr. Upledger indicated 6 major Meridians to take into account:

  - Pericardium *(see image)*
  - Lungs
  - Spleen
  - Heart
  - Kidneys
  - Liver

- During treatment, these 6 major Meridians will be considered merely as exit and entry channels.

- The flow of the Meridian will be evaluated for its:
  - functionality
  - quality
  - amount of energy
  - possible interruption (energy cyst)

  and the destructive emotionality will be released from the viscera associated with the Meridian.

- By creating a continuous flow from one hand to the other through the Meridian 'channel,' the release (emptying) of destructive energy will be achieved, while, at the same time, constructive energy will enter (filling).

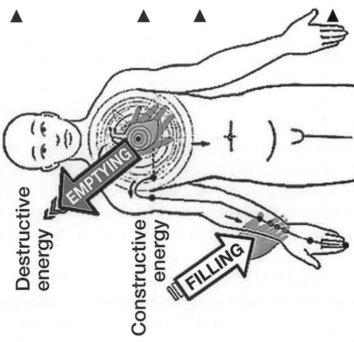

Fig. 13.13. Meridian emptying and filling technique

Meridian Emptying and Filling Technique

1. Use Arcing to locate the Energy Cyst.
2. Using intention to energetically empty and fill the meridian, release the destructive energy through intention and consequently dissipate the Energy Cyst; then replace it with a flow of constructive energy. For an unpaired organ (e.g., the pericardium), keep one hand on the organ and place the other alternately on all the distal points of the meridian. For a paired organ (e.g., the lungs), treat the organ and its distal points alternately, first on the right and then on the left.
3. Reassess the new situation in the organism with Arcing to make sure the Energy Cyst was successfully dissipated.

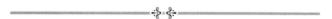

EXPERIENTIAL CONSIDERATIONS FOR AN INTEGRATED PERSPECTIVE

Among the privileges in my life was meeting the artist, writer, and geomant Marko Pogačnik while I was with another exceptional individual, my friend Ramona Sierra.

As is well known, charismatic people attract people with a similar energy. It seems as though they are destined to meet in order to exchange information, not on a conscious level but rather on the level of the collective unconscious. It was perhaps for this reason that I had the fortuitous occasion to witness the encounter between Marko and Ramona during a seminar on personal development titled "Earth Therapy."

Marko is internationally renowned for his use of geomancy, a discipline of art that has its roots in sixteenth-century Persia. He uses it as a tool to reveal the ancient wisdom of the Earth. He conducts seminars all over the world with the purpose of diffusing the healing process of Earth, and he collaborates with communities and companies in works of landscape restoration and redevelopment.

Marko developed the cosmograms (graphical archetypes carved in stone that energetically enrich his sculptures) and a method of Earth acupuncture that he calls lithopuncture. This technique consists of placing monoliths in the ground in correspondence with the landmarks of the energetic meridians of the Earth. He essentially listens to Earth, assesses it, and sees it as if it were a human organism. He then communicates with it through its energy and the images that it sends to him. He claims that the spirit of Earth lives in our society and is able to influence the reality we live in day by day. Earth, through its several manifestations and their respective names (Mother Earth, Triple Goddess, Black Virgin, Gaia, etc.), expresses its female nature through all the different civilizations, cultures, and religions—but this aspect is directly affected by the transformations of our planet that nowadays are becoming more and more intense.

Visions, dreams, and intuitions are only some of the means by which the Triple Goddess chooses to reveal herself to the artist. It's said that life always finds a way of saying what it needs to say. This expression means that the ways the Goddess chooses to manifest herself are different every time. They can be identified in natural manifestations as well as in their ability to influence all of creation, from the animal realm to the most intimate aspect of modern human sensitivity and consciousness.

Marko founded his philosophy of art on cosmogony, in particular referring to the vibration that is established between Earth and the human organism, which comes from Earth and returns to it. Through this echo of the birth of the universe, he seizes the messages that unveil interrelations with other living beings and the structural and emotional affinities that connect him with them. Through the cosmograms he carves into his artworks, he wants to transmit these messages, spreading positive qualities in the environment and creating an antagonist to the destructive inclinations of human beings.

Among his first literary works is *The Daughter of Gaia: Rebirth of the Divine Feminine,* in which the artist clarifies how the freedom of the heart connected with creative imagination and the perception and study of the Triple Goddess is able to create a bridge between worlds that would otherwise be destined never to meet: the world of human beings and that of the Divine Feminine. Another of his books is *Nature Spirits & Elemental Beings: Working with the Intelligence in Nature.*

Going back to the encounter between Marko and Ramona, I can say that it was a revelation to see two people so culturally different and yet so similar and empathic exchange information. In my role of interpreter for them and the other students attending the event, I felt like I was taking part in a world summit on the future of our planet.

At this point, I feel compelled to talk a little about Ramona Sierra to make you understand the caliber of this woman. She is a Native American, of Pueblo and Arapaho heritage, and her ancestors come from mountain villages north of New Mexico. She is a social worker and a CranioSacral Therapist and lives in Salt Lake City, Utah, where she directs Sierra Health Associates and Sierra EarthWorks, two organizations whose objective is to unite Western medical practice with the practices of holistic cultures. Her twenty years of experience in nonconventional medicine includes traditional indigenous healing practices.

Now you have a sense of the two protagonists in this encounter. The discussion touched upon the concept of earthworks, which draw from ethnic, psychological, and spiritual techniques to enhance the physical well-being of each living being. It also touched upon the concept of natural healing practices, with specific references to the techniques of releasing and dissipating energetic blockages (working with the chakras, the viscera, and the meridians), both in humans and in Earth. Other subjects were the use of drums as the sound of Mother Earth's heart and the energetic spots connecting East and West, including Trieste, my city.

My Own Journey

Since my first encounter with Dr. Upledger's CranioSacral Therapy, I have always had the impression that I was not just learning a technique for healing but setting out on an unusual and unexpected life journey. I first met Dr. Upledger in 1994, and he encouraged me to complete all the core courses for CST training in just one year and helped me in all the ways he could. Thanks to him, I also met figures of inestimable value who were fundamental for my personal growth, such as Ramona.

After first meeting her, and thanks to Dr. John (as I used to call him), I opened up more and more to a reality that may seem very different from the traditional path of development and training but actually draws a lot from it. My reality is made of many itineraries, each of them different from the others, each of them carrying a different and new message that was extremely useful for my training and my personal and professional growth. These are the messages I try to transmit to my students, my patients, and all the people with whom I share my life path.

I have had many amazing experiences of growth, like building a wheel of medicine with Ramona in Utah, going to the Blue Lagoon in Iceland, and, in 2004, traveling to Hawaii. Hawaii is still a virgin land with a very peculiar energy. The island chain, located along the nineteenth parallel, is surrounded by very deep waters—the ocean is 5,000 meters deep even at a close distance to the coasts. Here I swam with dolphins in the wild—a breathtaking experience!

Ramona and other shamans were with me, and together we connected with the spirit of the land of Hawaii. The lava that flows every day from the volcano to the ocean incessantly nourishes, expands, and transforms the islands. We walked on the youngest land of the planet.

My trip to Hawaii, like the other events, did not consist of tourist itineraries. They were experiences of profound growth that got me closer to the knowledge of the subtle energy of nature, which is present also in the individuals who are gifted with unconditional love and share it thanks to their wisdom.

Let us now jump ahead to 2009, when I experienced the most fundamental occurrences in my profession and concluded my cycle of studies. That year I took some Italian students to Florida, where they attended a course that I had the honor to conduct with Dr. Upledger at Upledger Institute International. Sharing with me his marvelous path as an Instructor was an incredible recognition. I will always keep the memory of that extraordinary gift.

Looking Back

Throughout my Life Cycle, I have been extremely lucky. I do not mean that I have been spared from the sufferings of life; I would not be human if that were the case. I am telling you this to encourage you to accept a concept I firmly believe in.

Even when I was going through periods of pain, loss, or grief, I always knew that there were people like Dr. Upledger, or Marko, or Ramona, working in their own way to bring a better energy to the entire planet and to all of us. I believe that by thinking about the joy some of my experiences gave me, I was able to dissipate several moments of inevitable sadness and discomfort in my life.

All of us can modify, transform, and improve with our will, as Assagioli taught us, the energetic level of our own life path, or at least part of it, by connecting with the positive energy of the emotions we have experienced, which fortunately are just as inevitable as the negative ones in life. This is how we can "make the world a touch better."

One More Point

In May 2000, a conference on destructive emotions and their social and individual potential took place in Dharamsala, India. Western and Eastern professors of psychiatry, psychology, developmental psychology, philosophy, philosophy of social science, neurobiology, biology, and epistemology took part in the meeting. Afterward, psychologist and science journalist Daniel Goleman wrote an essay about it in collaboration with Tenzin Gyatso, the fourteenth Dalai Lama.

From discussions that took place during the event, as reported by Goleman, emerged a consensus that destructive emotions can generate the following:

- conditions in which the chain of perception, cognitive process, and cognitive response is altered, producing dangerous effects on individuals and relationships;
- cognitive processes that are inadequate for processing perceptions and following logical steps, and that cause a scarce or incoherent assessment of the information;
- altered psychophysical states that are inadequate for recovering the necessary information from memory and for contextualizing triggering events;
- difficulties with social and individual behavior and in interactions with the others;
- anomalous patterns of neural activation and distinct psychophysical effects.[6]

In the West, the effects of destructive emotions often are defined as the "dysfunctional attributional style," whereas they are "mental afflictions" in the East. Both cultures hold that individuals require deep reflection in order to become aware of destructive emotions and be able to "diminish their influence on our inner life and, consequently, on our social behavior," as Goleman noted. However, the greatest challenge is "to nurture our positive and balanced emotions in order for them to become our main attributional style."[7]

Clinical Observations

After returning to Italy from England and living for some time in Padua, I began work in the northeastern port city of Trieste. At that time I was collaborating with a physician who referred to me some of his patients who, for one reason or another, were not getting good results from allopathic therapies.

One of these patients was a young woman from Udine, a city nearby. She complained of serious lumbar pain that prevented her from lying on her back for very long. Based on this premise, I imagined there would be some issues in treating her on the therapy table. As if this were not enough, she appeared to have an extremely grumpy temperament.

Our first encounter was not very encouraging, since she started criticizing me as soon as she entered my office. The first thing she said was that she considered me to be just another of the many therapists she had met. She believed I would not be able to help her in any way and would just refer her to my friends to help them make money off other people's misfortunes.

No one would be surprised to hear that this did not seem a good start to me, especially in terms of establishing the relationship of trust between patient and therapist that is so desirable in this field. However, this was only the beginning. Though she accepted treatment, she really did not want to lie down on the table. It took me a while, but I convinced her. Still expressing an annoyed attitude, she lay down but told me she had no intention of remaining in that position for long.

That was one of the few times when I did not know what to do to achieve good results at the end of the treatment.

I started by placing my hands on her feet. As I was listening to her internal rhythm, I was directed toward the woman's spleen and liver. At the same time, I visualized the image of a group of skinheads confronting the police in front of a bar I knew, called Pedrocchi, in Padua. The image surprised me; I wasn't sure how it was relevant. Did it come from my non-conscious or from my patient's? After all, I had left Padua not long before, but I did not know whether my patient was connected to that city in any way. And yet the image was more and more vivid. Why was it manifesting itself?

I asked the craniosacral rhythm to give an answer through the Significance Detector and decided that the visualization was not coming from me. At that point I had to ask my patient whether that city held any significance for her and start the Therapeutic Imagery and Dialogue. I was wary of triggering her surliness and skepticism, but it had to be done, so I asked her. She answered with a blunt "NO."

I stayed quiet, obviously a little disappointed, and kept my hands on her feet. Once again I was led toward the area of her spleen and liver, and she fell silent as well.

After some interminable minutes, miracle of miracles, she started talking, verbally expressing her thoughts. The first thing she said was, "It's my father's fault, that bastard, that I couldn't study in Padua!"

With the same anger and resentment, she told me she was the only female child in her family and that her brothers had always enjoyed privileges and liberties that she was denied only because they were male. In her family's tradition, women had limited choices about both personal and family matters. Daughters had the right to a primary education and, at most, to attend high school but not to enroll at a university.

She had wanted to study psychology at the University of Padua. Her parents had given her brother everything he needed to attend a university in Venice, but they had expected her to look after the house, get a job, and eventually make her own family, give birth to her own children, and stop working in order to devote her time to raising them, consequently becoming dependent on her children's father.

Because of all of that, she had decided not to marry and not to have children, especially to deprive her parents of the grandchildren they expected from her.

As she was expressing her frustration, she explained how she had experienced only personal sacrifice in her family. She'd had to give up on her freedom of choice and, consequently, on all the opportunities she could have taken, in direct contrast to her brothers. For her, not being able to attend university during the prime years of her youth meant she'd lost the biggest opportunity of her life.

After she finished telling me her story, she asked me how much time had passed while she was talking on the therapy table. When I told her it had been almost forty minutes, she immediately asked me, "Why doesn't my back hurt after lying down for so long?" She immediately got up, without even giving me the time to answer, saying the session was over. She paid and left.

I never saw her again, but I was happy about that experience, though it had been so peculiar. I had stayed all session with my hands on her feet, at first not knowing what to do. But as she had started talking, I found that I was drawn to that placement to work on the distal points of her liver and spleen meridians. I released all the entropic energy that was blocking the energy flow and, at the same time, sent syntropic energy to help the system reorganize. All of that was needed because, up until that moment, she had lived grieving the life she had lost.

By obliging the woman's resistance to having hands on her body, I had decided to intervene through the most distal point of the viscera involved in her emotions. By connecting with her liver and spleen meridians, I could still treat and dissipate the primary cause of her pain and her musculoskeletal system.

The musculoskeletal system tends to adapt to muscular restrictions as well as to pain and alterations of visceral organs. Over time, it modifies its position to compensate for the imbalance created by visceral dysfunctions and fascial restrictions. We often do not realize that a slow and progressive adaptation is automatically occurring in our body until we start to feel localized pain along the spine and cannot connect it to a specific cause. The spine starts to move and frequently modifies its curve, causing changes to the lumbar column. At first the adaptations made by our body in these cases prevent us from feeling the pain caused by the fascial tension, which is created because of visceral dysfunctions or pathologies. Nonetheless, the constant overwork of the spine within this adaptation and compensation eventually causes a pathology due to functional overload, which is then manifested through joint pain.

In order to correct or prevent this innate mechanism of our body, we must be aware of the primary cause of pain. Therefore, we must search out what generated it instead of focusing solely on the symptoms. By intervening with the organs that are suffering, we reduce the fascial tension that oppresses the spine.

Remember, structure and function are interconnected and the body is a unit. Several causes (both physiological and emotional) can trigger the skeletal system to reflect pain held in one or more viscera. One of the most common causes is the tension suffered by the system because of problems connected with internal organs. In this case, the spine might become rigid and be in constant pain in correspondence with the innervations that are connected with the dysfunctional organs.

During the session, my patient had told all of her story, more to herself than to me, thereby releasing most of her repressed emotions (anger, melancholy, resentment, isolation, frustration). In the end she had gotten up without pain thanks to the facilitation of the release of destructive energy carried out by the treatment.

⁃❊ A CST-CENTERED VISION ❊⁃

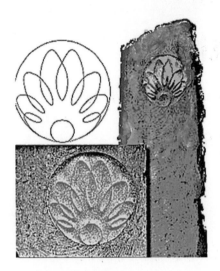

Fig. 13.14. Reproduction of cosmogram on the Cyprus stele of the *Hologram of Europe* installation, by Marko Pogačnik

Marko Pogačnik is a Slovenian artist who defines himself as a "geomant," a healer of the Earth. Many of his works are steles created for lithopuncture, a technique of Earth healing that treats our planet as a body and works in the same way as acupuncture on the human body in traditional Chinese medicine.

The steles are installed on specific energetic spots of the planet in correspondence with its chakras or with the points where its energetic meridians meet. In order to potentiate the effect and to inform the surrounding space of the virtuous qualities it lacks or the archetypical qualities that need to be revealed, the steles are carved with specific graphic symbols called "cosmograms."

Hologram of Europe is an artwork of thirty-four steles created by Pogačnik for the European Union on the occasion of the tenth anniversary of its establishment in order to irradiate in the space the quality of love.

I remember reading in a blog Pogačnik wrote to accompany the aforementioned work, "all gestures that define the apparition of form, whether it is visible or not, require a transformation; everything is interconnected and interweaves; inhaling is always followed by the exhaling of the eternal dance of life. That is how the cosmogram comes to life, vibrating, resounding, harmonizing, activating, synchronizing, balancing, unlocking, informing, melding, dialoguing in the multidimensional space of Life."

These aspects of Pogačnik's lithopuncture perfectly coincide with many of the concepts we have addressed so far. Moreover, the way the artist uses the energetic meridians of Earth (which correspond to the meridians that cross the poles of Earth only by analogy) to heal the planet on a qualitative level, through both cosmograms (intentions and will) and lithopuncture (therapeutic action), is extremely interesting.

CHAPTER 14

Small Deaths

Midrange Values on the Holmes and Rahe Stress Scale

If there is a solution, why do you worry? If there is no solution, why do you worry?

ARISTOTLE

We are now going to examine the twelve midrange stressors (points 19 through 30; see page 197) of the Holmes and Rahe Stress Scale. As discussed in chapter 8, psychiatrists Thomas Holmes and Richard Rahe gave each stressor a rating, measured in life change units (LCUs), as a measure of the stress it might cause in an individual's life. The midrange stressors comprise what we might call "small deaths": forced changes or radical modifications of an element in one's life, which might compromise the regular energy flow of our organism and/or generate Energy Cysts.

Among the most common small deaths that, due to physical and/or emotional symptoms, may require the intervention of a Facilitator are:

- accidents that inhibit the individual's functionality in a beloved sport
- events that initiate life changes
- traumas that cause physical disability
- loss of economic stability
- loss of a loved one
- loss of a job or the change of a workplace.

Since all the abovementioned situations are characterized by subjective and/or objective loss, we should bear in mind that the onset and persistence of physical symptoms, which can be different for each of us, may be associated with a trauma even if said trauma looks like nothing serious. It is precisely the apparent harmlessness of a situation that can cause us to underestimate its importance. And symptoms might derive from the individual's lack of awareness about the underlying cause or causes.

HOLMES AND RAHE STRESS SCALE: STRESSORS 19 TO 30

Rank	Stressor	Holmes and Rahe LCU Value
30	Trouble with boss	23
29	Revision of personal habits	24
28	Change in living conditions	25
27	Begin or end school/college	26
26	Spouse begins or stops working	26
25	Outstanding personal achievement	28
24	Problems with in-laws	28
23	Son or daughter leaving home	29
22	Change in responsibilities at work	29
21	Foreclosure of mortgage or loan	30
20	A large mortgage or loan	31
19	Change in number of arguments with spouse	35

Therefore, among the different possible causes of symptoms, the Facilitator should consider even the life changes that seem to be positive, since they could be hiding a stressor. For instance, a sentimental union certainly implies a change in the habits of everyday life, especially if the people involved move in together to start a new stage of their relationship. This event is obviously an extremely joyful one, but the efforts to adapt one's lifestyle to fit the new situation generally create a lot of stress.

Small deaths are cracks in our vital energy continuum. The more we have and the more we experience them as emotionally traumatic, the longer we will hold the destructive emotions in our physical, emotional, and spiritual body, wearing us out and getting us closer to biological death.

Our objective is not to encourage anyone to abstain from making decisions due to fear of change; that would be extremely wrong. In fact, fear itself can paralyze, and as we have seen, it is an emotion that can assume an extremely destructive connotation. Let us not forget that the flow of life resides in constant transformation, but we need to be aware of the situations we are facing and all the issues that could be connected to them.

It is crucial for the Facilitator to take into account the number, type, and potential impact of events taking place for the person who is asking for help. Most importantly, the Facilitator needs to understand how that person dealt with each change (small death) and whether the change has a traumatic connotation. All of this information is essential for a correct assessment, especially in the presence of a full-blown symptom.

A small death is an event of loss determined by a change that is not necessarily important but is obvious in our everyday life. The sense of loss arises from the awareness that we have lost the ability to access something or that something in our life has lost its former connotation. The sense of loss frequently is connected with the sense of deprivation, negation, dismay, or oblivion we experience in events that are somehow irreversible or disabling, and it is sometimes even able to deprive us of the possibility of accessing a familiar, and therefore reassuring, reality.

However, we should never forget *panta rhei* (everything flows). By consciously letting everything flow with the intention (will) of finding the proper means and moments for us to reflect on, address, and transform whatever blocked or cracked our vital energy continuum, we can at least avoid the increase of destructive energy that may compromise our future, thus influencing constructively and epigenetically our homeostasis and personal growth.

THE EMOTIONS OF SMALL DEATHS

Small deaths may be caused by objective losses that we internalize as subjective losses. They may be caused by changes we are subjected to or those we make voluntarily. Even in the latter case, the changes (social, personal, affective, economical, etc.) that affect the reality around us often make us feel the burden of responsibility for being their cause.

Addressing the emotions of small deaths, psychoanalyst Marina Valcarenghi wrote:

Things change and we change with them, while relationships transform and sometimes die out. What we can do is either find the courage to accept change and go on, cruel as it can be, or pretend nothing happened and keep reviving the past. This last option may be chosen for several and even reasonable reasons, such as financial security, the protection of one's family, reassuring habits, memories, the fear of doing the wrong thing, an addiction, a moral imperative, or uncertainty about the future. . . .

I do not believe there are right or wrong decisions, everyone tries to live as they want and as they can, but on a psychological level the fear of failing is a mistake to me. What we experienced in our lives is a part of ourselves, and every time an experience is concluded its worth does not get lost; an end is not a defeat, it is only the recognition that life is dynamic, has its own movement, and in that movement we find each other or go in opposite directions. A journey is not wrong only because it ends, a job is not a mistake only because we feel we need to do something else: everything we have seen, understood, and loved, everything that gave us joy or pain, and all the surprises of that journey, that job, that city, or that love will be engraved inside us forever, no matter what. Whether we leave or stay, melancholy will follow.[1]

In other words, *panta rhei,* and yet we continue to internalize all the many common life changes as objective and/or subjective losses or small deaths.

We now know that every emotion and feeling of a loss can be connected to the weakening of an organ where an Energy Cyst has formed. The more emotions we find connected to a specific situation, the more likely it is that one or more Energy Cysts were generated in the organism. The final, most apparent symptom is only the result of all the other anomalies caused by destructive emotions in the organs. Let us analyze them more specifically. As mentioned earlier, emotions are potentially destructive when there is an excess or lack of the following:

Emotion	Affected Organs
love (in a romantic relationship)	heart, lungs
fear (of death)	kidneys, lungs, heart
sluggishness/lethargy	spleen, kidneys
security (economic)	pericardium, spleen, liver
defensiveness (of family)	pericardium, spleen
fear (of making mistakes)	kidneys, heart, spleen
attachment (addiction)	lungs, spleen
uncertainty (about the future)	lungs, liver
fear (of failure)	lungs, spleen, liver
defeat (represented by an ending)	spleen, liver
pain (vs. joy)	lungs, heart
melancholy	spleen, lungs

To be able to face everyday life and the changes it brings as well as possible, it is crucial to be aware of the effect that every single change has on our homeostasis and vital energy continuum and to prevent the dysfunctions that the accumulation of unresolved traumatic situations might cause. Our awareness about the possible risks of changing the status of any aspect of our lives, in addition to the Facilitator's intervention to support our process of consciousness and self-healing, can help us in this regard.

How?

To understand the Facilitator's method of assessment, let us go back to Valcarenghi's article, in which, at the end, she mentions melancholy as the ultimate emotional manifestation. Melancholy is certainly connected with any objective or subjective loss that follows a change of status. The spleen is doubtless the organ most involved in the melancholy caused by the loss of a known situation. Nevertheless, as shown in the list of correlations between the organs and emotions above, the spleen is not the only organ cited; the Facilitator will know that the lungs, seat of sadness, also can be easily associated with melancholy. And, though acknowledging the eventuality of melancholy, we need not disregard the other traumatic emotions preceding the event that allowed the destructive energy of melancholy to settle, take root, and manifest, creating a breeding ground for Energy Cysts in the organism.

When we have to deal with a change of any kind, it is advisable to find immediately a way to process and resolve constructively the small death we are experiencing in order to reinforce our organism, prevent any possible dysfunction, and prepare in the best possible way to address the delicate stages following loss. The Facilitator can support us in processing the change we are going through to find a possible solution to the consequences that change may provoke.

The area of application of CST and SER when treating symptoms caused by loss is very wide. We must bear in mind that Facilitators do not treat just the symptom; rather, they search for its cause(s). As we have seen, the actual cause often does not reside in the most recent occurrences, and it may surprise us to find out what it is.

A Facilitator is likely to propose one of the techniques we have already encountered, the Therapeutic Imagery and Dialogue, to support us during the change or to deal with the cause(s) that generated our symptoms. Combined with the assessment used to evaluate the functionality, quality, and amount of energy that meridians contain, the Therapeutic Imagery and Dialogue technique allows us to locate the Energy Cyst. The localization and treatment of an Energy Cyst brings release of the emotions connected with the destructive energy that is trapped in the organs and viscera. At the same time, the Facilitator is enabled to foster the inherent positive resources of the patient, which can emerge even in scenarios of separation and/or loss, initiating the transformation of destructive situations into constructive potentials for the patient's present and future.

OBJECTIVITY AND SUBJECTIVITY IN LOSS

We have used the terms *objective* and *subjective* several times to define a loss, and we also have pointed out that an objective loss can be experienced emotionally and thus become subjective. In order to describe this transition a little better, we are going to rely on the pedagogic vision of Jesuit philosopher, psychologist, pedagogue, and psychoanalyst Eugeniusz Jendrzej.

Jendrzej noted that the postmodern world is characterized by losses: of a sense of historicity, of time, of the difference between reality and appearance, of a sense of mystery, and, most particular to our own discussion, of the ability to overcome the opposition between subject and object. He writes, "By 'subject' I mean the human individual in the becoming. 'Object,' on the other hand, is reality, it is the other, it is others, and the radically Other—God." He refers to the work of philosopher-theologian Bernard Lonergan, who defined *object* as two very different things: the object of the world of immediacy and the object of the world mediated by meaning. "The object of the world of immediacy," writes Jendrzej, "is neither named nor described; it is the world of the immediate experience of senses . . . [and] the sum of what is seen, heard, touched, tasted, smelled, or felt. . . . However, . . . reality is accessible not only through experiencing but also through comprehension, judgment, and decisions. The object of the world mediated by meaning is known not only through sensory experience of an individual but also through the internal and external experience of a cultural community and its way of reasoning."

Just as we have two meanings for the word *object,* Jendrzej notes, we have two meanings for the word *objectivity:* immediate objectivity and the objectivity of the world mediated by meaning. "Only the second is truly human objectivity. . . . It is a unity, but it is an articulated unity."

Pediatrician Donald Winnicott, among the very first psychoanalysts, based his theory of human development on two structures. The first structure consists of the succession of stages of interdependence, whereas the second is the gradual actualization of three fundamental tendencies of development: integration, personalization, and object relations. As Jendrzej writes, "Although both structures have two well-articulated poles—the pole of the subject and the pole of the environment (i.e., of objects)—it is the second structure that seems most suitable to illustrate more clearly how Winnicott reconciled the two poles."

He continues:

> The three fundamental tendencies of the maturation process are part of the entire life of the individual. They initially constitute an undifferentiated unit, then start to gradually differentiate and eventually integrate. The differentiation and integration occur between them and inside them, both on the pole of the subject (INTEGRATION) and on the pole of the environment (HOLDING). . . . Objects and phenomena are necessary in order for a relationship between the subject and the world to begin, and subsequently, little by little, they spread over the entire intermediate area between internal psychic reality and the external world,

i.e., the entire cultural field. The intermediate area, i.e., the potential space, constitutes the place of interchange between the subject and the objects, where subjectivity and objectivity interweave. The breadth, richness, and flexibility of such space may be considered the measure for authentic subjectivity and genuine objectivity. The depth and flexibility of the intermediate area vary depending on the single concrete individual.... Therefore the possible variations are as many as the people in the world.

The continuum constituted by these variations, Jendrzej notes, ranges from the integration of the subjective and objective poles to their division, varying in intensity up to even the point of excluding one of the poles. "Winnicott theorized the origin of subjective convictions about the possibility of contact with external reality. He called such convictions the philosophy of the 'real.'... Furthermore," Jendrzej concludes, "it is surprising how close Winnicott's mature subject is to Lonergan's 'existential subject'; how much both are capable of mediated contact with external reality and one's internal world; how both—as Winnicott would say—have a rich and flexible intermediate area, and how much for both—as Lonergan would say—objectivity is the consequence of authentic subjectivity."[2]

OBJECTIVITY AND SUBJECTIVITY IN BIOPHILOSOPHY

In living beings, objectivity is inevitably connected with subjectivity. In CST and SER, the same concept implies that physical traumas and dysfunctions are inevitably connected with an emotional component. Every objective loss must be connected with an emotion, which means that it is easy to relativize the objectivity of the loss, converting it into a subjective occurrence.

Vallori Rasini, a professor of philosophy at the University of Modena and Reggio Emilia in Italy, wrote a very interesting piece on what she calls the "anthropology of subjectivity," in which she defines the relationship between objective and subjective in science, especially biological sciences and natural medicine, which are the sciences of the living beings. We recommend reading the entire article (see the bibliography at the end of this book). But, in short, Rasini makes a case for the the introduction of subjectivity as a scientific principle "for research on organic beings in general, and not only in the fields of medicine and anthropology. This concept makes it impossible to make a clear division between the subjective aspect—the perspective of an observer—and the objective aspect of research."

Biological science, Rasini says, is a peculiar and much-debated science because of the theoretical and methodological difficulty that arises due to the subject being the same as the object. Sciences such as chemistry and physics can rely on the premise that the observed object is independent from the observing subject; the science of life cannot say the same. "In researching the living organism—it does not matter to which realm it belongs—true knowledge can be obtained only through a special approach: only by participating in life can it be understood; only the living can grasp the living, avoiding making it a mere object," she says. Objectification—removing the subjective component—makes nonliving "things" out of living beings, and that, claims Rasini, deprives them of their main characteristics and distances our knowledge about them from its "relation with life":

> In every biological act, in every vital event, we must recognize implies an indissoluble bond . . . between the subjective element and the objective element. After all, what is subjective affirms itself and is recognized as such only in the encounter with the objective, outside as well as inside itself. When it comes into contact with the environment, the organism proves its subjectivity in the form of opposition to the other; in biological phenomena of crisis and recovery, the subject finds their identity thanks to the opposition and the discontinuity of their own being. It is the "anti-logic" that governs the realm of the living. Every single action of a living being represents a sudden change, which does not testify to a constancy of functions but, on the contrary, their constant transformation, . . . Characteristic of every biological act is the ability, in relation to the world, to overcome the limitations imposed by biological functioning through the modification of the form of responses. . . .
>
> All this is due to the fact that every organism spends its life in a continuous oscillation, always at risk of crisis and a fall. The phenomenon of crisis represents a clear sign of subjectivity, and it is a typical process of living beings that consists of a fracture from what is considered the "regular" trend, characterized by the improvisation with which the turning point is determined and by the impossibility of explaining it in causal terms. . . .
>
> Therefore, since life implicates subjectivity, it is profoundly anti-logical, implying contradiction, paradox, and absurdity among its most essential modalities.[3]

SMALL DEATHS AS NECESSARY LOSSES

Small deaths are inherent to the Life Cycle. We would do well to see them as necessary losses, perhaps taking a lesson from the field of ecopsychology.

Ecopsychology was born at the beginning of the 1990s in California as a cross-discipline of psychology and ecology. The premises for its conception were the considerations and intuitions of American ecologist and philosopher James Hillman and American biologist and naturalist Edward Osborne Wilson. This field of study has a strong anthropological and philosophical connotation and is based on the identification of a correlation between the growing existential, individual, and social suffering and the worsening of environmental degradation. The augmentation of environmental degradation followed the quick process of urbanization that radically changed the lifestyle and habits of the majority of the world's population, consequently creating an increasing psychological discomfort. For this reason, ecopsychology tries to recover a unitary vision of humankind and environment. It promotes contact with nature to enhance psychological well-being and the attention to one's own inner reality. It highlights the inherent sense of belonging to the natural world to generate pleasure in one's care for environment and, on a social level, the push toward policies of sustainable development.

In an article discussing small deaths from the standpoint of ecopsychology, Italian psychologist Pamela D'Alisa wrote:

> All plants whose natural processes are not somehow blocked by the outside evolve gradually, constantly renewing themselves through small deaths. For example, a seed dies to produce the sprout, and a flower dies to produce the fruit, which, in turn, dies to produce a new seed. Whether it is a natural loss or a seasonal pruning, every plant has to periodically give up some parts of itself in order to get stronger and thrive. It is exactly what happens to us since we are living beings whose life is always characterized by growth and change. For this reason, we should not oppose transformation but rather slowly let go of everything that limits us and has come to an end in order to foster and facilitate our new maturation. Therefore, it is crucial to learn how to constantly and trustingly "die for ourselves." This expression refers not to our physical death but only to the symbolic death of anything that has become useless, superfluous, or damaging in our lives. . . . We all struggle trying to get rid of habits, relationships, ways of thinking, and behaviors that make us feel safe. They allow us to move in a world we know and think we control, even if they are not very beneficial to our well-being. "Pruning" is a form of art; we need to know what, how much, where, and when to cut. . . . We should then learn how to be confident in our decisions to "cut," while at the same time we need to recognize our own "green spots," the aspects of our lives that are ready to sprout and grow in the next future.[4]

Clinical Observations

While I was going through the medical history of one of my patients, he told me that his back had started to hurt in the lumbar area, and the pain was irradiating alternately to his legs.

Before starting the treatment, I asked him what his profession was in order to understand whether his body was being put under chronic physical stress, perhaps due to incorrect posture or to lifting excessive weight. He told me he was the manager of a food production company and that his job was more wearying on a mental level than on a physical level, but he had to go to his office seven days a week for almost the entire year.

The treatments began with forty-five-minute sessions twice a week. I worked on the connective tissue of the lumbar area and mobilized the lumbar vertebrae, the hip bones, and the sacrum, thus also influencing the innervations of the lower limbs. After the fourth treatment, my patient started to show some improvements, but they ceased just after another session during the fifth week. I decided to move to a subtler energetic plan and we started the SomatoEmotional Release. When we entered the Therapeutic Imagery and Dialogue, he revealed that both his grandfather, founder of the company he had taken over, and his father, who had inherited it before him, died at the age of fifty. He was forty-eight. He was afraid to die and, at the same time, was working a lot to ensure that his family would be financially secure if he did die when he turned fifty. In order to do so, he had started to distance himself from his own family, even though he was working to support them . . . and he felt lonely.

I recognized that his fear had generated a destructive chain reaction that was feeding his physical pain. Trying to communicate with his non-conscious through the Therapeutic Dialogue, we searched for a possible constructive transformation of his negativity in order to make him aware of his fear and consequently find an acceptable way of dealing with it and resolve it.

At the end of the third month of treatments, he was aware of the need to abandon his fear. At the same time, he realized that up until that moment his way of dealing with it—without resolving it—had been to overwork, not only to earn more money but especially to avoid thinking about death.

During those months I had been treating mostly his kidneys, the organs that usually withhold fear. Once we released the destructive energy trapped there, we addressed all the situations that had led to the creation of Energy Cysts, dealing with all the layers that had stratified in his organism, and allowed the sedimentation of the fear of change and loss (the fear of dying).

Much care was required to ask the patient to change his working and emotional state without causing yet another small death, which could add to the previous affective losses. During the following sessions, we used the Therapeutic Imagery and Dialogue to establish compromises he could commit to sustain, making the transformation possible. Through his non-conscious, he decided that he wanted to face the change gradually. He would start by finding some time for himself, at least half a day every week to take care of himself and his body through exercise and another half a day to spend some time with his family.

The compromise of finding an equal balance for all the parts involved proved to be the correct approach. My patient put the plan into action and, after three months, started showing up for our appointments without any back pain.

Now he receives periodical CST and SER treatments, usually every two months. He does so only to maintain his physical and emotional well-being and keep faith with a promise he made to himself—to take care of himself. He got rid of his fears before his fiftieth birthday, which he has now long passed by.

❧ A CST-CENTERED VISION ☙

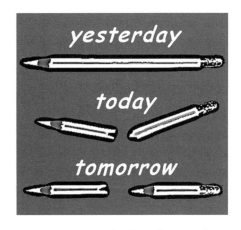

Fig. 14.1. Reproduction of *Yesterday, Today, Tomorrow,* by Lucille Clerc

Artist Lucille Clerc created *Yesterday, Today, Tomorrow* (fig. 14.1) shortly after the terrorist attack on the Parisian offices of the magazine *Charlie Hebdo.* The evident meaning of the image is that even when we have to deal with small deaths or even worse occurrences in which our vital energy continuum is interrupted, broken, or modified, it is always possible to find a way to enhance our potential to evolve into a new constructive situation.

We like to think that this also can happen thanks to the support of CST and SER. In fact, the image seems to communicate, *Do you think you broke us? Look! You just gave us a new opportunity.*

CHAPTER 15

Energetic Framework of the Human Body

Assessing with the Vector/Axis System

When I examine myself and my methods of thought, I come to the conclusion that the gift of fantasy has meant more to me than my talent for absorbing positive knowledge.

ALBERT EINSTEIN

Dr. Upledger was a visionary physician with the determination and courage to search for the meaning of his own intuitions, estimate their scientific veracity, convert them into theory, and convert theory into experimentation in order to achieve results that are applicable in practice.

We find better-known examples of this kind of mentality in Leonardo da Vinci, who wrote, "Practice must always be founded on sound theory." In fact, hundreds of years before the parameters of the scientific method were defined, da Vinci used intuition, systematical observations, experimentation, accurate and repeated measurements, theoretical models, and frequent attempts at mathematical generalization.

In order to get to the veracity of what his instinct told him, to implement experimentation in practical therapies, and to make the consequent evaluations, Dr. Upledger carried out a body of scientific research to validate the model he created and substantiated his intuition through systematic, theoretical, and practical protocols. He essentially made the most of the functionality of the two cerebral hemispheres.

One of his most singular intuitions, which later became one of the techniques Facilitators now employ, was his interpretation of the energetic framework of the human body, which he called the vector/axis system.

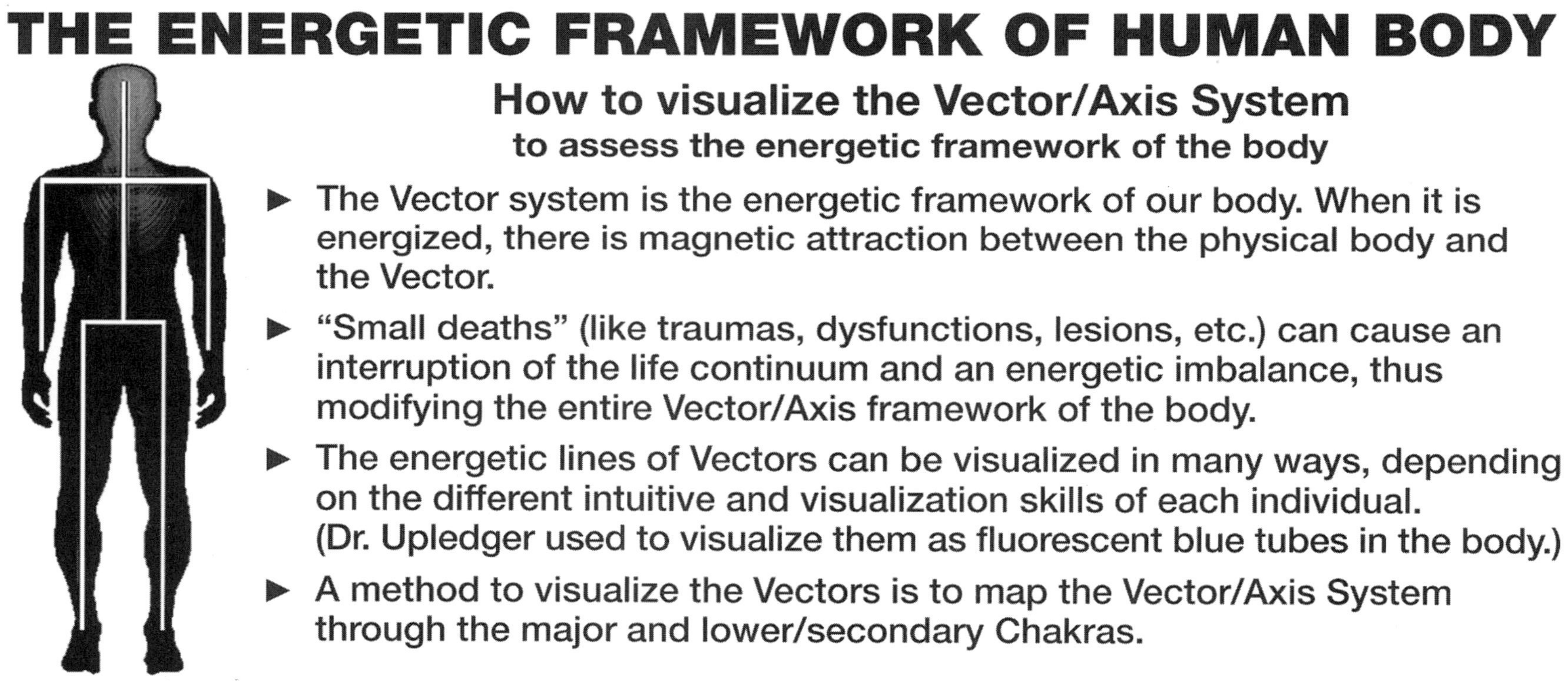

THE ENERGETIC FRAMEWORK OF HUMAN BODY

How to visualize the Vector/Axis System to assess the energetic framework of the body

▲ The Vector system is the energetic framework of our body. When it is energized, there is magnetic attraction between the physical body and the Vector.

▲ "Small deaths" (like traumas, dysfunctions, lesions, etc.) can cause an interruption of the life continuum and an energetic imbalance, thus modifying the entire Vector/Axis framework of the body.

▲ The energetic lines of Vectors can be visualized in many ways, depending on the different intuitive and visualization skills of each individual. (Dr. Upledger used to visualize them as fluorescent blue tubes in the body.)

▲ A method to visualize the Vectors is to map the Vector/Axis System through the major and lower/secondary Chakras.

Fig. 15.1. The energetic framework of the human body: vectors

THE CREATIVE PROCESS

As discussed previously, we generally attribute intuitive and creative peculiarities to the functions of the right hemisphere, while its activity of processing sensory stimuli also necessarily involves the left hemisphere and their interconnection through the corpus callosum.

Drawing from recent research in neuroscience, science writer and creativity consultant Giovanni Lucarelli synthesizes the key points of what actually happens in the human brain during the creative process:

> Three areas or, better yet, three "networks" . . . are involved in the various phases (clarification, conceptualization, processing, selection, application) of the creative process. . . .
>
> If we carry out activities that require focused attention . . . connections (the Executive Attention Network) are activated between the areas of the prefrontal cortex and the posterior part of the parietal lobe. . . .
>
> When we need to create mental images of past experiences, think about future projects, or imagine alternatives for a present scenario, the deep areas of the prefrontal cortex, the temporal lobe, and various regions (external and internal) of the parietal cortex are involved. This network of connections (the Imagination Network) is also involved in social relationships. . . .
>
> The third "cerebral circuit" (the Salience Network) constantly monitors both external events and the internal stream of consciousness and gives priority to the most salient bits of information to resolve a specific task, depending on the current circumstances. It involves the medial prefrontal cortex (the anterior cingulate cortex) and the anterior insular cortex. This "circuit" is also in charge of activating and alternating between the Executive Attention Network and the Imagination Network.[1]

In fact, Lucarelli continues, the mental processes that contribute to the creative process involve different areas of both cerebral hemispheres. He cites American psychologist Rex Jung, who noted that once a problem is defined, the executive attention network quiets, yielding space for imagination, intuition, and the formation of new ideas through the imagination network. After that, depending on the complexity of the task and environmental cues, the executive attention network and the salience network ramp up again.

THE INTUITIVE MIND

The word *intuition* has its root in the Latin prefix *in-*, "inward," and verb *tuēri*, "to look at"—in other words, it means "to look inward." Italian counselor and criminologist Marilena Cremaschini describes intuition as "the ability to translate our experiences and perceptions into action, making the choices that are adequate to achieve our wishes." She continues:

> Its function is to allow us to communicate with our unconscious and our Higher Self, which is nothing but our spiritual part, inner wisdom, consciousness, and "sixth sense."
>
> It is therefore the ability to properly perceive the information coming from the outside, decipher it, and assess it correctly according to the needs of a specific moment.[2]

Intuition can be seen as part of our "adapative unconscious": our individual, unique internalized wisdom that is shaped by everything we have learned, felt, thought, or expressed. Psychologist Howard Gardner, perhaps best known for his theory of multiple intelligences, notes that intuitive intelligence is necessary in order to become more receptive toward our own inner world. As the editorial team of the psychology blog *La Mente è Meravigliosa* (The Mind Is Wonderful) writes:

> Thanks to Howard Gardner, we know that there are many types of intelligence and that all of them are equal and useful. Intuitive intelligence in particular allows us to let emotions emerge in our consciousness in order to make quicker decisions or, at least, to have that type of "more intimate" information available so that we can contrast it against a more rational and convergent perspective.
>
> The messages our intuition sends us are sometimes extremely complex: sensations, forms, words. . . . It is our task to interpret them. The more freedom we give our mind, without prejudices or barriers, the more easily our intuition will emerge. Intuitive intelligence can be used every day, but only if we allow ourselves to think more freely and, at the same time, to be more receptive toward our own emotions.[3]

EIDETIC INTUITION, PHENOMENOLOGY, AND EVOLUTIONARY CREATIVITY

The term *eidetic* comes from the Greek words meaning "knowledge" and "to see." In fact, eidetic intuition is intellectual insight or grasp of the essence of things and phenomena—

the knowledge of their pure essence as a phenomenon belonging to consciousness.

The need to create is a peculiarity of consciousness, which, when active, is able to transform intuition into theory and theory into practice. The need to "create" based on what you see or intuit is a prerogative of being aware of lived experience (visual, auditory, tactile, perceptive, emotional, etc.). This happens when our consciousness is active, that is, when we pay attention to and process what happens both outside and inside us. As a natural consequence we feel the need to reveal the intuition that is derived from a stimulus by transposing it into reality. Therefore, a theory is born from intuition and the theory is subsequently transposed into practice.

The immediate knowledge of things and phenomena (observed or perceived) is actually intuitive before being scientific. This phenomenological reduction is the intuitive premise of science and finds a correlation in philosophy, whose objective is the completion of the essence of phenomena—in clear opposition to the Galilean logic that denies the essences—and psychology, which evaluates the ability to hold sensory perceptions and translate them into images.

Among the greatest representatives of eidetic intuition of the last century were philosophers Edmund G. A. Husserl (1859–1938) and Henri L. Bergson (1859–1941) and psychologist Wolfgang Metzger (1899–1979). Philosopher Maurice Merleau-Ponty (1908–1961) and physicist and philosopher Albert Einstein (1879–1955) were widely influenced by eidetic intuition and phenomenology, giving way to subsequent developments.

Edmund Husserl

Husserl was one of the major contributors to eidetic intuition and the founder of phenomenology, a philosophical current that studies how the things (phenomena) of the world manifest themselves into consciousness. The main subject analyzed by his philosophy is the relationship between theory and practice and between science and practical life. In his phenomenological concept of the world, perception is produced by the interweaving of current modes of givenness (manifestations of phenomena brought to consciousness) with the modes of givenness that are no longer present or not yet present. As one writer, explaining the concepts for the Italian educational forum Skuola.net (*skuola* means "school"), put it:

> Consciousness is always aware of the infinity of its possible experiences. It knows that there is an infinite number of possible horizons, without actually needing to travel the infinity of possible horizons. Consciousness constantly presumes the existence of a "unitary horizon" that embraces all possible horizons: the "universal horizon" or "world horizon." . . . The life of our consciousness is a constant anticipation of the possibility of realization.[4]

Albert Einstein

Not only was Einstein a contemporary of Husserl, but he also discussed his phenomenology. Giorgio Jules Mastrobisi, a researcher at the Albert Einstein Archives of Jerusalem, provides a documentation about this discussion and Einstein's considerations through the study of some of his unpublished writings. Mastrobisi tells us:

> Husserl's inevitable search for the hidden meaning of the "vision of essence" represented his huge effort to try to grasp the theoretical element that was indispensable for his work. In light of this research, Einstein engaged in a confrontation with Husserl's phenomenology, giving body to a series of considerations that seem to follow Husserl's from the perspective of the conceptual and terminological structure. . . . Einstein believed, "It is not possible to establish a difference between sensory impressions and representations, or at least, it is not possible with absolute certainty." . . . However, when facing the theoretical task of setting such a differentiation, he had to give up, thus implying the existence of a world of "sensory experiences that fall into the category of peculiar psychic experiences." Therefore, scientific thinking meant as simply "considering an object and going further" needs to go back to a preliminary "there is" on the ground of the sensible and the experiential world, just as they manifest themselves in our life and to our body. Nevertheless, "this body must not be considered as an information machine but rather as the actual body we call our own, the sentinel monitoring our words and actions." . . .
>
> This is the sense of a true transcendental philosophy and Husserl's pure phenomenology, which can be proposed as a "scientific hermeneutics."[5]

INTUITION AND EMOTION

Dr. Upledger dialogued with the Higher Self and the world of intuitions and hidden or expressed realities and phenomena, developing sensations and images into ideas, theories, and creative representations to produce a practical protocol for Facilitators. What about emotions?

During CST and SER treatments, a Facilitator encounters a patient's nonconscious in the Third Space, which both the Facilitator and the patient are able to reach through the Therapeutic Imagery and Dialogue. This space is where intuition is disclosed, implying healing. It is where the spiritual, energetic, and emotional bodies manifest themselves as fundamental resources for the development of a creative and transformational hypothesis that envisions improvement through change. In that space, Dr. Upledger visualized the vectors that compose the energetic framework of the human body.

We have now analyzed different philosophical perspectives on the subject of intuition. Let us now delve into the opinions of the scientific world.

INTUITIVE INTELLIGENCE AND ADAPTIVE UNCONSCIOUS

We have already mentioned emotional intelligence. With a view to the interconnection and interrelation of all phenomena, we are now going to analyze intuitive intelligence as well.

Let's begin with communications psychologist Francesca Cilento, a professor at the Catholic University of the Sacred Heart in Milan, who set forth a scientific perspective on intuitive intelligence and the role of emotions in developmental growth:

> Intuitive intelligence works side by side with rational thinking in the management of everyday choices, remaining in the background and relying on the guidance of emotions. . . . Intuitive intelligence is an intellectual ability that is widely employed . . . in the background and in parallel to analytical reasoning, which is merely sequential and generally quite slow and tiring. . . . In fact, intuitive intelligence and analytical intelligence operate simultaneously since every decision, rational as it may be, always has an intuitive foundation. The intuitive system functions through the mental representation of "chance" to estimate the likeliness that an event might occur. . . . It is easy to confuse intuitive intelligence with emotional intelligence, and that happens because making a choice with our intuition also means letting our feelings guide us. . . . Neuroscience considers intuition to be founded on the gathering and analysis of sensory information. Some scientists call it "adaptive unconscious," meaning that the most gifted individuals are those who are able to detect the smallest environmental variations and adapt accordingly in the best possible way. In this vision, emotion would act as a bridge between the environment and the individual, and that would be its key role. Intuition contributes to happiness by creating a pathway to our dreams and deepest needs, subsequently allowing us to make the most satisfying choices.[6]

A study by a research group from Drexel University—founded in Philadelphia as the Drexel Institute of Art, Science, and Industry and later developed into the current university and affiliated with the well-known Academy of Natural Sciences of Philadelphia—showed how intuitive intelligence solves problems more easily and in more strategically correct ways than deductive analytical reasoning. Describing the study, science writer Simone Valesini noted:

John Kounios, one of the researchers from Drexel University taking part in this study, explains that analytical, conscious reasoning can sometimes prove to be rushed or inaccurate, causing us to make mistakes when trying to solve a problem. On the contrary, since intuition is unconscious and automatic, it cannot by its very nature be rushed. . . . Analytical reasoning proceeds through gradual degrees and therefore provides some of the information that helps build a possible response even before the reasoning has been completed, which may lead us to make an error. Unlike the reasoning process, the intuitive process gives all or nothing; before producing a result, it does not provide any kind of information on a conscious level. . . . As Kounios illustrates, deadlines create in the individual a subtle sensation of anxiety, which can transform instinctive reasoning in analytical reasoning. . . . It is for this reason that we need to have more flexible deadlines if we are searching for creative ideas. A deadline that cannot be postponed at all tends to bring actual results, but they are rarely creative results.[7]

The scientific field is investigating the neurobiology of intuition to a greater and greater degree, creating a true neurobiology discipline. Two of the most renowned figures in its field of application are cognitive psychologist Robin M. Hogarth, who is also an economist and research professor at Pompeu Fabra University in Barcelona, and scientific journalist and sociologist Malcolm Gladwell. The scientific foundation for the study of the neurobiology of intuition mostly comes from Dr. Keiji Tanaka, a Japanese neuroscientist and research professor at the RIKEN Center for Brain Science, and Portuguese neurologist, neuroscientist, and psychologist Antonio Damasio.

The studies of these key figures tell us the following:

Intuition opens dimensions that are otherwise invisible to us, enabling us to contact a part of ourselves that operates in the deepest meanders of subconscious. It sometimes seems to be something so foreign to us that we often perceive it as something neither much scientific nor much logical. . . . However, it is incorrect to think so. . . . Medical researcher Jonas Salk, known for developing the polio vaccine, wrote about the necessity to always consider our sixth sense in everyday life. . . .

During some experimentations with medical imaging on the neurobiology of intuition, it was observed that the area most involved in the intuitive process was the precuneus, a small portion of the superior parietal lobe located between the cerebral hemispheres. The precuneus is also connected with episodic memory, visual-spatial processes, and, what is even more interesting, our consciousness. . . . Another area that is activated when we respond intuitively is the ventromedial prefrontal cortex . . . which holds information about past rewards as well as the negative consequences of mistakes.... The relevance of this area in our decisions ... is based on the fact that it leads us to respond in accordance with our emotions.... Scientific studies on neurobiology of intuition also concern the caudate nucleus, a structure included in basal ganglia, which are connected with learning processes, habits, and automatic behaviors.... It stimulates the impulse of the sixth sense to help us make quick, almost automatic decisions based on experience and what we have previously learned.[8]

ANALYSIS CREATES PARALYSIS

"Analysis creates paralysis" is an expression Dr. Upledger used to repeat during his classes when students wanted to dissect all the details of a discussion—thus using the left hemisphere excessively—rather than initially just grasp the sense of a concept he was trying to convey on an intuitive level.

Cognitive scientist Sian L. Beilock, now president of Dartmouth College, would probably agree with him. In a 2017 interview with Alexandra Wolfe, of the *Wall Street Journal*, on the topic of paralysis by analysis, she talked about the relation between stressors (including analytical/intellectual stress) and some of the most common cognitive or motor blockages in everyday events. However, this concept has much more ancient roots, since it takes inspiration from one of the most well-known fables written by Aesop, Greek writer of the sixth century BCE, the one about the cat and the fox.

Nowadays, we often talk about insight and problem solving, and psychologists, neurologists, sociologists, pedagogists, and anthropologists feverishly engage in discussions on the influence of these behaviors on everyday life, which risk causing us to become paralyzed. Fortunately, in this debate and in all situations that are difficult to understand or address, we can rely on the great intuitions of great individuals, who have lived and will always live in all epochs. Experts in various scientific or humanistic disciplines are always here to help us with their eurekas or their constructive, determining solutions for all the different scenarios that life brings, whether these solutions are concrete or spiritual, and whether they are applicable in ordinary circumstances or extraordinary ones.

TWO BASIC PRINCIPLES FOR THE ENERGETIC FRAMEWORK OF THE HUMAN BODY

So far we have partially analyzed the topics of energy, the law of conservation of energy, and, in more depth, polarity. Before discussing the vector/axis system as the energetic framework of the human body, let us analyze a little more the energetic field of the individual.

The energetic field of the human body complies with the laws of the entire Universe, in particular the "laws of polarity" and the "law of conservation of energy." All the Universe, including the smallest particles, is permeated with energy. The whole material and spiritual world is based on energy, which forms a "framework" of the Universe, constantly circulating and transforming into a multitude of different forms with different qualities. The human energetic "framework" is extremely complex and constantly interacts with the Universe. . . . Some of the ancient peoples of Asia thought that the individual is continually cooperating with the Universe, and if there is even just a slight crack in the harmony of this cooperation, people get sick; when the crack is significant, the energetic imbalance can lead to death. In order to manage a person's energy, ancient healers got to know the energetic human anatomy and its interaction with the Universe. . . . They considered seven energetic centers in the human body . . . five of which are located along the inside of the spine, whereas the other two are in the head. . . . Eastern healers established an outline of the cosmic energy that penetrates the crown and goes through the spine and the coccyx to reach

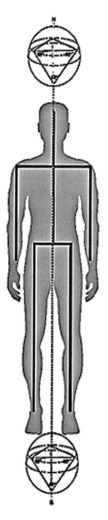

Fig. 15.2. Vector/axis system and polarity

the soles, whereas the energy of the Earth goes through the feet and reaches the head. An energetic scale is established in the organism, harmoniously distributing the "yang" and the "yin" in every organ and cell. The human body is like a magnet in which every particle is regulated by the signs plus and minus.[9]

We are examining polarity and chakras to trace a beginning outline of what the energetic framework of the human body is. This framework can be visualized through vectors, which we have mentioned in this text as well.

Vectors have their own landmarks in the human body, which correspond to the major chakras and some of the lower ones. They are aligned on an axis that follows the law of polarity. For this reason, in order to delineate techniques of energetic treatment of the human body, from now on we will be talking about the vector/axis system as it was visualized and theorized by Dr. Upledger.

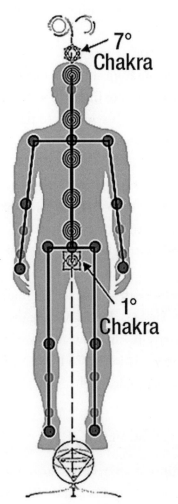

Fig. 15.3. Polarity and map of the vector/axis system, with major and minor chakras

HOW TO MAP THE VECTOR/AXIS SYSTEM

The hands are essentially a CST and SER therapist's eyes.

During SER seminars, some students had trouble visualizing or perceiving the vector/axis system. Consequently, it was extremely hard for them to carry out a treatment employing the vectors. One of the reasons behind this difficulty could be that when absorbing/assimilating new information, the general tendency is to rely almost exclusively on the left hemisphere of the brain. Therefore, both in the seminars and in this text, exploration of the connection between the two hemispheres and the corpus callosum is a preparatory subject that should enable us to use the right hemisphere as a tool to give shape to what is apparently difficult to perceive/sense solely through the hands.

As an aid to the visualization of the vectors, we can use an analogy with the meridians and parallels of the Earth. Taking polarity as a reference (like the North Pole and the South Pole of the planet) and using the chakras as landmarks, we can start to map the vectors. Imagine that each person has a polarity whose north is the middle of the crown, directed toward the seventh chakra, and whose south is at the opposite pole of a straight line descending the body from the seventh chakra, passing through the five major central chakras, proceeding in the direction of the first chakra (pubic region), and stopping at the iliac bones. Then imagine this straight vertical line being crossed by two horizontal straight lines, one going from shoulder to shoulder and the other from hip to hip. This completes the basic map; see figure 15.4.

A useful method to visualize the entire vector/axis system is to trace a map using the seven major chakras and some of the twenty-one lower chakras (those that are most directly connected with the organs involved in CST and SER).

Imagine a two-dimensional map of the chakras in which the first and the seventh chakras are used only as directional poles; the first chakra indicates the downward direction (root) and the seventh chakra indicates the upward direction (crown). Now connect the first and the seventh chakras with a straight line passing through all the other major chakras. This is how we get the first vectorial axis, the central one.

Each of the lower or secondary chakras (note that they can be single or paired) corresponds energetically to one of the major chakras. By connecting these secondary chakras both horizontally and perpendicularly to the central axis, we are able to obtain a complete map of the vector/axis system, which in CST and SER constitutes the energetic framework of the human body; see figure 15.4.

HOW DO WE USE THESE VECTORS?

This is the question Dr. Upledger asked himself after he visualized (or sensed or perceived) the vector system in which energy moves in CST and SER treatments. In

Energetic Framework of the Human Body 219

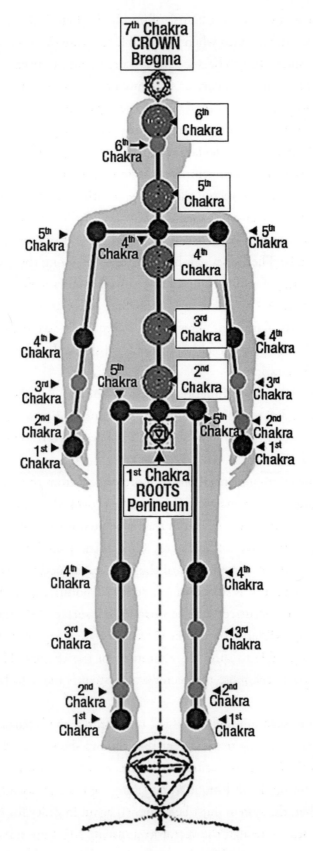

Fig. 15.4. Map of the vector/axis system through the major and minor chakras

fact, his experimentation over the course of hundreds of clinical cases started exactly from this question, and it ended when he was able to create the working protocol that helps Facilitators successfully rebalance any misalignment in the energetic framework of the human body, restore the correct structure of the vector/axis system, and allow the energy flow to go back to normal within the organism.

That said, in CST and SER treatments, it is not enough to just implement the realignment technique on the deviation of the vector/axis system, even if there are immediate improvements. The Facilitator also must search for the cause of the deviation or misalignment of the vector and remove it; otherwise there is the actual risk of not resolving the issue and inducing a state of well-being that is only temporary.

What could be the possible cause of the misalignment of one or more vectors in relation to their axis? The causes can be multiple, but among the most common we find are the suffering of an organ or an unresolved traumatic factor/emotion/event that created an active lesion, an Energy Cyst, which is deviating or blocking the vital energy flow in a particular vector. The vector consequently adapts to the dysfunction and assumes a deviated position (either broken or dislocated), which then affects the entire energetic framework.

Energy Cysts, somatic dysfunctions, physical trauma, emotional disorders, and everything we have defined as a small death interrupt or distort the alignment and continuity of the energetic system and sometimes are expressed through an evident postural dysfunction.

Therefore, the misalignment of one or more vectors from their axis and the subsequent interruption of the energetic flow can be provoked by an Energy Cyst. We must locate it to find the cause or causes that generated it to be able to dissipate it.

Let us imagine the effect of an Energy Cyst in the vector system as if it were a stone falling in a body of water. Up until the impact, the body of water has a linear surface; after the impact, it is subjected to a series of modifications altering both the area where the impact occurred and the surrounding surface. We know that Energy Cysts have their own vibrations and, like chakras, create energy vortexes (that in this case are antagonists) able to shift the alignment of the vectors. The more Energy Cysts in an organism, the more the vector/axis system is likely to be compromised (see fig. 15.5).

It is essential to keep in mind that if the treatment of the vector/axis system only realigns the vectors, and the reassessment that follows shows that the system is not able to maintain the correct structure, it becomes necessary to search for the Energy Cyst that is preventing the technique from having a good and lasting result and dissipate it. After that, the system must be realigned again in order for it to last.

Moreover, when we realign the vector/axis system, it is important to respect the time needed for vectors to settle and fuse. Rushing the end of the treatment allows

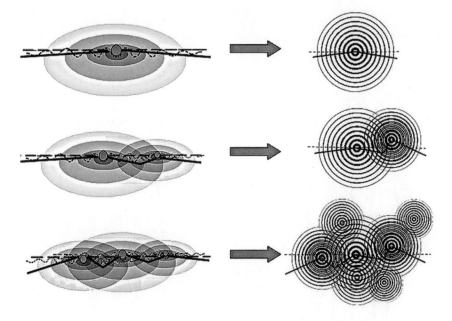

Fig. 15.5. Wave expansion generated by Energy Cysts

the vectors to assume a position that is only temporary, even after the dissipation of the Energy Cyst, since remnants of the situation could remain in the Cellular Memory.

ALIGNING VECTORS TO THEIR AXIS

Let's look at two techniques Facilitators can use to align vectors to their axis. The first technique asks you to visualize the vectors. If you cannot perceive the vectors visually, you can use touch.

Energetic Visualization and Mobilization

1. Stand in front of the patient and place your hands on their feet, keeping your eyes half closed so you can visualize the vectors.
2. Raise the patient's lower limbs slowly and move them slightly in the direction of the head (diagonally or following a straight line) with the aim of putting the part of the vector that is disjointed from its axis back into its place.
3. Mobilize the upper limbs, moving them in the correct direction to reconnect each vector with its axis.
4. Do the same with the rest of the body, wherever you detect a misalignment or a bending of a vector, using the body as a magnet to attract each vector toward its axis. Use slow and gentle movements of traction, compression, rotation, or a combination of these until there are no more deviations of vectors from their axis.

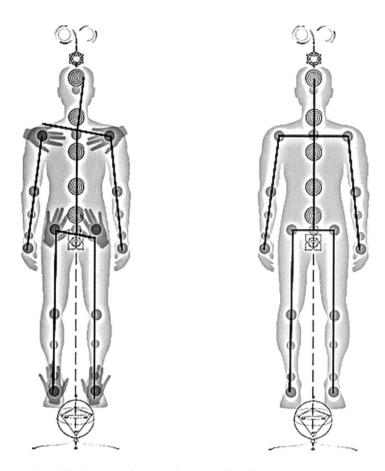

Fig. 15.6. Vectors along their axis before being realigned (left) and vectors along their axis after being realigned (right)

Energetic Touch and Mobilization

This technique can be carried out either through touch by placing your hands on the patient's body or through energy perception by keeping your hands at a close distance from the body and moving them as though you were scanning it to visualize the vectors from above the patient's body.

If you cannot perceive the vectors visually, you can use touch.

1. Stand in front of the patient, close your eyes, and place your hands on their feet. Imagine sending energy from your hands in the direction of their hips, and assess the continuity of the energy flow to detect possible blockages or obstacles.
2. If you perceive a blockage, keep sending energy along the axis with your intention until the energy flows without any restriction.
3. Repeat the exercise for each vector of the body until energy flows regularly everywhere.

If vectors resist realignment, or if they are realigned but then once again diverge from the correct alignment, search for the emotional component or dysfunction that caused the vector deviation or the Energy Cyst that led to a blockage, using the information offered by the emotional correlations of the organs, meridians, and chakras involved in the points of blockage. Use the Significance Detector to choose the issue you want to work on. Always rely on the instructions of the patient's non-conscious.

If you perceive the presence of Energy Cysts when assessing the system, you can use Therapeutic Imagery and Dialogue (page 39) or the technique of filling and emptying the meridians (page 188) to restore the correct vector/axis alignment in a stable way.

After dissipating any Energy Cysts, it will be much easier to realign the compromised vector durably on its axis.

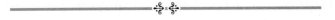

FROM DR. UPLEDGER'S OBSERVATIONS TO A NEW METHOD

Among his patients, Dr. Upledger reported cases of vector lines emanating from the body (for example, through the physical limit of the shoulders) but still forming ninety-degree angles at the intersection with the main axis. Even in these cases, there was a dysfunction.

His guidelines for Facilitators synthesize the technique to realign the vectors as follows:

1. Assess the vector/axis alignment in the system.
2. Use the physical body as a magnet to mobilize the system.
3. Mobilize the vector slowly, giving it the time to realign.

As noted above, if the vector does not readjust or does not maintain the correct position after the alignment technique, it is necessary to find the dysfunction that is determining the anomaly and treat it, or find the Energy Cyst and release it.

After realignment of the vector/axis system, it is immediately possible to see an improvement, and the patient perceives a better proprioception, which the Treccani *Dizionario di Medicina* defines as:

> The overall functions in charge of controlling the position and movement of the body through the information detected by peripheral receptors called

proprioceptors (the receptors of the muscle spindles, the golgi tendon organs, the receptors of the joint capsules, proprioceptive reflexes). The information coming from the proprioceptors enters the spinal cord at the level of the dorsal horns. Here the afferent fibers have synapses with local neurons and form proprioceptive reflex arcs; other branches climb the entire spinal cord to reach the cerebral centers in charge of the regulation of movements, such as the brainstem and the cerebellum. Such information is processed inside the spinal reflexes that maintain the correct posture and oppose gravity.[10]

After employing the assessment and rebalance techniques on the vectors, Dr. Upledger was able to see the improvements in his patients, "They are very much aware of the positive effects of vector/axis integration and alignment when these techniques are performed on them, and they keep reporting a sense of 'improved correctness' and 'better body awareness,'" which actually corresponds to proprioception.

Dr. Upledger, ever the good educator, wanted every Facilitator to learn and implement his method but also to experiment with it through new research, discoveries, intuitions, and applications in order to improve it and surpass it. As he wrote in *SomatoEmotional Release and Beyond*, "When you practice this technique, it develops and expands your sensory limits. An unknown universe awaits further exploration."[11]

Bearing in mind Dr. Upledger's instructions and the therapeutic objective, in the next chapter we will analyze the assessment and treatment of the vector/axis system with another method that is both eidetic and empirical, relying on the logistic references and also the energetic peculiarities of chakras.

CONSIDERATIONS

One of the biggest challenges I faced as a CST and SER Instructor was teaching the first Italian SER1 seminar to vision-impaired members of the Italian Blind Union.

During the first three days of the course, I thought it best not to address the vectors. However, when I explained my doubts to my assistants, who on that occasion not only were CST students of mine but also had worked with blind people for years, they reassured and encouraged me to address the topic with the students.

When I finished explaining the topic to the class, giving verbal instructions on the initial placement of the hands to employ this technique, I was surprised to find that the students found it all clear and to see them start to practice, following one of the approaches from Dr. Upledger's *SomatoEmotional Release and Beyond* that I had illustrated.

The students placed their hands at a minimal distance from the body, starting from the feet and moving toward the head. When they found the crack and/or deviation of a vector, they started to move the vector, using energy to bring it back to its axis. They used only hand movements and did not touch or move the body.

Unbelievable, and yet true! I must confess that my assistants and I were all extremely glad for this outcome.

Since then, I have always proposed the method of perceiving and mobilizing vectors as "shining lines" (as Dr. Upledger used to see them) or, for those who have difficulties in imagining them, through other forms of subjective visualization.

Clinical Observations

In collaboration with a maxillofacial surgeon, I had been treating a patient for over a year who had suffered a cranial fracture in a car crash. During one of our sessions, the patient told me that his wife, who was in the car with him during the accident, had suffered a lesion to one of her lumbar vertebrae. She had gone through surgery and been implanted with some medical screws, but her body kept rejecting them. Other surgical procedures had followed the first one, but the outcome was always the same.

In addition to her obvious discomfort, she was constantly feeling severe back pain. For this reason, my patient had decided to ask if I could assess her problem and treat her. I agreed to meet his wife in my office for a consultation, and she accepted.

She was a tall, thin woman of thirty-five, and she looked a little scared. She was certainly quite fatigued. I invited her to sit on the chair in front of my desk, and as she was telling me about the aftermath of her first surgery, she started to cry and did not stop until she finished her story.

She admitted that after being dismissed from the hospital, she happened to look at her image in the mirror and saw it "cut in half" at the waist, with her torso dislocated laterally from the lower part of her body.

She told me that the screws the surgery had implanted kept bothering her. Her life had become an ordeal because of the severe pain. Moreover, she told me that the doctor who had performed the surgical procedure and kept seeing her regularly absolutely forbade her from searching for alternative treatments or remedies to alleviate her pain as a replacement for the physiotherapeutic sessions he had prescribed to her. If she did, he had said that he would refuse to look after her situation.

That was a red flag. What should I do? The decision was my patient's, but I obviously felt a great responsibility in this respect.

She told me she trusted me, especially after having seen the positive results of the treatments her husband had gone through with me. She therefore felt perfectly aware of the choice she was about to make, and she was ready to ignore her doctor's advice.

However, I kept asking myself whether it was appropriate for me to treat her against the opinion of the doctor who was supervising her recovery. I must admit that this was probably one of the few times I would have preferred not to treat a person who was asking for my help. What kind of treatment could I propose? I realized I was blocking myself. So, as I invited the patient to lie down on the therapy table, I simply started praying for everything to work out in the best way possible for my patient's sake.

I started the treatment by placing my hands on the patient's feet, and I automatically thought of the most energetic technique I knew.

From the most distal point of her energetic framework, I started to connect with her vectors and send energy from the soles of the feet toward the pelvic area. I was worried, but after a few seconds I started perceiving the exact disconnect the patient had described when she told me that she saw herself as cut in half at the waist. By following the longitudinal axis of the vector system, I visualized the central vector completely dislocated from its axis up to the corpus callosum.

I started to realign the vector to its axis. I was worried because I was encountering a strong resistance. Meanwhile, the patient flinched as if she had been shocked, and her body made a sound as if it had been manipulated with osteopathy. I flinched too as I looked at my patient in wonder, observing her reaction. Very calmly, she asked me what had happened and what had caused the noise she had heard coming from her body. I did not know what to say, and I muttered something about a realignment that I realize now was probably completely unintelligible.

Anyway, surprised and not scared at all, she asked me whether she could stand up. When I said she could, she stood up and immediately went to the mirror that was hanging on one of the walls of the office. She burst into tears as she looked at herself. I started to worry again, but I tried to keep a reassuring composure on the outside. She turned to me and told me that it was the first time since her surgery that she could see her body perfectly aligned.

She thanked me, got dressed, and left.

She came back the following week and told me that she had gone to the surgeon for a checkup. After an evaluation, the specialist expressed his contentment regarding the improvements he was finally observing. At that point, she told him she had been treated with CranioSacral Therapy and would like to tell him about it.

He stopped her instead and told her, "I don't know what you did or what kind of treatment you received, and I don't even want to know. But quit physiotherapy and continue with whatever you did. Then come back for a follow-up so I can evaluate your progress."

It goes without saying that the patient was extremely happy—and I was too.

I treated her for a few months more, dissipating the entropic energy that had gathered in her organism after the trauma of the incident and the surgical procedure. Afterward, she recovered completely and went back to her usual everyday life.

I think this was the most striking experience I had in my work with vectors. It helped me understand how hugely an energetic treatment can influence the organism.

Thank you, Dr. John!

CHAPTER 16

Chakras

Energetic Landmarks for Mapping the Vector/Axis System

If you want to find the secrets of the universe, think in terms of energy, frequency, and vibration.

ATTRIBUTED TO NIKOLA TESLA

We have seen that in traditional Chinese medicine, each organ of the body concerns one specific meridian. The same goes for chakras, which have an energetic and emotional component that is connected on a physical level to a specific organ. These correspondences constitute a further assessment method for Facilitators to use in the search for an anomaly or dysfunction within the organism and the restoration and stabilization of the normal physiological functions, including the energetic and emotional balancing of the individual. Bearing in mind the objective of this text, we also must note that the function of chakras is to allow us to access the cognition of the energetic framework of the human body (vector/axis system). We actually need this framework to support us in situations of change, loss, abandonment, separation, and bereavement, which are all scenarios that could compromise our vital energy continuum.

MAJOR AND LOWER/SECONDARY CHAKRAS AND RELATED ANATOMY

In Assam Bihar's *The Seven Chakras,* we read, "Chakras are energy and awareness centers in the human body.... The primary chakras are seven, but there are many other sides ... that 'ideally' correspond with acupuncture meridian points.... Each of them oversees certain organs.... In the West they are called by number or refer to the center or to the physical plexus concerned."[1]

Mapping the Vector/Axis System with Major and Secondary Chakras

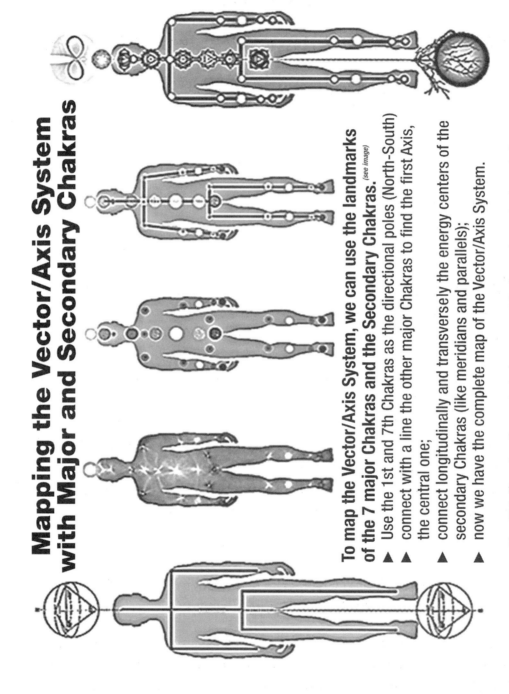

To map the Vector/Axis System, we can use the landmarks of the 7 major Chakras and the Secondary Chakras. *(see image)*

▲ Use the 1st and 7th Chakras as the directional poles (North-South)
▲ connect with a line the other major Chakras to find the first Axis, the central one;
▲ connect longitudinally and transversely the energy centers of the secondary Chakras (like meridians and parallels);
▲ now we have the complete map of the Vector/Axis System.

Fig. 16.1. Mapping the vector/axis system with the major and minor chakras

We will focus on the choice of the appropriate chakras to perfect the mapping of the vector/axis system as far as it is pertinent to CST and SER. If an Energy Cyst located along a vector interrupts its energy flow or causes the vector to deviate from its axis, we can turn to the characteristics of the chakras that constitute the landmarks for that vector in order to establish its energetic nature.

To help us identify the type of energy we may run across, we are going to briefly list the seven major chakras and their physical and emotional correspondences in the human body. For each major chakra (a primary landmark of the system), we will note some of the corresponding lower chakras (secondary landmarks), which can be helpful in the mapping of the vector/axis system.

FIRST CHAKRA

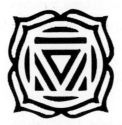

Also called: Root chakra
Color: Red
Musical note: C
Primary landmark: Perineum or pubis/coccyx
Secondary landmarks: One in the sole of each foot and one in the palm of each hand
Organs involved: Adrenal glands, kidneys, bladder, spinal column, rectum

The energy of the first chakra is also called kundalini in Sanskrit. It relates to the will of survival, the satisfaction of instincts and primary needs, and the physical aspect of sexuality aimed at reproduction.

On a physical level, it is connected with the adrenal glands and the secretion of adrenaline and corticosteroids, which ensure adaptability in situations of danger (fight-or-flight response) and the ability to adapt to intense effort.

SECOND CHAKRA

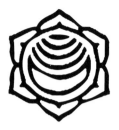

Also called: Sacral or sexual chakra
Color: Orange
Musical note: D
Primary landmark: Infraumbilical/between the navel and the pubic bone
Secondary landmarks: One in each ankle and one in each wrist
Organs involved: Gonads, reproductive organs, sciatic nerve

The second chakra relates to sexuality and its emotional component, creativity, the sense of beauty, and self-esteem.

On a physical level, it is connected with the genitals and their influence on the development of sexual characteristics. It is also associated with disorders of the kidneys and blood circulation and to some dysfunctions of the immune system.

THIRD CHAKRA

Also called: Solar plexus chakra
Color: Yellow
Musical note: E
Primary landmark: Pit of the stomach/solar plexus
Secondary landmarks: One at the center of each tibia and one at the center of each forearm
Organs involved: Liver, gallbladder, spleen, stomach, pancreas, duodenum, small intestine, transverse colon

The third chakra relates to the desire for power and the will to manipulate the world to find a place in society. It is able to assimilate and transform what life presents.

On a physical level, it is connected with digestive functions and especially with the pancreas, the exocrine gland that also contains endocrine cells responsible for the production of insulin and glucagon.

FOURTH CHAKRA

Also called: Heart chakra
Color: Green
Musical note: F
Primary landmark: Halfway between the spinal cord and heart
Secondary landmarks: One behind each knee and inside each elbow and one connected to the thymus gland
Organs involved: Heart, thymus, bronchi, lungs

The fourth chakra relates to love, the ability to love unconditionally, empathy, and healing. It is the point of convergence and the energy center of the sky-earth axis.

The main organ it is connected with is the heart, but the thymus gland also has a strong influence (until puberty). The fourth chakra is also connected with the vagus nerve, the immune system, and the endocrine organs that manage the production of atrial natriuretic factor (ANF), a hormone produced by specialized cells of the myocardium. It is involved in the control of the homeostatic balance of water, sodium, and potassium in the organism and in the control of lipid balance in the circulatory system. It also reduces the amount of lipids in the kidneys by lowering blood pressure.

FIFTH CHAKRA

Also called: Throat chakra
Color: Light blue/blue
Musical note: G
Primary landmark: In the center of the throat
Secondary landmarks: One under each collarbone, between the medial and the lateral epiphysis, and one connected to each anterior upper iliac ridge
Organs involved: Throat, thyroid, tonsils, larynx, vocal cords, esophagus

The fifth chakra relates to communication skills and creative expression in forms such as music, dance, art, and rhythm in general.

On a physical level, it is connected with the thyroid gland, which is the inner clock regulating growth and metabolism.

SIXTH CHAKRA

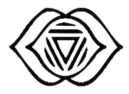

Also called: Third eye chakra
Color: Indigo/purple
Musical note: A
Primary landmark: In the middle of the forehead, on the glabella
Secondary landmark: A central one behind the eyes
Organs involved: Hypophysis (pituitary gland), brain, eyes, ears, nose

The sixth chakra relates to the ability to understand vibrational nonsensory reality; therefore, it relates to intuition and the vision of entities that normally cannot be perceived. It is connected with the third eye.

On a physical level, it is connected with the hypophysis, which influences all the other endocrine glands of the organism.

SEVENTH CHAKRA

Also called: Crown chakra
Color: Violet/white light/golden light
Musical note: B
Primary landmark: Aligned with the coronal suture at the center of the fontanelle (in the bregma)
Secondary landmarks: None
Organs involved: Epiphysis cerebri (pineal gland), brain

The seventh chakra is considered the seat of illumination, where the individual Self merges with the cosmic universal Self, the channel of the Higher Self; it accommodates mystical experiences of peace and bliss.

On a physical level, it is connected with the pineal gland, whose function relates to our adaptability to nighttime and daytime, development, growth, and aging in general.

SOME ORGANS WE HAVE NOT YET CONSIDERED

We have already examined some of the vital organs that are connected with the meridians. We are now going to introduce the anatomical functions and energetic characteristics of some of the other organs correlated to the chakras. Working through this selection of organs and systems serves to provide an essential and coherent view of the most important organic structures involved in the subjects of this text. Once we have considered all the main structures involved, we will be able to focus more consciously on the emotionality that is connected with each organ and/or system and its function in CST and SER treatments when dealing with situations of loss, death, small deaths, separations, abandonment, and bereavement.

Spinal Cord

The spinal cord, like the medulla oblongata, plays a role in protecting the brain from the pain coming from serious physical traumas by blocking the conduction of nerve impulses up to the brain stem.

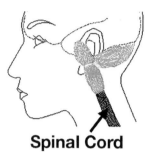

Fig. 16.2. Spinal cord

Hypophysis

The pituitary gland (or hypophysis) interprets cosmic symbols received from the universe through the pineal gland and translates them into concrete action. It can assume functions that concern the hippocampus and memory and contributes to problem-solving skills.

It balances dysfunctions of the endocrine system and problems connected with the brain, the spinal cord, and the immune system. Its posterior part plays a crucial role in renal functions.

Hypothalamus

This organ is the protagonist of the stress axis, also known as the hypothalamus/pituitary gland/adrenal cortex. It regulates and influences sleeping patterns (along with the reticular system), hunger, thirst, emotional and sexual behavior, body temperature, the endocrine glands, and the activation of the autonomic nervous system; it also regulates testosterone and plays a role in addiction.

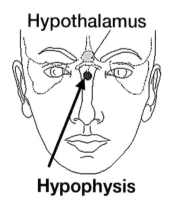

Fig. 16.3. Hypophysis and hypothalamus

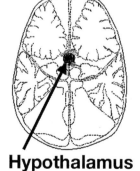

Fig. 16.4. Hypothalamus

Pineal Gland

The pineal body contains three magnetic crystals that allegedly point north, like an inner compass. Traumatic factors connected with electromagnetic pollution disturb the pineal gland. It orchestrates the integration of the body with the mind and the spirit. It also helps determine which energies gain access to the inside of the physical body. The pineal gland relates to the center—a structure connected with the hippocampus and the insular cortex of the brain—to control the third eye (sixth chakra) and the channeling process, thus acting as one of the greatest intermediaries between the universe and the earthly body. The center is a small anatomical structure that until recently has always been little considered. It is located inside the brain and is connected to the hippocampi and the insula. The main function of the center is to receive, filter, and convey the energetic connections between cosmic energy and the organs of our body.

The pineal gland is connected with the pituitary gland, which operates to create earthly harmony. It is a mediator between individual consciousness and the whole. It gets us closer to a type of spiritual wisdom that is useful to our conscious awareness. It reacts to light in the healing process.

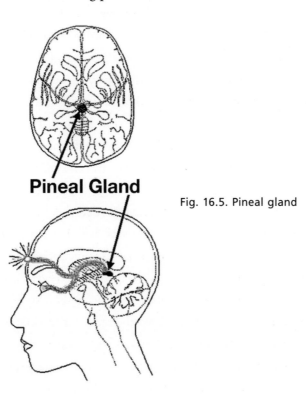

Fig. 16.5. Pineal gland

THE ROLE OF CHAKRAS IN WESTERN CULTURE

In traditional yogic disciplines, chakras are treated with techniques meant to rebalance or reharmonize them. In CST and SER, we employ the chakras solely as an energetic reference to work on the vector/axis system. We believe it is essential to learn the energetic connection of chakras in the human body and their correlation to the emotions that might be withheld in the organs.

To go into a bit more detail, we are now going to rely on texts written by scholars, instructors, and experts of yoga. We do not want to linger over the seven major chakras since information about them abounds in the literature on the subject. Rather, we will substantiate the choice of the secondary (or lower) chakras. As we have seen, secondary chakras, while generally less well known, are quite useful for tracing the map of the vector/axis system and gathering instructions and suggestions about the physical and emotional nature of an anomaly that has caused a misalignment of a vector from its axis.

Before we get started, let us first briefly mention the origins of chakras. They were first described in writing in texts dating back to before the fifth century that document tantric religious traditions of northern India. Most readers probably know that the term *chakra* is a Western adaptation derived from Sanskrit, the official Indian language that corresponds to ancient Greek and Latin as a matrix for modern Indo-European and Indian languages. The Sanskrit term that *chakra* derives from means "wheel," "disk," or "circle," all shapes that resemble the chakras.

In Indian religious tradition, chakras represent a mystical diagram that could be superposed to a mandala, symbolizing both the unity of existence and the centers that host the elements of the subtle body (or yogic body, the academic definition created by André Padoux to distinguish it from the transmigrant body). In the original tantric traditions that generated yoga and ayurvedic medicine, in Hinduism, and in Buddhism, they are centers where the divine energy and the energy of creation reside.

Many Indologists and Western scholars studied chakras through Indian philosophy, religion, and other cultural contexts. Some regarded them as mystical diagrams; some as tools to define different religious systems of different eras; some as reference in the context of practices that concern spiritual ascent; and others as an element of practices and rites meant to preserve good health in the body and balance in the spirit (also in beliefs that include reincarnation and/or metempsychosis).

Among the most famous Westerners who studied the doctrine of chakras, introduced it, and spread it outside the Eastern cultures is Sir John Woodroffe (1865–1936), a British Orientalist writer also known by the pseudonym Arthur Avalon. He was one of the first translators of an Indian text in Sanskrit on this subject and was also cited by psychologist Carl Jung.

Jung studied in depth the energetic charge of the chakras and saw in their potential an archetypical correlation with the unconscious life of the individual. He associated them with the source of psychosomatic disorders in cases of dysfunctions. In addition, he claimed that Western culture had not yet developed the awakening of cosmic consciousness, and he found some correspondences between the various levels of chakras and the levels of the identification and development process of individual consciousness with the Higher Self.[2]

Mircea Eliade (1907–1986), Romanian philosopher, historian, and writer, was one of Jung's students. He had a deep knowledge of Eastern philosophy, studied ancient texts directly from Sanskrit versions, and brought to the Western world the most important philosophic concepts of Indian religion, along with its practices and rituals. He considered chakras to be centers that represent yogic states and allow us to access transphysiological experiences, which would be inaccessible without a spiritual ascent.[3]

Charles Webster Leadbeater (1854–1934), British bishop, theosophist, occultist, and founder of the Liberal Catholic Church, was a controversial—and for some inconvenient—figure. He lived and studied in India for many years before returning to British society in London, where he continued to practice rituals and ceremonies that involved the subtle bodies and relied on the chakras and their triple nature, mandalas, and mantras. As writer Diego Fayenz describes some of Leadbeater's considerations:

> In the human psychophysical organism, we can notice a precise relationship between moral qualities, the development of latent powers, and the power centers or chakras. . . . Theosophical schemes representing the occult structure of man and the world and their respective planes and bodies can have similar properties when they are taken as meditation mandalas since they offer to those who meditate the ability to visualize archetypical realities existing in consciousness, thus establishing through intuition a psychological relationship between spiritual reality, the external scheme (mandala), and the individual.[4]

Rudolf Joseph Lorenz Steiner (1861–1925), founder of anthroposophy (a doctrine derived from theosophy), attributed to chakras the peculiarity of being the tools of perception for the astral body, just like the five senses for the physical body. According to Steiner, this function of the chakras becomes possible only after a person has done work to evolve spiritually and awaken the primary functions of the chakras. In his texts, Steiner provides instructions to activate the chakras, which, from his viewpoint, constitute power centers for opening up to inner development and the perception of the subtle worlds.

Contemporary Italian journalist Gabriele Burrini provides a brief introduction to the history of the chakras leading up to Steiner's anthroposophical interpretation:

> The wave of the New Age movement brought a wide and specific interest in chakras for purposes connected with health. In fact, chakras are energetic centers

whose activation can restore the natural psychophysical harmony of the human body when it is eroded by everyday tension and stress. This is the path chosen by Reiki, crystal healing, chakra chromotherapy, and aura balancing, in which generally a therapist/guru activates the chakras of the "patients" through the touch of their hands or by placing specific crystals or beams of light on their bodies. Indian yoga employs chakras very differently, since it regards them as stages of an inner path toward liberation, made by meditation on the scriptures, liturgical recitations of mantras, and self-regulation of breath and posture—a mystical or "mental" path opening human soul to the communication with the Absolute. . . . This "mental" path of the chakras belongs to Buddhism as well, even though it is absent in the Small Vehicle (Theravâda) and appears only in tantric Buddhism Vajrayâna, which developed in the 7th century and spread mostly in Tibet. . . . How can we recover the "internal map" or "fascinating geography of soul" connected with the world of spiritual archetype? One of the answers is the personal interpretation of the chakra system given by Rudolf Steiner in *Initiation and Its Results* and *An Outline of Esoteric Science*.[5]

So far, we have cited just some of the most authoritative figures who brought the practices involving chakras to the attention of the Western world. We could summarize the easily deducible conclusion of these paragraphs through the words of professor David G. White: "In fact, there is no 'standard' system of the *cakras*. Every school, sometimes every teacher within each school, has had their own *cakra* system."[6]

MEDICINE, YOGA, AND CHAKRAS

Nowadays, yoga is a common practice in the West and is generally well respected by the Western medical establishment. Western medicine also often takes interest in practices involving chakras—which are not so far removed from Leadbeater's and Steiner's initiation practices—to benefit human health.

We can return to the field of neuroscience and quote Candace B. Pert again, this time specifically in regard to chakras:

A bearded yogi dressed in white and wearing a turban showed up at my office one day to ask me if endorphins were concentrated along the spine in a way that corresponded to the Hindu chakras. The chakras, he explained, were centers of "subtle energy" that governed basic physical and metaphysical functions from sexuality to higher consciousness. I had no idea what he was talking about, but, trying to be helpful, I pulled out a diagram that depicted how there were two chains of nerve bundles located on either side of the spinal cord, each rich with many of the information-carrying peptides. He placed his own chakra map over my drawing and together we saw how the systems overlapped.[7]

THE LOWER CHAKRAS: DIVERSE COMMENTARIES

Let us now go through some specific details on the lower/secondary/minor chakras, with the aid of a selection of excerpts taken from articles and essays by various authors—some less known than others but interesting nonetheless—who offered their knowledge to associations, schools, websites, or blogs. Each of them adds, specifies, or confirms something about what we have said on the subject of chakras through a descriptive contribution, a personal view, and/or criticism.

Daniela Stranieri and Roberto Tulli for the association L'isolache non c'è (Neverland): "According to ancient Eastern traditions, chakras are 144,000 for some, or 88,000 or even 145 for others. This is due to the fact that there is no human way of calculating exact data in this respect. . . . Anterior chakras are usually connected with the sphere of emotionality, whereas the posterior ones are connected with will; those of the head are connected with reasoning. It is possible to have good physical health only if emotionality, will, and reasoning are all perfectly balanced.[8]

Annica on the blog *Sezione Aurea*: "Each Chakra is located in a specific sector of the body that contains a certain number of organs. For example, the 3rd Chakra includes the stomach, the small intestine, the large intestine, the liver, and the gallbladder, the spleen, and the pancreas, and each of these organs and viscera corresponds to a Meridian. . . . Therefore, anything concerning these Meridians concerns the 3rd Chakra as well."[9]

Gabriele Bettoschi on the website Lifegate: "Many emotional, psychological, and physical disorders can be explained through the energy flowing in our bodies. . . . By crossing, energy flows create actual energetic centers that have been called chakras since 3,000 years ago. . . . Each chakra is directly associated with a specific organ or endocrine gland of the physical body. The total number of the energy centers is very high—some ancient Hindu texts count more than 10,000 of them. . . . Quantum physics recently gave valid scientific support, succeeding in explaining chakras through the theory of vibrational energy. . . . This physical theory allows us to consider the physiological system invisible to human beings that was developed in ancient Hindu culture. . . . According to ayurvedic medicine, these centers are responsible for the overall project and quality of our life and indicate the areas where our vital functions are imbalanced."[10]

Felice Pascale for the nonprofit organization Dhyana: "Chakras are not only an expression of energy but also a connection with the universe since they are the union of spirit and matter manifesting as consciousness. . . . Chakras are energy and cyclicity constantly rotating. Although they cannot close, they may be blocked, causing imbalance and energetic disorders. . . . Studies highlight that illness represents the effort of the body toward the resolution of a deeper and more intimate malaise. Therefore, illness manifests not the dysfunction but rather the actions taken to resolve the dysfunction."[11]

The blog *Ascoltare la Vita* (Listen to Life): "We could say that chakras are points of intersection between different energetic levels of the individual, especially between physical, psychological-emotional, and spiritual levels. . . . Even though we cannot see the chakras, they can be recognized along our vertebral column from our posture and physical behaviors. . . . The system must be open to take and give energy. If functions are not balanced, the system becomes overloaded or empty. . . . Cultural conditioning, childhood trauma, restrictive or fatiguing habits, emotional or physical wounds, a way of thinking based merely on common places, and lack of attention all deprive us of our confidence and take us away from our center, causing us to develop defense strategies that later become chronic patterns. . . . The major chakras are seven, a sacred number; seven like the colors of the rainbow and the musical notes. . . . If one or more of the seven chakras are muted or dominate the others with their tone or color, there is no harmony but rather a cacophony; no homeostasis, but illness. . . . It means that some parts of us are disconnected. . . . The symptom is therefore energetic information about the disconnected part."[12]

The website Tradizione Sacra: "In ancient representations, chakras were depicted as flowers on a tree that symbolize the spinal cord since they accumulate the vivifying forces of a serpent-like flow originating from the area of the coccyx. Each chakra has two functions, an internal one and an external one, which means that they are responsible for a part of the body and provide a connection between this area and the surrounding environment. . . . Each energy center is not only the source of a certain type of energy but also surrounds the individual with energy, creating an ethereal, astral layer that can be 'denser' or 'subtler' and contains the mind, the desires, the perception of causality, and the soul."[13]

The blog *Moonboulevard:* "The lower or secondary chakras . . . are 21, located in correspondence with each eye, behind each ear, at the crossing of collarbones, in correspondence with the thymus, above each breast, in correspondence with the solar plexus, in correspondence with the stomach, two at the level of the spleen, on the liver, on the palm of the hands, in correspondence with gonads, behind each knee, under the soles of the feet. These chakras form at the meeting of 14 nadis, which represent a sort of subtle network of channels (*nadi* in Sanskrit means 'channel' or 'vein') whose function is to connect and convey vital energies (prana) through various subtle centers (chakras) of the human body to nourish different parts. The nadis cross along the column of the major and secondary chakras, which are preferential centers that allow contact between the material and the energetic body."[14]

Christopher Wallis (aka Hareesh) on his website: "The theory of the subtle body and its energy centers called *cakras* . . . comes from the tradition of Tantrik Yoga, which flourished from 600–1300 CE, and is still alive today. In mature Tantrik Yoga (after the year 900 or so), *every one* of the many branches of the tradition articulated a different chakra system. . . . Five-chakra systems, six-chakras systems, seven, nine, ten, twelve, twenty-one and more chakras are taught, depending on what text and lineage you're looking at. . . . Now, I know what you're thinking—'But which system is right? How many chakras are there really?' And that brings us to our first major misunderstanding. The chakras aren't like organs in the physical body; they aren't fixed facts that we can study like doctors study neural ganglia (with which the chakras were confused in the nineteenth century). The energy body . . . is an extraordinarily fluid reality, as we should expect of anything nonphysical and supersensuous. The energy body can present, experientially speaking, with any number of energy centers, depending on the person and the yogic practice they're performing. . . . All associations of the chakras with psychological states is a modern Western innovation that started with Carl Jung. . . . So when it comes to the chakras . . . tell your yoga students that every book on the chakras presents only one possible model."[15]

ALIGNING VECTORS TO THEIR AXIS WITH THE CHAKRAS

The preceding chapter offers two techniques for aligning vectors to their axis. Now we will look at yet another, whose objective is to align the vectors to their axis with the aid of chakras. When we identify an Energy Cyst that is causing a misalignment or disconnect of the vector lines, we can use the instructions offered by the physical and emotional nature of the chakra that corresponds to the location of said Energy Cyst and proceed with its dissipation.

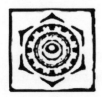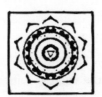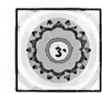

Fig. 16.6. The seven major chakras

With this technique, we may employ chakras on a solely energetic level:

- to visualize and map the vector/axis system
- to follow their rotating movement with our intention, as if they were handles that can move and realign a vector to its axis
- as magnets to anchor a vector to the energetic center of a chakra (which corresponds to the correct original landmark) from which the vector is misaligned;
- to identify the nature of one or more Energy Cysts in the organism, based on the related chakra's particular energy

The technique can be broken down into two phases, which we'll look at separately.

Visualization, Assessment, and Mobilization of Vectors through the Chakras: Phase One

As a Facilitator, it is useful to memorize the correspondences of the chakras so that as soon as you locate the misalignment of a vector, you can work on the specific energy of the chakras and meridians involved and thus dissipate the Energy Cysts in the body.

1. Use the first and seventh major chakras as directional poles to visualize the central axis and check its alignment (which should be a straight line between the poles).
2. Use all the other major and lower chakras to complete the map of the system (see fig. 16.7).
3. Place your hands on the two lower chakras of the feet to perceive and assess the position and alignment of the vectors in the vector/axis system.
4. Keeping your hands on the patient's feet, mobilize the vectors to cement the main axis—from the first to the seventh chakras—and use the energetic center of each chakra as a magnet to anchor it.
5. Proceed along the track of the secondary chakras of the lower limbs, first on the right side and then on the left, while you keep aligning the vectors to their axis. Pay attention especially to the junctions of the vectors at the level of the hips.
6. Do the same with the upper limbs and the scapular junctions.
7. Finally, place your hands on the sides of the head, at the level of the sixth chakra, and reassess the junctions and the alignment of the vectors with the central axis.

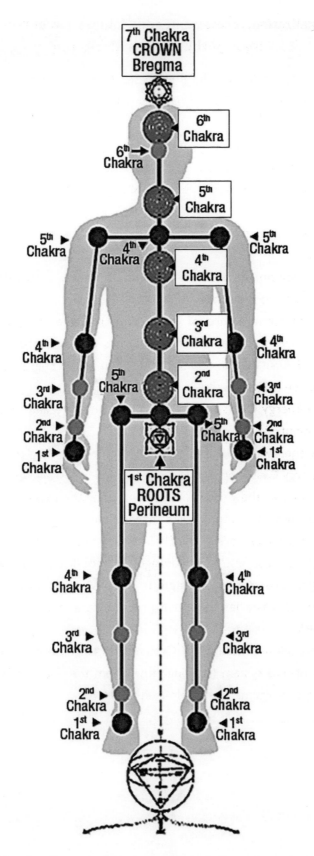

Fig. 16.7. Mapping the vector/axis system through the major and minor chakras

Visualization, Assessment, and Mobilization of Vectors through the Chakras: Phase Two

After the reassessment following the first phase, if one or more vectors still tend to misalign, we need to search for a deeper Energy Cyst, which has likely emerged after the release in phase one.

For the purposes of illustration, we will simulate the position of an Energy Cyst at the level of the fifth chakra, the throat chakra. The white arrows indicate the direction of the anomalous dislocation (see fig. 16.8).

1. Map and assess the vector/axis system again, as in the first phase, starting from the feet station.
2. Identify the position of the deviation, misalignment, or break of any of the vectors in relation to their axis.
3. Identify the energetic nature of the chakra(s) where the point(s) of break/misalignment/deviation of one or more vectors was detected.
4. Work on this information to locate the position of the Energy Cyst(s), using the Arcing technique (page 33).
5. Dissipate the Energy Cyst(s) using Therapeutic Imagery and Dialogue (page 39) or meridian emptying/filling (page 188).
6. Stabilize the energy flow in the meridian(s) corresponding to the chakra with which the Energy Cyst is energetically connected.
7. Realign energetically the vector/axis system, using the major and lower chakras as handles to move the vectors like magnets and make them adhere to their axis in the energetic centers of the chakras (see figs. 16.8 and 16.9). Remember that the vectors must first be encouraged to mobilize by inviting them to orientate on their axis. You will be able to perceive their movement, which can be fluid, with no obstacles; slow, with resistance in some spots; or still, then suddenly quick.
8. After the dissipation of the Energy Cyst(s) and realignment of the vectors, reassess the vector/axis system (starting either from the head or from the feet) to ensure that the realignment is stable (see fig. 16.10).

Chakras

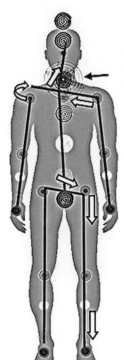

Fig. 16.8. Misalignment of vectors caused by an Energy Cyst at the level of the fifth chakra

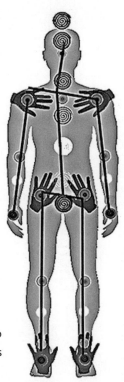

Fig. 16.9. Using chakras to realign the vectors

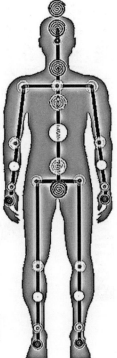

Fig. 16.10. The vector/axis system after realignment

Bodily Treatment with Energetic-Postural Assessment
Mobilization of Vector/Axis System
with the aid of the energetic map of Chakras

▲ Postural assessment of the Vector/Axis System
▲ Energetic assessment of Vectors through Chakras
▲ Energetic mobilization of Vectors
▲ Identification of the Energy Cyst
▲ Dissipation of the Energy Cyst
▲ Reassessment of the Vector/Axis System

Energy Cyst corresponding to the Throat Chakra

To realign the Vectors, we will work on the landmarks of lower Chakras and complete the dissipation of the Energy Cyst

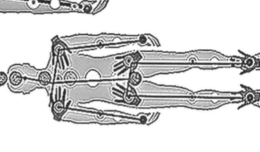

Fig. 16.11. Vector/axis system realignment through the chakras

Clinical Observations

One of my patients had a passion for cycling and defined himself as an amateur cyclist. Knowing that I am an osteopath and used to be a sports masseur for several cyclists and cycling teams in Great Britain, he asked for my help.

He told me that one morning, as he was cycling through a crossroad, a car did not give him the right-of-way when it should have and hit him. Though it was a mild bump, it knocked him off balance and he fell. He was bruised here and there, and later the arm and leg he had fallen on became quite painful.

The driver who hit him was on the phone at the moment of the accident and consequently did not realize what had happened. He continued on his way without stopping, leaving my patient there on the street.

My patient, who was a postman, lost a month of work because of the accident. Although the affected leg and arm were not fractured or broken, they kept hurting and swelling so much that the pain caused him to completely change his posture to compensate. Consequently, he was now feeling a series of undefined aches in most of his bony structure.

But the worst thing, he told me, was that he could not participate in a cycling race he had been training for. To train for this race, he had actually neglected most other aspects of his life. He said he was resigned to it, but it seemed to me that his stoic attitude was simply a facade.

I invited him to lie down on the therapy table. Even before he lay down, I distinctly saw that his body was out of axis.

Once he was on the table, I treated him with manipulative osteopathic techniques that seemed to give him relief. However, though I saw that his bony structure was realigned when assessing his posture, his body was still giving me conflicting signals on an energetic level.

I went on with the treatment and started assessing the vector/axis system.

I realized that some vectors of the patient's energetic framework were not aligned with their axes, so I used the Arcing technique to search for Energy Cysts in the patient's organism. I found two Energy Cysts that were causing a deviation of a vector in the proximity of the solar plexus chakra. That chakra is connected with the energy of anger that is held in the liver and the energy of disillusion held in the spleen.

I started treating the meridians of the liver and spleen, voiding them of the excessive energy they held, dissipating the Energy Cysts, and consequently rebalancing the third chakra.

After the implementation of these techniques, it was easy to realign the vector/axis system and make it stay that way for the long term. Finally, I had the impression that the physical and energetic frameworks were aligned and balanced.

After the treatment, the patient told me he was feeling reinvigorated and relieved. He had actually been extremely angered at the car driver, who prevented him from participating in the race, but he did not want to admit it in order to keep up his facade of making the best of a bad situation. He had realized that being abandoned on the ground without aid or comfort made him feel like the victim of an incredible injustice.

Before leaving my office, he told me he recognized that up until that moment, he had imposed on himself an extremely severe training, maybe too severe for an amateur. He decided he would let himself train a little less intensely, giving more space to his other interests.

CHAPTER 17

CST and SER in Grief

Support for the Living

We must be willing to get rid of the life we've planned, so as to have the life that is waiting for us.

JOSEPH CAMPBELL

We are going to examine more in depth the anatomy, physiology, functions, and emotions connected with the organs and systems most involved in grief. Our analysis will go hand in hand with CST and SER; therefore, it will be foundational for the Facilitator's treatments.

Before going through the main organs and systems involved in processes of separation, loss, death, small deaths, abandonment, and bereavement, we will offer a brief description of our anatomical-physiological perspective through the immortal words of the unforgettable neurologist Rita Levi-Montalcini (1909–2012), the first woman to be admitted to the Pontifical Academy of Sciences, who was awarded the 1986 Nobel Prize in Physiology or Medicine:

> Everybody says that the brain is the most complex organ in the human body, and, as a physician, I could agree. Nevertheless, as a woman, I assure you that there is nothing more complex than the heart, whose mechanisms continue not to be fully understood. In the reasoning of the brain there is logic, in the reasoning of the heart there are emotions.[1]

DEFINITIONS OF GRIEF

Traumatic grief follows a critical event, such as a death or sudden meaningful loss that was not expected or predicted. This type of grief is particularly complex to process. However, though it shares the same characteristics and relative consequences of psychological and emotional trauma, if it is addressed adequately, it will develop accordingly, and its processing will not last too long.

Complex (or complicated) grief, though not common, occurs when an individual is not able or does not have the chance to process and accept rationally a loss or its emotional and relational meaning. Consequently, the individual's discomfort never leaves, and emotional pain is amplified and becomes acute and constant, endangering the person's physical and psychological health and, in the most extreme cases, causing a psychopathology. This aspect of grief needs to be addressed with the intervention of external specialists who must help and guide the individual in the grieving process, transforming the scenario of acute psychological and emotional suffering into a grief that is processed naturally on a physiological level in the correct time.

Serious grief refers to a loss with a strong social or cultural meaning, in which the subject is involved along with an entire group of people, and the scenario of grief (e.g., a natural catastrophe, terrorist attack, etc.) takes on an unequivocal burden of pain. It often requires both an individual and a collective processing, with common practices on a cultural, religious, and/or ritual level.

Mild grief and half mourning designate the time needed to observe cultural and social traditions during the period reserved for mourning. From an anthropological point of view, this occurs both on a subjective level (for the person who is directly involved in the loss and consequent grief) and on a more general level (for those who are involved indirectly).

Micro-grief is the stage following a stressful and sudden change (a small death) that forces individuals to transform their lifestyle and has a strong impact on them, generating great suffering.

ANATOMY AND PHYSIOLOGY OF GRIEF

In our examination of loss, stress, and trauma, we are getting closer and closer to the subject of the loss of losses, death. We already know that death does not exist for the living since the living experience death only through the traumatic emotions connected with the fear of death or through the grieving process.

Later in this chapter, we will see how Dr. Upledger's CST and SER deal with the trauma experienced by those who are going through this particular moment of their existence, and we will clarify the role a Facilitator can play when intervening with individuals who have not processed grief adequately. We can never reiterate enough that grief is a common circumstance of everyone's Life Cycle since it represents the phase following an objective/subjective loss and the consequent trauma. In a case where the grieving process was not addressed or completed, the Facilitator might have to restore the functionality of the patient's specific organs and systems, releasing the destructive/entropic energy that is contained in them, which is energetically inhibiting the individual's process of self-realization during the path of their Life Cycle.

First, though, we need to introduce the organs and systems that are most involved in the various types of grief, on both a functional and an emotional level. Then the reader will be able to identify the consequences of grief on a person's health.

Fifth Diaphragm

The fifth diaphragm involves the ninth, tenth, and eleventh cranial nerves. It manages arterial blood flow in the head, venous drainage, and drainage of cerebrospinal fluid through the jugular veins. The fifth diaphragm must be released to restore the functionality of all the other structures involved.

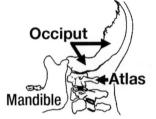

Fig. 17.1. Occiput and atlas

Compression Triad

The bony structures involved in what is defined in CST as the compression triad (or depression triad) are the sphenobasilar synchondrosis, the fifth diaphragm, and the L5–S1 junction. If more than one of these three joints is dysfunctional, it is necessary to work on all of them to restore their functionality.

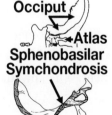

Fig. 17.2. Compression triad

Vagus System

The vagus system is part of the autonomic nervous system, whose mediator is the vagus nerve. The vagus nerve is the tenth cranial nerve and is the longest in the the human body. It innervates all the fascia surrounding the viscera. The vagal system includes all the organs and viscera that are crossed by the vagus nerve and pertains to the parasympathetic nervous system (which in turn is part of the autonomic nervous system). The vagus system is likewise responsible for the functionality of all the organs connected with constructive and destructive emotions.

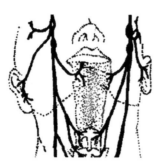

Fig. 17.3. Vagus system

Third Ventricle

This biological structure is the second most involved in experiences of grief. In fact, the third ventricle could be defined as "the heart of the brain." It withholds emotions in general and sadness specifically.

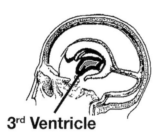

Fig. 17.4. Third ventricle

Amygdala

When an individual is unconscious (e.g., anesthetized or comatose), the amygdala can "see and feel" what the individual would see and feel if they were conscious, and these paired organs withhold the fear of that moment. The amygdala can be treated with the technique of Direction of Energy technique (page 143).

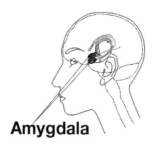

Fig. 17.5. Amygdala

Fornix

The fornix is the fundamental structure of the limbic system. Its fibers originate in the hippocampus. It helps the two hemispheres cooperate with each other and constitutes the main seat of trust.

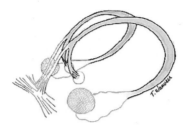

Fig. 17.6. Fornix

Hippocampus

The hippocampus is located inside the temporal lobes, which deal with recent memory and emotional fear. It relates directly to the olfactory nerve, the first nerve that forms in the embryonic stage and reaches the limbic system without interacting with the reticular system. The hippocampus holds the emotional memory of olfactory events, especially those connected with fear. Dysfunctions of the hippocampus are the main cause for anxiety.

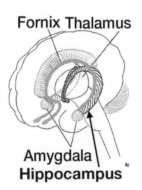

Fig. 17.7. Hippocampus

Medulla Oblongata

One of the functions of the medulla oblongata is to protect the brain by blocking excessive information and impulses—pain in particular—that come from the peripheral nervous system. One possible dysfunction of the medulla oblongata manifests through obsessive and/or compulsive behavior in response to an excess of impulses that are not stopped before arriving to the brain.

The medulla oblongata is connected with the cerebellum, which can inhibit SER as a defense when the medulla oblongata decodes the experience of SER as premature for the patient. That is why it is essential to have a direct and honest dialogue with the cerebellum and the medulla oblongata during SER.

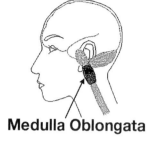

Fig. 17.8. Medulla oblongata

The medulla oblongata holds the experience of past, present, and future, making them available to the structure that Dr. Upledger called "center."

Cerebral Cortex

This is the gray matter covering both hemispheres. It is constituted by six layers, each with a specific function. The cerebral cortex manages the instincts (limbic system).

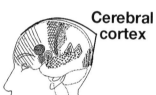

Fig. 17.9. Cerebral cortex

Locus Coeruleus

Located in the brain stem, the locus coeruleus is part of the pons and constitutes the floor of the fourth ventricle. When an event activates a series of physiological changes, the locus coeruleus releases noradrenaline and norepinephrine. That is why it sometimes plays a role in emotions involving anger, pleasure, and aggressiveness.

The locus coeruleus is involved in memory and sleep (or rest) processes, the perception of pain, anxiety, and the regulation of mood and appetite.

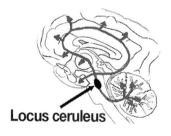

Fig. 17.10. Locus coeruleus

Thalamus

The thalamus detains about 50 percent of the pain perceived by the system, thus protecting the brain. It holds the key to the record/experience of the second half of life. It is functional in long-term memory and stimulates the conception of the first memory of our existence.

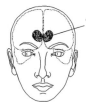

Fig. 17.11. Thalamus

Cerebellum

The cerebellum is the most ancient part of our central nervous system and is involved in our perception of loss and death through the vagus nerve. This structure authorizes the emergence of memory into consciousness when it is useful for our health and personal development.

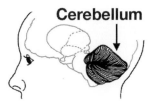

Fig. 17.12. Cerebellum

Vagus Nerve

The vagus nerve, or tenth cranial nerve, innervates all the viscera, which is why it is sometimes called the "parasympathetic queen." As part of the parasympathetic system, it manages the control and regulation of the human organism in the phases of

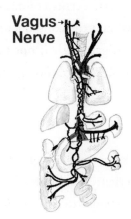

Fig. 17.13. Vagus nerve

rest, sleep, digestion, and assimilation and elimination of nutrients even when the organism is not ready to take action.

The vagus system has a huge influence on cardiac functionality and breathing.

Its nuclei are inserted in the medulla oblongata, which filters the information directed to the brain. This includes the memories about the interruptions of the vital energy continuum, which, as traumatic events, can cause dysfunctions to the vagus system.

The vagus nerve also has several interactions with the RAS, which consequently can cause palpitations, nausea, and so on.

Limbic System

The limbic system (of the mammalian brain) is the seat of our emotions and can be accessed through the intention and one of the cranial vault holds. After employing the hold, when the individual's emotionality is expressed, we can access the neocortex to find a constructive solution to dissipate and transform the destructive energy caused by trauma.

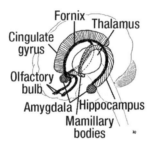

Fig. 17.14. Limbic system

ASPECTS OF GRIEF

We are going to continue our analysis of the various typologies of grief by exploring its aspects and connotations from different perspectives: neurobiology, philosophy, anthropology, psychology, and psychotherapy. We must always keep in mind that we are still exploring the emotional side of traumatic events connected with a loss and observations on the ways they can be managed and the consequent outcomes. This is such a wide topic that it is impossible to investigate fully if not through the attestations of neurobiologists, authors, philosophers, and psychologists and the explanations of their approaches in this respect.

Neurobiology of Grief

Neurobiology mainly studies the neural structures involved in the emotional response to a specific significant event experienced subjectively and the biological modifications occurring in the organism in response to said event.

Virginia Valentino, psychologist, cognitive behavioral psychotherapist, and EMDR therapist specifically dealing with PTSD (post-traumatic stress disorder) patients, writes:

> The combined activation of a series of subcortical and cortical cerebral structures is typical of emotions. . . . Each structure plays a specific and differentiated role depending on the type of emotion involved. . . . In addition to well-known structural and functional investigation systems such as fMRI and PET, these roles are now studied also through an even more innovative technology, diffusion tensor imaging . . . which assesses fiber circuits and their functioning. . . . We now consider the structures of the limbic lobe as crucial cerebral structures for emotional processing and regulation . . . whereas the structure that represents the ultimate neurological basis for emotional states is the amygdala . . . which sends several connecting pathways to the hypothalamus and the brain stem that are essential to activate vegetative and endocrine motor reactions connected with the emotion. . . . The amygdala is activated by extremely intense emotional experiences, especially when the emotional tone is markedly negative, but it is also involved in the decoding of noteworthy social information. . . . Behaviors involving either the inhibition or the liberation of specific attitudes and the modulation of internal states are selected according to the information about the environmental, sociocultural, and interpersonal context.[2]

Contemporary Western Philosophy of Grief

Bearing in mind that grief is a reaction to not just death but to any event that involves loss, we are going to briefly examine the opinions of some philosophers in this respect and their analysis of bereavement and loss in the Western world.

Umberto Galimberti, a professor of philosophy and critic and translator of the work of German philosopher and psychiatrist Karl Jaspers (1883–1969), defines grief as "the psychological state following the loss of a meaningful object that used to be an integral part of existence. Said object could be external, like in the case of the death of another person, a geographical separation, or leaving a place, or internal, such as the loss of an opportunity, the loss of one's own social image, a personal failure, or similar occurrences." He notes:

> Usually, suffering requires thoughtfulness and grief requires processing, but in our society, which gives value mostly to extroversion and efficiency, thoughtfulness and privacy are viewed with suspicion, and the grieving process is immediately suppressed by an action taken with the purpose of erasing loss and pain. Nonetheless, actions are not able to accomplish this objective, since it should be the soul's task to address pain and integrate it by accepting it in one's own life.[3]

Roberto Garaventa, another professor of philosophy, analyzes grief primarily as the response to the occurrence of an absence, which is a sort of contemplation of the nothingness that is imposed on the individual after a void takes the place of something that used to be present in our perception and experience. That is almost like Aristotle's theory of *horror vacui,* according to which all nature—and consequently also human nature—rejects emptiness and lives or survives attempting to fill it. In the critical analysis we are going to cite, Garaventa focuses on Karl Jaspers's work:

> According to Jaspers, nihilism is psychologically an inescapable stage of life that aspires to become aware of itself. All that is dead, all that appears definitive, . . . must in fact be questioned if a new form of life is to rise. . . . "Being-beyond-being," "super-being," "authentic being" . . . it is only this kind of nothingness (identified with the being of Transcendence) that is able to give meaning to the individual's life outside the possibility of the nothing of nihilism and the nothing of death.[4]

Mario Mapelli, philosopher, psychologist, and professor of communication psychology, proposes his philosophical-pedagogical perspective on grief by defining it as an "educational modality in the exercise of life experience." Here is a brief excerpt of his own explanation of this perspective:

> Grief is a constructive occurrence in the life of all individuals, an existential condition that we all go through. It is a change that is suffered, not searched for. . . . The objective of pedagogic reflection and practice is to offer spaces and tools to interpret change, so that our existence does not keep changing without us. . . . In John Dewey's reflection, experience is the bridge-concept between the events scattered in everyone's existence and their potential educational meaning. All experiences are located in continuum and cannot be conceived as existing by themselves. . . . Dramatic events interrupting the usual everyday linearity introduce in the individual's biography discontinuity, which forces them to find new meaning (crucial moments of personality reorganization, such as peak experiences or landmark events). Karl Jaspers defined as "limit situations" the experiences that force the subject to address their own historical-cultural conditioning (death, guilt, fight, pain). In situations of acute pain and discomfort, we tend to make ourselves emotionally impenetrable and close in ourselves to defend ourselves from the outside world. Processing implies a cognitive and emotional effort that the individual needs to make by themselves, and it takes time; it implies the possibility of postponing action. The educational space must take the shape of a place of retreat and transformation. . . . Every transformation implies a "passage of

state" and therefore contemplates within it the death of what we used to be. We all resisted to an infinite number of "small deaths" connected with disappointment, abandonment, and renouncement. "Transforming death into life" is the processing task of an education that treasures the subjectivation of the individual in their search for meaning. Experiences concerning loss take root in an original experiential and emotional ground. If coming out from our mother's womb is an observable and circumscribed event, the psychological birth of the individual is a slow development happening on an inner level through relational meditation. It is only through the succession of experiences of separation and reconstruction, frustration and satisfaction, loss and recovery that the child starts to become aware of its own existence as an autonomous entity. The processes that are involved in the processing of the original separation are reactivated in all the existential phases of change. . . . Grief can be seen as the restoration of our own internal world. . . . Grief is first a time we live and experience, a suspended time of profound internal transformation.[5]

Anthropology of Grief

The English term *grief* derives from the Latin verb *gravo* (burden). The Italian term *lutto* derives from the Latin verb *lugeo* (mourn). The grieving process depends both on the personality of the individual and on the incidence of the sociocultural models they are aware of (e.g., philosophical models, religious models, etc.). Anthropology explores the scenarios of grief in different societies, ethnicities, and cultures, documenting traditional ritual practices in various historical and geographical contexts.

When it comes to the death of a loved one, anthropologists generally agree on the existence of two main aspects of grief. The first is the ritual dimension, whose objective is mostly to exorcise loss itself, death, and the fear of dying (Western concept); the second is the celebration of life, in which death is perceived as a natural and integral part of life, even when it is framed by threatening connotations that connect it to extreme situations (Eastern concept).

The communal context in which grief is addressed is the main focus of anthropology in this context. In the Western world, grief is more easily addressed as a private issue, whereas in the Eastern world and much of the southern hemisphere, grief is seen as a more communal type of suffering.

Following the death of a loved one, the period of mourning is addressed in so many different ways that it is unimaginable to summarize them here.

Faced with the infinite variety of expressions of grief, ranging from extreme anguish to strict self-control, it is reasonable to investigate the relationship between the suffering caused by death and the expressions that culture dictates, conditioning the reality of feelings through its norms. Psychology generally regards emotions as profound and universal biopsychological processes with a constant substratum that is not conditioned by the sociocultural environment. The anguish and work that grief represents, with its tendency to oscillate between denial and acceptance of the event, should therefore be universal. Anthropology has recently started to address emotions, not so much as deep processes and their respective physiological manifestations, but more as the "discourse," the symbolic forms through which emotions are expressed, described, and managed. The concepts associated with emotions mimic external cultural patterns and reflect on an ideological level the forms of social relationships.[6]

Other scenarios of grief may emerge in wider communal contexts, though they can be equally personal. One need only think of the radical life changes caused by collective and sociocultural losses, with a consequent modification of the habits of an entire community, such as those arising from wars, mass murders, racial and religious purges, loss of charismatic leaders, territorial changes, and natural catastrophes.

To sum up, we could say that grief is commonly defined as the period in which a slow and painful process of acceptance/internalization of loss (and its context) occurs. During this process, individuals experience conflict while searching for a redefinition of their own identity.

To explain it in a more anthropological way, unconscious cultural and social sediments cause thoughts and feelings to emerge and activate a defense mechanism against loss.

In the contemporary Western world and its technology-dominated culture, we observe more and more cases of removal of bereavement and death, as well as the tendency to trivialize the traumatic charge of these events, which can be identified with the stage of denial.

Another evident and often inevitable tendency of contemporary Western society is to reduce grief almost entirely to an individual psychological phenomenon. That is exactly the opposite of the cultural habits of times and/or societies in which all the people were and/or are used to taking part in another person's grieving process and witnessing it as a community, giving their support to the individual.

Unlike the current Western context, other cultures, conventionally defined as "traditional," require that the community assists the dying and the grieving and takes care of the ritual conventions that are meant to restore the balance of social relationships that has been threatened by loss. In this way, the individual and the cultural components integrate with each other and are able to interact.

Therefore, grief is a situation identifiable through different spatiotemporal, environmental, and cultural coordinates. The time and rhythm of grief, the places designated for the activities connected with it, the acceptance of individual and/or collective responsibilities, the type of social relationships and role models this context dictates, and the roles proposed as an alternative to the latter are determined by the sociocultural context in which loss takes place.

Every aspect of grief always brings us to consider at least some of the objective conditions and responses connected with the needs of those who are suffering from loss:

- biophysical response
- psychological response (repetitions, explanations, reconstructions)
- emotional response (alternations of means of communication, avoidance, invectives)
- behavioral reactions (change in personality, change of perspectives and attitudes in the social environment)

Even post-traumatic stress disorder (PTSD), which was specifically noted by Dr. Upledger and the therapists of the Upledger Institute International's staff in the Upledger CranioSacral Immersion Report, is relevant to some of the abovementioned scenarios.[7]

KÜBLER-ROSS'S FIVE STAGES OF GRIEF

One of the best-known analyses of the behavior of people in mourning is that of Swiss psychologist Elisabeth Kübler-Ross, whose studies led her to become the founder of psychothanatology (or psychological thanatology). This field focuses on the stages of the grieving process in order to understand how to offer psychological support both to the terminally ill in the process preceding death and to the relatives and loved ones of a dying or deceased person during their grieving process.

Kübler-Ross describes the grieving process as divided into five stages that everyone has to go through when they are forced to deal with:

- a difficult objective loss or separation (situations/scenarios representing grief)
- the diagnosis of a serious physical pathology (bereavement as a subjective loss that will change permanently the individual's health and approach to life)
- a diagnosis announcing a person's own imminent death (the loss of losses)

We are now going to examine the five stages of grief as they are presented in thanatology with an eye to CST and SER and everything we have evaluated so far.

For each stage, we are going to consider the most involved organs, systems, meridians, and chakras, without ever forgetting the following:

- The body is a unit.
- Structure and function are interconnected.
- The whole is greater than the sum of its parts.

Stage 1: Denial (Rejection)

In this first stage, denial is the defense mechanism that prevents any objective examination of the reality of the event. It is caused by the individual's perception, which makes such reality seem unbearable. The individual is not able to process or accept the loss or even come up with possible strategies to overcome the trauma. This first stage can result in shock and stupefaction, but in the worst and most pathological cases, the individual may suppress the trauma completely.

Organs and systems:	Reticular system, pericardium, heart, kidneys
Meridians:	Kidneys (to dissipate shock and fear)
	Heart (to dissipate the emotions of shock)
	Pericardium and heart (for deep pain)
	Lungs (to restore the life continuum and dissipate pain and fear)
Chakras:	First (to remedy uprooting and restore the functions of the kidneys and adrenal glands)
	Fourth (to dissipate the pain connected to emotional pain and restore renal homeostasis)
	Sixth (to widen perspectives)
	Seventh (to reconnect with the Higher Self)

Stage 2: Anger

Anger can be expressed in different ways by different individuals, the most common being the usually immediate outburst toward other people (even loved ones), toward a higher entity, or even toward themselves.

This stage is extremely delicate on the relational level because it might coincide with a cry for help or, on the contrary, with a complete withdrawal. Nevertheless, the stage of anger hides another functional mechanism, in this case one that prevents the individual from facing the sense of sadness or deep fear that inevitably emerges after a loss.

Organs and systems:	Liver, amygdala, fifth diaphragm
Meridian:	Liver (to dissipate anger)
Chakras:	Third (to dissipate the effects of anger)
	Fifth (to restore communication with the external world and inhibit the implosion)
	Seventh (to restore communication with the Higher Self)

Stage 3: Bargaining (Negotiation, Compromise)

In the third stage, the individual starts to assume a planning attitude, motivated solely by the hope for a positive solution. According to their personal values, they may use all their energies in promises, compromises, and negotiations with themselves, someone else, or a higher entity since they are prone to believe in the prospect—often delusive—of a favorable and positive outcome that could fix the present situation.

In this stage, the individual may make resolutions like *If I get back what I have lost—health, a relationship, the chance to have a long life, etc.—I promise I will . . .*

This is also the stage in which individuals try to take control of their own life by fixing what can actually be fixed, even if their endeavor causes a profound sadness and they still do not deal with the problem, wishing instead for a return to way things were before the trauma.

Organs and systems:	Lungs, spleen, third ventricle
Meridians:	Lungs (to restore the energy flow)
	Spleen (to dissipate disappointment)
Chakras:	Second (to reactivate energy and restore self-esteem)
	Third (to gain confidence in oneself or others)
	Fourth (to dissipate sadness)

Stage 4: Depression

The stage of depression is actually the first real moment of awareness of loss, whether that loss is occurring, has occurred, or is about to occur, and it precedes the solution of grief. It is often characterized by an increase in physical and/or emotional pain. In this stage, the obvious irreversible nature of the loss and the consequent and inevitable new life situations/scenarios that will follow are not denied anymore.

Depression can manifest in two different ways, both characterized by a renewed awareness of the situation. The first is acknowledgment of every objective aspect of the loss (e.g., powerlessness, loss of social relationships, loss of the previous aspect of the body). The second arises from anticipation of other possible losses that could be encountered in the future as a consequence of the loss that has occurred. The individual acknowledges for the first time that it is useless to resist, and depression takes the place of the emotions of the previous stages, which now look pointless in the process of dealing with the loss. The more the individual recognizes that the loss is not reversible, the more they experience the depressive stage.

Organs and systems:	Limbic system, compression triad
Meridian:	Liver (to reactivate the energy of trust, dynamism, and courage)
Chakra:	Sixth (to reactivate the ability to envision the future)

Stage 5: Acceptance

In the last stage, individuals have processed the new life situation/scenario; they are now aware of their own condition and accept it. Should remnants of the previous stages partially persist or tend to come back, they lose their intensity.

This stage has a strong communicative component and is also called restitution stage since the individual takes care of everything that needs to be and can be fixed both on a practical and an inner/spiritual level. It is the stage in which everything is arranged in a present space/place in order to gain access to a future space/place.

Organ and system:	Cerebral cortex
Meridians:	Kidneys (to dissipate fear)
	Pericardium (to open the heart)
Chakra:	Seventh (to reconnect on a spiritual level)

According to thanatology, the development of a grieving process is positive when an individual passes through the five stages in succession. It is extremely rare, however, for this path to be linear. Especially at the beginning of the process or until the fourth stage, it is more common for someone who is grieving to go back and forth from one stage to another.

In undeveloped grief, the stages become chronically cyclical because they are badly handled or the individual is stuck in one of the first four stages. This condition usually occurs when individuals are afraid, sometimes even on an unconscious level, that they will not be able to deal with future emotions, which are generally connected with the following stage. For example, they may prefer to remain in an angry state that they already know and control (known scenario) rather than face a sadness that they think they will not be able to handle (unknown situation/phase).

Even more frequently, individuals are afraid to overcome the depressive stage, which can last even for years, because they know that by doing so they will have to take full responsibility for their own life. In fact, for some, getting through this stage means being forced to admit that they cannot any longer depend on someone else to deal with their psychical and emotional needs and that they have to end any psychological and emotional dependence in order to go on.

It is interesting to note that Kübler-Ross, in her everyday clinical experience with patients and their families in contexts of death during life, came to the conclusion that death is not the end of everything. She offered her personal reasoning on that in her book *Death Is of Vital Importance: On Life, Death, and Life after Death*.

THERAPEUTIC INTERVENTION IN THE GRIEVING PROCESS

We are now going to introduce the working method Facilitators should use when addressing grief with patients and their families through CST and SER, always bearing in mind that grief is mainly the product of a trauma due to an objective or subjective loss; as such, in some cases it might be expressed through some pathological aspects that need to be dealt with.

CST therapists can intervene and give their support in any stage of the grieving process, which, as we have seen, can be considered in cases of small deaths (small losses or changes of state), separation and/or abandonment (in any phase of the Life Cycle), or objective/subjective loss (including physiological losses).

The Facilitator's intervention can be extremely useful, especially with individuals who have not processed one or more stages of the grieving process and have subsequently allowed destructive consequences to ensue, or in cases that require external support during any of the stages of grief.

When the grieving process is insufficient or does not develop at all, the Facilitator may have to restore the functionality of specific organs and systems in the patient's body in order to release the destructive energy they contain and allow the patient to proceed on their path toward self-realization.

Those who proceed gradually in processing grief and consciously reach the last stage—whether they do so with the help of a Facilitator or by themselves—will likely avoid any regression and experience milder setbacks during the earlier stages. If patients are supported as they face and come to accept sadness due to a loss (third stage) in order to successfully process it, it will be almost impossible for them to revert to an earlier phase, like denial. By doing so and following their own natural rhythm, they will reach the stage of acceptance; pain will diminish, transform into a new constructive opportunity, and disappear.

However, remember that grief is witnessed and experienced not only by those who suffer the objective loss of a loved one or an important relationship. Other conditions, such as degenerative diseases or terminal illnesses, can feel exactly like an irreversible loss, even when they are not associated with a loss in the individual's personal sensory sphere.

Supporting Grieving Families with CST and SER

In a family, the emotional display of grief might reflect various hierarchical dimensions established within the family unit itself, behaviors or affect prescribed by the family's community or society, or concepts about life and death shared and accepted by the whole family.

It is the Facilitator's task to identify the specificity of the environment in which each person expresses grief and then assess the emotionality and treat it, taking into account the interactions in the family unit. By following the correct approach and listening, the Facilitator can carry out the therapeutic action:

- supporting the family in assisting their loved one until the person's death
- facilitating the grieving process of those who outlive their loved one to help them find a new balance
- supporting those who were subjected to the abandonment of or separation from someone who used to have a significant role within the family

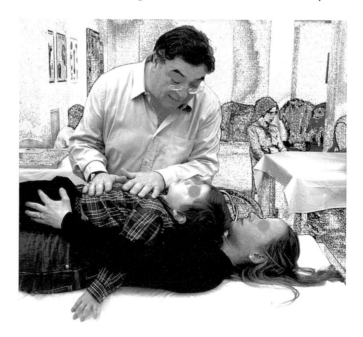

Fig. 17.15. CranioSacral Therapy to support the family unit

Grief, Separation, and Loss
The Experience of Death for the Living

▲ The experience of death for the living is represented by the period in which the person is grieving.

▲ The most common causes of grief are:
  – an irreversible loss;
  – a separation (from a loved person);
  – being abandoned.

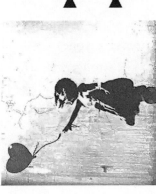

M.K. Banksy

▲ CST deals with grief as a TRAUMA (traumatic event) that might lead to a pathological outcome.

▲ The elaboration of grief is subjective and mainly depends on:
  – the personality of the single individual;
  – conscious sociocultural models (religious, philosophical, etc.).

▲ The intervention of the CST Facilitor might be helpful to:
  – subjects who have not elaborated their grief (causing the permanence of destructive consequences;
  – individual grieving processes;
  – the grieving process of a family.

Fig. 17.16. Training course slide: CST and SER support to bereavement

Ten Key Points

1. Pay great attention to what sort of help you were asked for and which member of the family asked for your help.
2. Explain to the grieving family the role of CST and SER Facilitators.
3. Communicate simply and frankly, using clear and unequivocal words, and do not judge.
4. Access your experience, personal skills, and abilities.
5. Do not comment; only make the situation explicit.
6. Remember that life means transforming constructively.
7. Remember that everything is possible; nothing is predictable. It is possible to win even at the last instant of the last second of the last minute.
8. Do not interfere or get involved in the living state of the family, but empathize with them (practice empathy, not sympathy).
9. Call emotions by their names and never trivialize them.
10. Listen. Do *not* assume.

Correct Approach: Happiness Is a Birthright

As Facilitators, when helping people who are going through a period of their Life Cycle involving grief due to a loss/separation/abandonment, we must care for patients with respect and remind them that happiness is a birthright that no one—except ourselves sometimes—can take away from us. Already inside each individual are all the tools needed to fight destructive feelings and emotions. By using the same frequency and energy, we are all able to make useful emotions and resources emerge to constructively benefit our own life and the lives of others.

In life changes, the real change lies in the correct attitude, not in the loss.

In their work, Facilitators should always rely on the correct attitude while considering the following factors we have analyzed:

- The Ego is one of the greatest obstacles in the Facilitator's work. We must give up our Ego, which is a childish modality, in order to rely completely on our Higher Self.
- Each loss, separation, abandonment, and bereavement needs to be dealt with and processed correctly. Loss can become an opportunity for anyone.
- The more unsolved traumas found in an individual, the stronger the stress associated with life changes. Work on ourselves can help us transmit indirectly what we have learned, even to the people around us.

CELEBRATION OF LIFE THROUGH GRIEF

In some Eastern and African communities, the grieving process is faced and experienced as a celebration of the lives of "those who are not with us here this day." Their constructive aspects and actions, both as individuals and as part of the community, are relived and remembered by others. That is a way to pass on the heritage of the deceased, made not of material goods but of examples and lessons, anecdotes, and moments of peaceful affection—all things that are useful to support the good life and peace of those who live and to awaken gratefulness for the journey they have shared with those who passed away.

Clinical Observations

My students and I treated patients at the hospital La Mandria of Padua, in a unit for people who were seriously incapacitated. One of our patients here was a woman who had been hospitalized for ten years, having been diagnosed with a permanent vegetative coma caused by postoperative complications. As opposed to other patients of that hospital wing, this woman had a particularly severe expression on her face, and for that reason few were eager to treat her. Even after treating her with the Still Point to relax her fascial system and parasympathetic nervous system, she continued to look tense and austere.

The patient's daughter was a police officer who used to constantly assist her. She had visited her every day prior to the coma.

Once, while I was treating the patient, I arced with the Arcing technique and found an Energy Cyst in the area of the pericardium. In that moment I came up with the idea to treat the woman through her daughter, using the Therapeutic Imagery and Dialogue.

I explained to her daughter how I wanted to proceed, telling her that I wanted to communicate with her mother through her. The daughter would sit on a chair by the bed and place her hands on the mother's pericardium area (the pericardium and heart chakra); at the same time, I would place my hands on the daughter's thighs (one of the listening stations of CST) and listen to the craniosacral rhythm while I asked the mother some questions. The mother, who obviously was not able to talk because of her condition, would answer through her daughter's voice.

When I proposed the treatment to the daughter, I was not sure I could actually do it. But after the first approach with this technique, the daughter said she was astounded by how natural this "thing"—as she called it—felt to her. Suddenly, the daughter started telling me about some of her mother's most private and intimate life experiences, which she herself had never heard about. Through her daughter, the mother said she had felt torn apart by a choice she should have made before the coma occurred.

Afterward, the daughter told me that her mother had been estranged from her hometown because she had gotten pregnant when she was very young. Since she did not want to have an abortion, she had moved to another region, where she delivered her child, which was the daughter I was talking to. Shortly after that, she had started living with a man who took care of both her and the daughter.

What the daughter did not know, and what we discovered during the treatment, was that her mother had been in another relationship and had wanted to leave her partner to move in with the other man, but she thought it was morally unjust to leave the partner who had done so much for her and her daughter. Moreover, her daughter was extremely fond of the man and considered him her father figure. The mother realized that if she did not want to abandon her current partner, she had to cut ties with the other man.

During this period of emotional stress, she had undergone a surgical operation that should have been just a routine procedure. Her daughter had gone to the hospital with her and trustfully waited for the surgery to end. Unfortunately, her mother had come out of the operation room in a vegetative coma.

During the treatment that was facilitating the communication between the mother and the daughter, we saw that the more the dialogue developed, the more the mother's face relaxed.

The daughter was astonished by what she was being able to do and, even more, by the fact that she was discovering in such a way a part of her mother's life that was so intimate and secret.

The last thing the mother communicated through her daughter was that the coma helped her avoid making any difficult decision about her life, but she had one single wish, which now had become true, and it was to confess everything to her daughter.

At the end of the session, the daughter was psychologically broken down, but her mother's face was almost radiant. Her muscles were relaxed, and as soon as her daughter, who had participated in this process of transformation, realized that she was seeing her mother's expression free of the grimness that had characterized it for so long, she became more serene as well.

Both women had gone through a transformation, finding in an unconventional situation the way to rebuild their relationship, even if it was in a different and unexpected life scenario.

❧ A CST-CENTRED VISION ❧

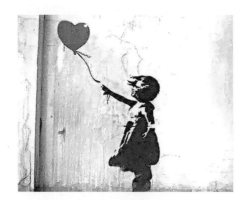

Fig. 17.17. Photograph of *There Is Always Hope,* by Banksy

Banksy is the pseudonym of an artist who is considered one of the greatest street art "writers." His piece *There Is Always Hope* (fig. 17.17) was made to symbolize the fight (of ideals and solidarity) to support those who are subjected to mass murders and wars all over the world (such as in Palestine, Syria, or other Middle Eastern countries). In the context of CST and SER, it offers a new perspective on energetic continuity to those who are grieving; the heart balloon is flying away, but it floats in the sky, bringing a message of unconditional love.

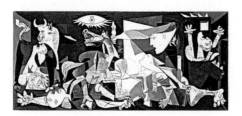

Fig. 17.18. Reproduction of *Guernica,* by Pablo Picasso

Picasso's cubist *Guernica* (fig. 17.18) depicts the scene of devastation following the Nazi aerial bombardment of Guernica, a city in the Basque region of Spain, during World War II. He created the piece to commemorate the victims of that carnage. It ranks among the most meaningful artworks to represent the concept of collective loss changing the life of a community. It also can symbolize the internal scenario of the individual who goes through these terrible experiences.

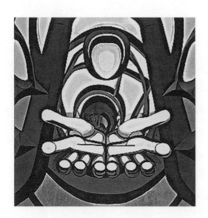

Fig. 17.19. Reproduction of *Our Present Image,* by David Alfaro Siqueiros

David Alfaro Siqueiros was a Latin American muralist, a forerunner of modern street artists. He painted many murals portraying realistically social topics with a strong political connotation. *Our Present Image* (fig. 17.19) shows symbolically and passionately a scenario of suffering and subjective privation and loss. Though representing the idea of loss connected with unjust events, it contains an element of an exhortation to recover personal dignity. Situations culminating with grief often burden us with a pain that stuns us, annihilates us, and bends us until we give up our dignity. In these cases, it is necessary to take action!

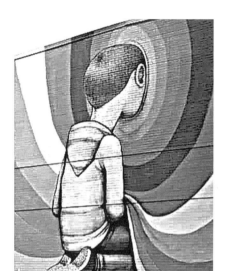

Fig. 17.20. Mural, Montreal, Canada, 2014, by Julien Malland (aka Seth Globepainter)

Julien Malland is a French artist who calls himself "Globepainter" because he leaves his graffiti in cities all over the globe. Each work is inspired by the specific social and cultural context of the place. His street art aims to provoke a spontaneous process of social reaction in people who need to communicate feelings and emotions suffocated by commercialization and technology.

His 2014 mural in Montreal (fig. 17.20) reminds us that the rhythm imposed by everyday life is often dictated by an excessive accumulation of external stimuli and information. It does not leave space for the reflection that is necessary to process the crucial events of our lives. Our cultural and social environment may thus sway us from our actual subjective vision.

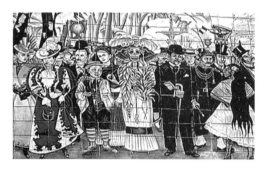

Fig. 17.21. *Dream of a Sunday Afternoon,* by Diego Rivera

Diego Rivera's *Dream of a Sunday Afternoon* (fig. 17.21) is a dreamlike representation of the artist as a child walking in Alameda Central Park in Mexico City with various figures, among them the most famous and controversial of Mexico's political and social elite. In the middle of the group, the figure standing out is Death.

The experience of loss and grief marks the lives of all of us. The sociocultural context we live in can determine our reaction and the importance we give to these experiences. Rivera highlights the equalizing power of death, which used to be a central theme in medieval danse macabre; death makes everyone the same, regardless of social roles and classes.

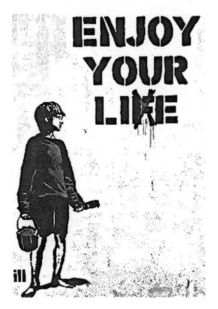

Fig. 17.22. *Enjoy Your Life*, by Banksy

The title Banksy's *Enjoy Your Life* (fig. 17.22) is a play on the words *life* and *lie*. The *f* is erased to transform the first into the second and give a whole other meaning to the statement. It provocatively implies that many people do not want to face reality and just prefer to deny the obvious. Banksy's work fits well with the first stage of grief—denial—as described by Elisabeth Kübler-Ross in her thanatology.

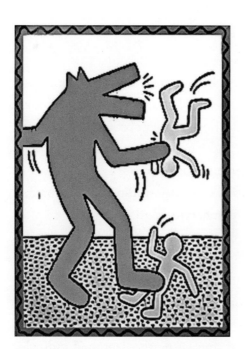

Fig. 17.23. Untitled work by Keith Haring

Keith Haring was one of the most well-known street artists. His visual language, almost cartoonlike, was universally recognized as among the most meaningful of the twentieth century. The doglike character in fig. 17.23, which he called his "doodle," was born as his distinguishing element, which then became his signature. This piece gave vent to his own anger. He died young, of AIDS.

Haring's piece reminds us that anger can devastate people and things. We often experience it as a discharge system or a defense mechanism, but it can turn against us, preventing us from being lucid and understanding what objectives we should pursue. In a patient, it is almost always a form of expression hiding other feelings or emotions (such as fear or a cry for help).

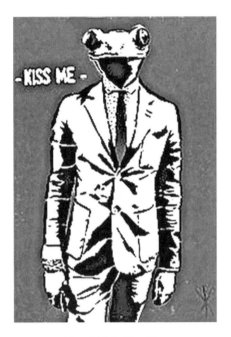

Fig. 17.24. *Kiss Me*, by Mr. Savethewall

Kiss Me (fig. 17.24) is an emblematic image: "If you kiss me, I won't be a frog anymore—I will become a handsome prince."

That is how street artist Pierpaolo Peretta, aka Mr. Savethewall, provocatively describes bargaining and negotiation. Sometimes, in order to achieve an objective, we might ask ourselves or others to do something we would normally never be willing to do or ask someone to do, thus going against our own nature, without understanding objective reality or not wanting to see it, and chasing illusions. When following this path, we cannot have any certainty about achieving a positive outcome.

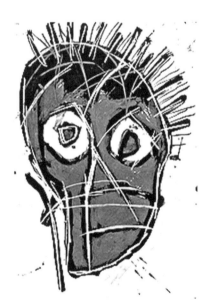

Fig. 17.25. Untitled work by Jean Michel Basquiat

The expressive power of Basquiat's murals, just like Haring's, brings street art to art exhibitions all over the world. He started his artistic production after a serious accident brought him to take an interest in anatomy, introducing many anatomical elements to his artworks. He worked in Andy Warhol's Factory studio. He died prematurely due to a heroin overdose.

Depression transforms our perception of ourselves and reality. It becomes a way of giving up in any life situation, allowing passiveness, stupefaction, and oblivion to prevail. Basquiat's image in figure 17.25 bears no title, which is a good way of translating the depressed individual's state of mind—without purpose.

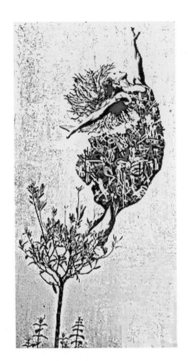

Fig. 17.26. *Dancer,* by Martin Whatson

In his mural *Dancer* (fig. 17.26), Norwegian street artist Martin Whatson represents elevation. The dancing woman is leaping upward in a complete harmony of form and gestures. Her dress is covered in colors and graffiti-like drawings and letters. This image reminds of us the liberation of the fifth stage of grief, the stage of acceptance, which is the stage of consciousness and awareness. Now we are able to renew our vital energy continuum. We have found our way and projected ourselves on it, wearing all the colors of the previous stages, which are transformed in experiences necessary for our transcendence.

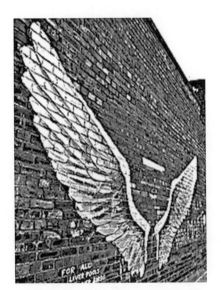

Fig. 17.27. *For All Liverpool's Liver Birds,* by Paul Curtis

Big green wings (fig. 17.27) were painted on a wall in Liverpool, a city whose symbol is a fantastic bird, the Liver Bird. Street artist Paul Curtis wanted them to be an encouragement to all the inhabitants of the city of Liverpool to metaphorically fly. It is an invitation to be photographed in front of the wings in order to take flight as a Liver Bird. Curtis's image reiterates that anyone can overcome the stages of grief and enter a new dimension of their lives, using their wings and flying over the most destructive scenarios in order to see a wider exterior and interior panorama and all the wonderful possibilities they have.

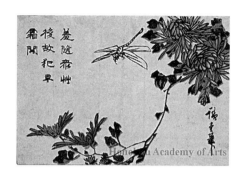

Fig. 17.28. *Dragonfly and Chrysanthemums,* by Utagawa Hiroshige

Japanese artist Utagawa Hiroshige's chrysanthemum painting (fig. 17.28) is part of the series Hana zukushi mitate fukurokuju, which means "gods of good fortune represented as flowers." In his work, Hiroshige expresses an intimacy with nature that is almost religious. We want to dedicate this painting full of good omens for the future to all those who are going through a phase of their Life Cycle in which they feel forced to face an important change, a loss, or a grieving process.

CHAPTER 18

Entropy and Syntropy
Therapeutic Energy in CST and SER

You see things; and you say, "Why?"
But I dream things that never were; and I say "Why not?"
GEORGE BERNARD SHAW

To introduce the concept of dissipating Energy Cysts, and more precisely the concept of releasing the destructive (entropic) energy in favor of the constructive (syntropic) energy through the method of SER, which we have partially described, we need to linger a moment on how the Facilitator uses syntropic energy to dissipate Energy Cysts. Therefore, we also need to introduce the concepts of entropic energy and syntropic (and/or extropic) energy.

ENTROPY

The term *entropy* comes from the Greek prefix *en* (inside) and the noun *tropē* (transformation). It is defined as the quantity representing the increase of disorder in a

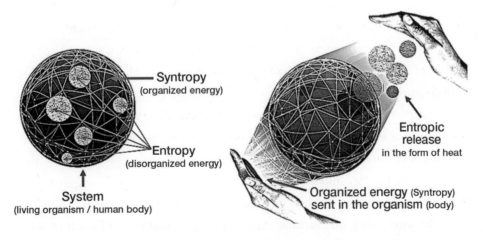

Fig. 18.1. Graphic representation of the release of the entropic energy held in an Energy Cyst

physical transformation due to the random distribution of the available energy—or, to put it more simply, the degree of disorder or randomness in a system.

Let us look at the aspects of entropy in various fields and disciplines.

Thermodynamics

Entropy equates to the second law of thermodynamics, a branch of physics that studies energy transformations and transfers between material systems.

> In a transformation, entropy actually does not always increase in the system involved; the metabolic processes occurring inside cells—which are open systems where exchanges of matter and energy with the external environment are possible . . . increase order (the physical quantity called "negentropy") instead of creating disorder. We should now clarify the distinction between an isolated system, a closed system, and an open system. . . . An isolated system is a portion of the universe that is not involved in exchanges of matter or energy with the outside. . . . A system is closed when it does not exchange matter with the outside, but it is able to exchange energy. . . . A system is called open if it is able to exchange both matter and energy with the outside. The human body is an example of an open system since it is characterized by a constant exchange of water, mineral salts, organic compounds, gas, and heat with the external or internal environment.[1]

After explaining these concepts, geologist and essayist Antonio Vecchia synthesized the principles of thermodynamics as follows:

> The variation of entropy in a system is directly proportional to the amount of heat received by the system and inversely proportional to the temperature of the system. . . . The law of conservation of energy, which is derived from the first principle of thermodynamics, states that energy cannot be created or destroyed, only transformed from one form to another. From that we can deduce that the total energy of an isolated system remains constant despite the chemical and physical transformation it may be subjected to. . . . The second principle of thermodynamics states that when a spontaneous process occurs in the universe, there is always an increase of entropy. Please note that the increase of entropy refers in this case to the entire universe, not only to the system we are analyzing. . . . If the first principle takes energy into account only on a quantitative level, stating that in an isolated system the total quantity of energy is maintained, the second completes it in the sense that it affirms that energy also has a quality and that it tends to spontaneously degrade in transformations, gradually going from more refined to less refined forms.[2]

Philosophy

As an extension of the second principle of thermodynamics, philosophy regards entropy as the intrinsic tendency of a system to irreversibly lose some of its order and qualities.[3]

Chemistry

In chemistry, the definition of entropy drawn from the second principle of thermodynamics demands more detail. As opposed to the concept of disorder we find in physics, some chemical transformations of the state of matter in which entropy increases actually bring the perception of an improved order (e.g., the crystallization of a liquid). Then, entropy should be defined rather as the degree of energy dispersion and not as the degree of disorder. The need for a differentiated definition is substantiated by chemical and physical examples showing how the entropy of isolated systems increases in correspondence with the relative number of microscopic states of each system.[4]

Physiology

We have seen that the human body is an open system, just like every single cell. Physicist Fausto Bersani Greggio, who studies environmental and biological electromagnetism and collaborates with the Italian National Institute of Nuclear Physics, explains in an article how the human body reacts to external stimuli:

> The trace of entropy is recognizable in human physiology when interactions with the external environment cause modifications within the organism or some of its parts. . . . Sensory organs represent the biological foundation of perception. . . . Their function is to record the changes that occur in the environment and communicate them to the brain. . . . Each of these organs works through a "transduction," which is the transformation of one specific type of energy found in the environment (e.g., light or sound waves) into neural signals, another type of energy. . . . When transduction occurs, our perceptive system transforms ordered energy—for example electromagnetic or sound waves, which contain information about the surrounding universe—into nerve impulses, a less ordered language, but the only one our brain can understand.
>
> This degenerative connotation entails the loss of the original information coming from the stimulus and prevents any further chance for it to produce work [a hallmark of entropy].[5]

Physics

Mirroring the degradation of information caused by transduction in physiology, when energy undergoes transformation, some of the energy is inevitably lost due to the inefficiencies of the process, according to principles of physics. That lost energy is dispersed into the environment and becomes unavailable to produce work—and that is entropy.

In most systems, the process is irreversible; the energy cannot be recovered and used for work. That is because the energy disperses randomly and becomes disordred, and it is difficult (if not impossible) to convert it back to a more organized form of energy.

As French physicist Olivier Costa de Beauregard explains:

The higher the number of particles constituting a system, the higher the probability that the disorganized states outnumber the organized states. A system is more likely to pass from a state of order to disorganization than the opposite since there are no restrictions ensuring its organized structure.... Within classic physics, events [involving a restoration of the initial physical state] are not impossible, but they are unlikely, and the improbability of their occurrence increases with the number of the particles involved and the microscopic configuration available. This brought many physicists to talk about a "thermodynamic arrow of time" connected with the increase in entropy.... The difference between past and future exists in any process, and it is not a prerogative of complex systems only, but it depends decisively on the initial conditions.... An isolated system is extremely likely to pass from a state of low entropy to a state of higher entropy, whereas it is highly improbable for it to go through a "fluctuation" that brings the entire system to a lower level of entropy through the inversion of the motion of all the particles. It is crucial to underline that the second law is valid in isolated systems ... but no system is actually isolated in nature; therefore, we often witness morphogenetic processes causing systems to maintain or even improve their degree of order and structure through constant exchanges of matter and energy with the surrounding environment.... The process bringing energy to more structured states is characterized by another quantity, "negentropy" or "information." "Entropy" and "information" can therefore be considered the two sides of energy ... and they are quantities strictly interrelated due to the principle of conservation of energy. In fact, they are connected with each other by the simple law that establishes that in an isolated system the sum of entropy and information is constant. We can expect a similar relation even in an open system."[6]

Psychotherapy

We can draw parallels between the law of entropy in physics and what happens in the individual on a psychological level. For the individual, any element that can be assimilated represents negative entropy, or negentropy, meaning it is a well-organized state of matter going through degradation. The classic example is digestion. But our brain, too, assimilates organic elements—the chemical compounds that stimulate the cells of our brain to initiate neural responses. And our neurons exchange energy, connecting through synapses to form neural networks.

However, as Roberto Minotti, a Gestalt psychologist and psychotherapist, notes, in the brain, "the organic level moves to an immaterial dimension, transforming biology into psychology. Our thoughts and memories cannot be observed, and yet they do exist; therefore we could say that our brain transforms visible chemical substances in invisible mental representations." He continues:

> Only our mind is able to assimilate structured forms and produce even more structured ones; it assimilates order and produces an order that is more complex and structured than the original. . . . The activity of human brain seems therefore to elude the second principle of thermodynamics, which states that order produces disorder, and follow different energetic and physical principles. If we consider the concept of irreversibility that is described by entropy (the "arrow of time"), only human mind can travel in time, observing past events, projecting future ones, and simultaneously remaining in the present. It operates reversible flows of energy in the form of representations, such as memories and images, connecting cerebral areas that handle the three temporal dimensions. The irreversibility of the energy of matter, with its tendency to go from order to disorder seems, to be overruled by the reversibility of thinking, which goes from order to order.[7]

Quantum Physics

The term *quantum entanglement*, sometimes replaced by the more descriptive expression *quantum correlation,* designates the quantum state of a physical system in which two particles can communicate in space and time, exchanging information. It essentially is the way quantum physics describes a long-distance relationship (with no spatiotemporal limitations) between two systems. Researchers of the technical and scientific committee of Upledger Institute International have validated some techniques proposed by Kenneth Koles, an acupuncturist, expert in Eastern medicine, researcher, and CST Instructor, based on quantum entanglement in the application of CST and SER.

According to Roberto Minotti, mentioned earlier:

> Quantum entanglement is one of the most fascinating properties of quantum mechanics. Within this connection between particles, if one of the two particles involved is subjected to an energetic modification, this affects also the other particle. The distance between the particles is irrelevant; they could be light-years away

from each other. Anyway, what is even more surprising is that the particles become "entangled" only if they have been previously produced by a specific process that tied them irreversibly. In other words, the exchange of energy between the particles occurs simultaneously if the two systems have interacted with each other for a certain period of time.[8]

Writing for *Wired* magazine in 2019, when the first image of quantum entanglement was obtained by a team of physicists from the University of Glasgow, journalist Viola Rita noted:

> Quantum entanglement does not have an equivalent phenomenon in classic physics and implies that in certain conditions the state of a system (e.g., a particle) cannot be described as a single state but rather as the superposition of several systems, so that the measurement of one influences the others. . . . Researchers found a method to photograph what happens in quantum entanglement through a camera that is able to capture the images of the photons at the same time. . . . The pictures they obtained show that these particles, although separated and far apart, moved in the same way. In practice, they were entangled. . . .
>
> Since quantum mechanics predicts entanglement, a phenomenon that is incompatible with physical reality, it constitutes a paradox, and the theories we have are incomplete because there are hidden variables explaining it.[9]

Considering the instantaneous effect of quantum entanglement, in which any modification of particle A on a quantum level immediately affects particle B on a quantum level, in a measurable way, Albert Einstein himself called phenomenon "spooky." We close our necessarily brief review by citing physicist Luigi Maximilian

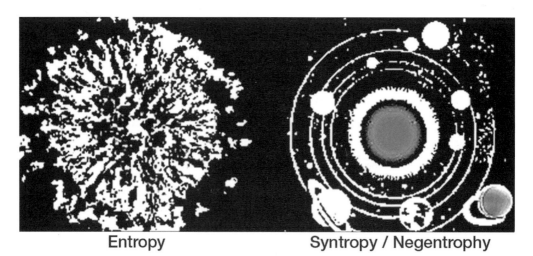

Fig. 18.2. Entropy and syntropy/negentropy

Caligiuri: "If we are not willing to reasonably believe that the reality we experience is made exclusively of our interaction with the world that surrounds us as we perceive it or measure it, then we must accept the possibility that quantum interaction at a distance between entangled particles is transmitted at a speed faster than the speed of light in vacuum."[10]

NEGENTROPY, SYNTROPY, AND EXTROPY

Although all these terms indicate a change of state starting from chaos and entropic disorganization, *syntropy* and *negentropy* have an analogous meaning, whereas *extropy* defines a concept that develops differently. Let us see how.

Negentropy

The term *negentropy* comes from the abbreviation of the expression "neg(ative) entropy." If entropy leads to chaos and disorder, negentropy describes the return of an unorganized system to order.

Syntropy

Syntropy has the same meaning as *negentropy*, but while *negentropy* applies to all physical phenomena, whether organic or inorganic, *syntropy* more specifically applies to biological organisms. When mentioning syntropy, it is only right to mention also Luigi Fantappiè, the mathematician who first proposed the theory of syntropy in 1942 in a paper titled, somewhat ambiguously, "The Unified Theory of the Physical and Biological World." (French physicist, historian, and Nobel Prize winner Louis-Victor Pierre Raymond de Broglie called Fantappié "a distinguished scientist and thinker, an attentive and helpful professor, and a limpid science communicator.")[11]

We can start our analysis of entropic, syntropic, and balancing phenomena with an article by Antonella Vannini, who tells us that Fantappiè "noted that all physical and chemical phenomena that are caused by past events are governed by the principle of entropy, whereas the phenomena that are attracted to future events (attractors) are governed by a principle symmetrical to entropy, called 'syntropy' by Fantappiè."

The reader will remember our earlier discussion of the second law of thermodynamics, which describes entropy: In any transformation or transfer of energy (such as the conversion of heat to work), some of that energy is lost (as heat) and disperses in the environment. Vannini writes:

> After the dissipated energy spread uniformly (e.g., no more heat changes), the balance that is created prevents energy from being further converted into work. This state of balance is also known as thermal death. On the contrary, syntropic

phenomena are characterized by the tendency to concentrate energy, create differentiation and order, and preserve the system from thermal death. Fantappiè immediately noticed the coincidence of the properties of syntropic phenomena and the typical qualities of living beings. . . .

On the one hand, he proved that diverging waves whose causes are in the past correspond to chemical and physical phenomena complying to the law of entropy; on the other, he proved that converging waves whose causes are in the future correspond to a new category of phenomena that comply to a principle symmetrical to entropy. Fantappiè called this principle "syntropy."[12]

Fantappiè worked with Italian physicist Giuseppe Arcidiacono to develop a model of the universe in which there are three fundamental types of phenomena:

Entropic phenomena: Phenomena in which entropy prevails, moving from order to disorder, or from complex to simple states, eventually leading to a balance.

Syntropic phenomena: Phenomena in which syntropy prevails, with constructive connotations, moving toward greater complexity and differentiation.

Balance phenomena, in which entropic and syntropic components are balanced. As Vannini describes them, "In these phenomena there is no syntropic differentiation or entropic leveling. They are in the middle between determinism (causes in the past) and indeterminism (attractors, which are causes in the future)."[13]

Exploring the ramifications of this concept, theoretical physicist Ignazio Licata explains:

What we observe in quantum processes consists in elementary transitions, such as the emission-absorption of particles. Relativistic symmetry compels us to consider "forward" and "backward" transitions . . . , which means considering the phenomenon of quantum nonlocality, the ability of quantum objects to exchange active information . . . without energy exchange in specific states of coherence. This is a different context for Fantappiè's suggestion, and in fact several physicists and biologists have suggested the possibility for quantum entanglement to play a role in guaranteeing the necessary conditions for the complexity of some biological processes. . . . Not long before his death, Fantappiè stated, "What is unexplainable in one universe can find its logical place in another universe associated with a greater number of 'degrees of freedom.' . . . Our spiritual self allows us the entire chain of universes, but some of us limit with their prejudices their own degrees of freedom, thinking they have nothing else than the freedom of material mobility." . . . The essential lesson in Fantappiè's words is the idea that physics and biology, the universe and the molecule, must meet on a deep level.... This tension toward a wider comprehension of reality is the link between the questions of modern science and Fantappiè's unified vision.[14]

Extropy

Although the terms *extropy* and *syntropy* are used in pretty much the same way in CST and SER, the concepts that further develop from extropy are different from those connected with syntropy. In fact, they are much closer to negentropy and sensibly more distant to Fantappiè's degrees of freedom, which we believe are more congruous with the work of the Facilitator.

The perspective on reality suggested by extropy is more relativistic, and though it is propositional, it is inevitably connected with the current of thought that gave birth to the transhumanist cultural movement. Trying to express these concepts in the most objective way possible, we are again going to use the opinions and explanations of competent authors and encourage the reader to do further research on the subject.

In 1988, then philosophy students Tom W. Bell (aka Tom Morrow) and Max T. O'Connor (aka Max More) coined the term *extropy*. They defined the term as meaning the extent of a living or organizational system's intelligence, functional order, vitality, and capacity and drive for improvement. More wrote a series of what he called "extropian principles" with the purpose of defining the objectives of extropianism, the evolving transhumanist philosophy. As he defined it:

> Extropianism is a "transhumanist" philosophy. The Extropian Principles define a specific version or "brand" of transhumanist thinking. Like humanists, transhumanists favor reason, progress, and values centered on our well-being rather than on an external religious authority. Transhumanists take humanism further by challenging human limits by means of science and technology combined with critical and creative thinking. We challenge the inevitability of aging and death, and we seek continuing enhancements to our intellectual abilities, our physical capacities, and our emotional development. We see humanity as a transitory stage in the evolutionary development of intelligence. We advocate using science to accelerate our move from human to a transhuman or posthuman condition.[15]

Yet another perspective on extropy is given by Kevin Kelly, environmentalist, writer, photographer, and cofounder of the magazine *Wired*:

> Extropy is neither wave nor particle, nor pure energy. It is an immaterial force that is very much like information.... The best we can say is that extropy resembles, but is not equivalent to, information.

We can not make an exact informational definition of extropy because we don't really know what information is. In fact the term "information" covers several contradictory concepts that should have their own terms. We use information to mean (1) a bunch of bits, or (2) a meaningful signal. When entropy (disorder) increases, it produces "more information" as in more bits. But when entropy decreases, it is the same as a rise in extropy (negative entropy) which produces "more information" as in more structured meaningful bits. Until we clarify our language the term information is more metaphor than anything else.[16]

ENTROPY AND SYNTROPY IN THE FACILITATOR'S PRACTICE

We know that Dr. Upledger himself never defined transhumanist or extropian, though he used the term *extropy* several times when teaching CST and SER. We also know that as a curious, sensitive, and open-minded academic, Dr. Upledger adopted terminology that could help him get across concepts to his students, and we believe that he adopted the term *extropic* only to match the term *syntropy* with a more neutral, actualized, and/or laic vision, one that could be more easily accepted. As regards the concept of extropy, there has been a particular focus on the extropy as information, as Kevin Kelly categorized it above. On an energetic level, information assumes a particular importance in the work of CST and SER.

Let us briefly go through what is useful to know for the restoration of the vital energy continuum that Facilitators carry out in their work.

Entropy

Entropy: *en = inside* and *tropos = transformation/tendency*

Entropy can be defined as the gradual degeneration of a system toward the maximum disorder (until thermal death).

When a trauma occurs in a biological structure, the organized energy becomes disorganized, and the physiological structure adapts to that disorganization. If the structure is not properly treated and complications ensue due to the increase and/or retention of entropic energy, the physiological structure can further proceed on its path toward chaos, which sometimes ends in death or coma.

Syntropy

Syntropy: *syn = together/converging* and *tropos = transformation/tendency*

Syntropy can be defined as the energy that converges toward attractors, increasing the complexity, differentiation, structure, and order of a system.

Syntropy is constructive energy. Constructive emotions (love, joy, happiness, etc.) that generate the adequate conditions to receive syntropic energy foster a healthy dispersion of the entropic energy caused by trauma. With the permission of the patient's Higher Self and through the Facilitator's hands, syntropic energy dissipates entropy.

Energy Cysts as Entropic Dysfunctions

The retention of destructive energy creates an entropic area that Dr. Upledger defined as an Energy Cyst. An Energy Cyst is therefore an entropic dysfunction.

Destructive emotions (fear, hate, anger, guilt, etc.) are the conditions that foster the retention of entropic energy and accommodate and encourage the sedimentation of trauma. On an energetic level, the sedimentation of a trauma can form an Energy Cyst.

It is as if the Energy Cyst stores the emotion caused by the trauma, holding it in the memory and in the organism to feed, maintain, exacerbate, and develop the destructive entropic condition. The areas of increased entropy (Energy Cysts) may originate from a wide range of destructive issues or situations (toxic, karmic, viral, traumatic, etc.). Even physical traumas might involve an emotional component that fosters entropic energy.

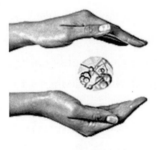

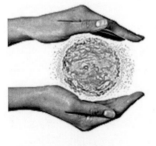

Fig. 18.3. Release of entropic energy retained by an Energy Cyst through the aptonomic touch

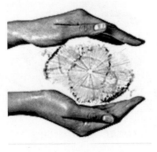

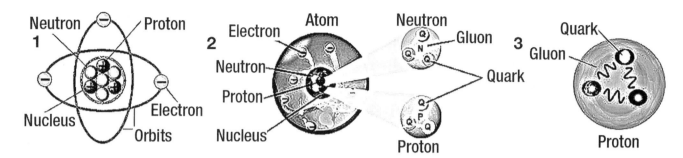

Fig. 18.4. The structure of an atom

Entropic energy withheld in the organism as an Energy Cyst can be gradually released through the aptonomic touch of the Facilitator, until the Energy Cyst is dissipated.

Therapeutic Energy

Every atom in a therapist's tissues (or the tissues of any organism, for that matter) has a nucleus made up of neutrons and protons. The nucleus is surrounded by electrons, which circle the nucleus in various orbits

An atom may release neutrons and protons, in pairs, from its nucleus. Paired neutrons and protons form nucleons. Each nucleon is highly energized.

The brain continues to control and direct these highly energized nucleons via specific nerve channels. These channels direct the nucleons to the internal aspect of the therapist's skin. When the therapist's brain decides that the treatment from the therapist shall be entered into the client's body at a specific location in or on that body, the nucleons then pass through the skin of the therapist and, from there, through the skin of the client.

After the therapist's nucleons enter the client's body, they are somehow directed by the combined intelligence of both therapist and client to travel to the problem site. When the nucleons reach the problem site (which could be a tumor, a cyst, a fibrosis, an osseous distortion, and/or an inflammation center), the positive energy of the

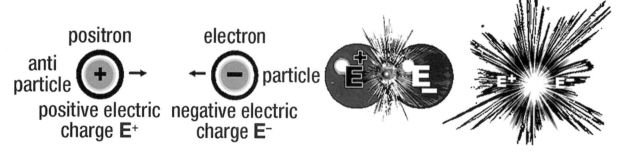

Fig. 18.5. From atom to energy

nucleon pulls the negatively charged electrons away from the atoms at the problem site within the client. When these electrons are pulled away, their atoms disintegrate.

As the atoms at the problem site disappear and the problem dissipates, the hands of the therapist can feel the problem (tumor, the cyst, the fibrotic tissue, osseous distortion, inflammations, etc) disappear as well.

Keep in mind that any material insulation between the therapist's skin and the client's skin will interfere with the passage of nucleons and their energies into the client's body. Some of the nucleons' energy will be used up to pass through the material, thereby reducing the therapeutic effect. For this reason, the insulation should be removed before treatment begins. The area of uninsulated, skin-to-skin touch can be quite small, perhaps only large enough to allow the touch of three or four therapeutically intended fingers.

THERAPEUTIC SIDE OF ENTANGLEMENT

Having explained what entanglement is from the perspective of quantum mechanics, we would like to define it from a therapeutic perspective in order to better appreciate the self-healing action of the individual through the Facilitator's work.

Gioacchino Pagliaro, psychologist, psychotherapist, and founder of the International Research Association on Entanglement in Medicine and Psychology (AIREMP), seems to support a view that is strongly similar to the therapeutic standpoint of Dr. Upledger:

> The human organism is composed of biological systems made of cells, which are made of molecules, which are made of atoms, which are made of photons—and therefore energy. Any material form has a vibrant immaterial manifestation. Since matter is energy, it vibrates, transmits, and receives information. The human organism is constituted by this energy/information that interacts with the entire universe and with the Mind [i.e., the Self, extended to a higher mental level]. All material entities are interrelated and connected with each other, depend on each other through their energy, and are part of the Mind. Thanks to the level of interconnection and interdependence of subatomic reality, characterized by nonlocality and nonlocal communication, subatomic particles interact with each other in our organism and with the universe, simultaneously creating the reality of entanglement. In the reality of entanglement, where space and time are conventions considered as illusions, there is no separation between living and nonliving entities, but there is a wide system of vibrational fields and nonlocal communication. Therefore, in the human organism, there would be not only molecular communication but also a communication with the outside and the inside that is

made of vibrations, resonance, and entanglement. The sense of separation of the human being from the environment and the universe, supported even by some recent theories of quantum physics, would be only an illusion, probably a mistake of the perception/representation of reality due to the conditioning of the culture of materialism.[17]

Clinical Observations

I am going to describe the clinical case that, so far, has been the most peculiar in my working experience.

I received a letter from a maxillofacial surgeon, who wrote to me after contacting Dr. Upledger about one of his patients. He lived fifty kilometers from my city, and Dr. Upledger had given him my name because I was the nearest person who was qualified to follow his patient.

In his letter, the surgeon asked me to treat his patient, who had gone through a car accident in which his skull had been virtually smashed. He knew of the Upledger method and was sure that this type of treatment could help his patient and, consequently, even him in his work of restoration of the patient's skull.

When I accepted, he sent me images of his patient's skull. I can only say that I had never seen and will never see again a cranium of a live person fractured in so many parts. It is enough for you to know that upon the impact of the accident, an eye ended up in his throat.

From the images, I understood that I had a huge challenge ahead.

Before the car crash, the patient had been a professional basketball player and an esteemed business and insurance counselor. When he woke up after a coma of about six months, he could barely remember four words and had to learn how to speak again and try to restore his cognitive and mnemonic functions with the help of both a speech therapist and a psychotherapist.

Not only had his skull suffered huge damage, but his body also was not in good shape.

I worked with him while he was still being supervised by his surgeon, employing techniques to stimulate the physiological release of tension in the intracranial membranes. The hardest challenge consisted in the fact that his cranium had been rebuilt with various artificial components; nevertheless, I could still feel his intracranial movements.

According to the maxillofacial surgeon, I "only" had to restore the maximum natural mobility of the cranial membranes and joints so that he could subsequently "put the finishing touch" to the restoration of the patient's skull. I did it, and I must say that the patient responded very effectively, also because he was a man of great strength and with a strong willpower.

The surgeon was satisfied with the results and was able to complete his work on the cranium. The patient was extremely glad as well, and he asked me to keep working with him for all the other dysfunctions and traumas caused by the accident.

I proceeded with my work with him. Moving to his ankles and vertebral column, I manipulated the abdominal cavity, from which the spleen had been removed, and we went through some SER techniques. The treatment sessions were regular, on a weekly basis, for more than a year, and we even became friends. I found it hard to remain empathetic (and not sympathetic) during the treatments, and I must say that I had rarely met a person who could address his self-healing so tenaciously.

After his long convalescence, the patient eventually went back to work. He did not go back to professional sports, but he never stopped exercising. His family, who was involved in the accident as well, split up, but he remained an attentive and affectionate father to his son, who decided to start practicing sports, as his father used to.

❧ A CST-CENTERED VISION ❧

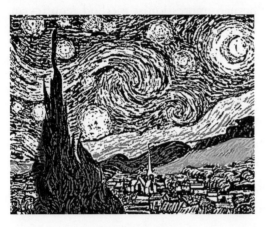

Fig. 18.6. Reproduction of *Starry Night,* by Vincent van Gogh

In the famous *Starry Night* painting by the troubled Dutch painter Vincent van Gogh (fig. 18.6), it is easy to perceive every visible part whirling. The image seems to vibrate in the immensity of the cosmic movement, as if all shapes in the scene were macrocosms compressed in microcosms that explode to manifest a unified, organized, and recognizable vision.

The brushstrokes in this painting are so distinctly separated that they form a single, indivisible scene. They perform particularly well as a representation of entropy transforming into syntropy thanks to the organization of energy. As Dr. Upledger said—making a surprisingly striking analogy with the technique Van Gogh used to create this image—during treatment, the Facilitator carries out a disgregation and asks the whole (the organism) to reorganize in a more functional way.

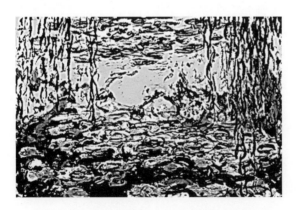

Fig. 18.7. Reproduction of *Water Lilies,* by Claude Monet

Claude Monet's *Water Lilies* (fig. 18.7) is one in a series of oil paintings depicting water lilies that Monet painted between 1897 and 1926 in a house in Giverny, between the Seine and the Epte. The perspective is at close range, so it is not possible to discern other elements of the landscape. The attention of the observer is drawn solely to the play of lights, the colors of the flowers, and the water.

As described in this chapter, in a CST treatment, nucleons pass from the therapist into the patient's body. The syntropic energy sent by the therapist transforms the entropic dysfunction and dissolves it. In Monet's painting, the representation of water is like the organism of the patient that receives the transformation; it is no longer the surface that reflects the harmony of the landscape but has become the landscape itself.

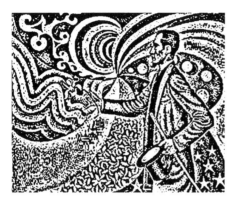

Fig. 18.8. Reproduction of *Portrait of Félix Fénéon,* by Paul Signac

"The neo-impressionist method requires an exceptional delicacy of the eye." Thus wrote French art critic Félix Fénéon about the work of Paul Signac, a neo-impressionist painter credited, with Georges Seurat, of developing the technique known as pointillism. If we observe pointillist paintings, it is impossible not to realize that the image in its whole is formed by small points of color. This technique reminds us of the way every atom and particle of our organism can play a fundamental role and how the CST therapist's touch has an "exceptional delicacy" of perception.

CHAPTER 19

Major Stressors

Critical Events on the Holmes and Rahe Stress Scale

I am convinced that life is 10 percent what happens to me and 90 percent how I react to it.

CHARLES R. SWINDOLL

This part of the Holmes and Rahe Stress Scale (points 1 to 18) completes the entire social adjustment scale. It includes the major stressors, which have the highest life change unit (LCU) scores.

The main anatomical elements involved with this level of stress are those we have already correlated with the emotions of fear and anxiety:

- the RAS, which in turn involves the trigeminal nerve (fifth cranial nerve) and the temporomandibular joints, or masticatory apparatus, which is fundamental for survival
- the vagus system (tenth cranial nerve)
- the HPA stress axis (hypothalamic-pituitary-adrenal axis), which regulates our organism's ability to adapt to stress; is activated by physical, emotional, and social stimuli or stressors; and activates the secretion of neurotransmitters, neurohormones, and other substances.

Shock of any kind activates the RAS, which is why any initial thought or decision made while the shock is occurring is determined and conditioned by the RAS.

HOLMES AND RAHE STRESS SCALE: STRESSORS 1 TO 18

Rank	Stressor	Holmes and Rahe LCU Value
18	Change to a different line of work	36
17	Death of close friend	37
16	Change in financial state	38
15	Business readjustment (mergers, failures, etc.)	39
14	Gain of new family member (birth, marriage of son or daughter)	39
13	Sex difficulties	39
12	Pregnancy	40
11	Change in health of family member	44
10	Retirement	45
9	Marital reconciliation or reconciliation with partner	45
8	Fired at work	47
7	Marriage	50
6	Personal injury or illness	53
5	Death of close family member	63
4	Jail term	63
3	Marital separation or separation from partner	65
2	Divorce	73
1	Death of a spouse or partner	100

THE HYPOTHALAMIC-PITUITARY-ADRENAL (HPA) AXIS

With the sympathetic and parasympathetic branches of the autonomic nervous system—which are activated through the release of adrenaline and noradrenaline—the HPA axis is the main effector of the individual response to stress in situations that are potentially dangerous.

On such occasions, the organism must avail itself of energetic resources that it has stored and distributed in specific areas of the body. These are primarily simple sugars, which will power the upper and lower limbs in order to prepare them for the most

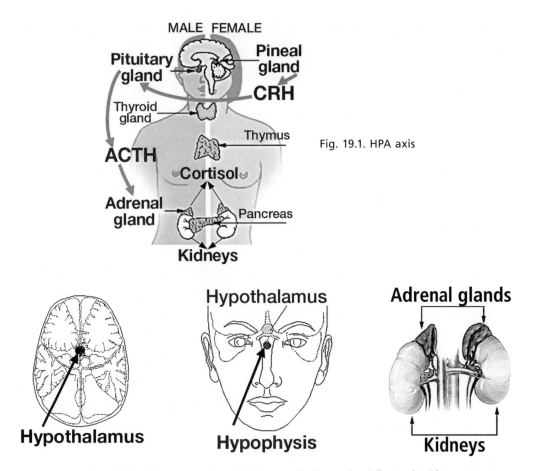

Fig. 19.1. HPA axis

Fig. 19.2. HPA organs: hypothalamus, pituitary gland (hypophysis), adrenal glands and kidneys

effective defense strategy (fight or flight). Moreover, the organism must momentarily stop other processes, such as the accumulation of more energy, that are useful under normal conditions but can prove to be damaging in an emergency situation.

The function of the HPA axis is made possible by the release of hormones that reach specific organs through blood circulation and facilitate the use of energy. These hormones belong to the group of corticosteroids; they are corticotropin-releasing hormone (CRH), cortisol, and adrenocorticotropic hormone (ACTH). In order to react quickly to potentially dangerous situations, the HPA axis has to be in direct contact with the sensory organs that convey information coming from the external world. The signals coming from sensory organs (ears and eyes) reach the hypothalamus, which releases CRH almost immediately (the process lasts a few seconds). CRH is secreted in the median eminence and sent to the hypophysis, where it induces the secretion of ACTH and its release in the bloodstream, which brings it to the adrenal cortex to induce the release of cortisol. In turn, cortisol increases the production of glycogen, maintains the balance of bodily fluids, and reinforces the immune response.[1]

Let us analyze perspectives on the HPA axis from cognitive psychotherapists, osteopaths, clinical psychologists, and chiropractors.

HPA Axis in Cognitive Psychotherapy

Discussing the neuroendocrinology of the stress response, a team of cognitive psychotherapists from the Beck Institute in Rome had this to say:

> Various cerebral networks modulate the activity of the HPA axis. More specifically, the neurons in the PVN [paraventricular nucleus of the hypothalamus] receive an inhibiting control from the hippocampus and the prefrontal cortex (PFC), whereas the amygdala and the brain stem exercise control on an excitatory level. Moreover, the glucocorticoids themselves exercise a negative feedback control on the HPA axis by regulating the neurons of the PVN and the hippocampus. It was proven that high exposure to glucocorticoids negatively affects the neurons of the hippocampus, decreasing the dendritic branches, eliminating dendritic spines, and reducing neurogenesis. In PTSD patients, the feedback control system of the HPA is compromised, and the basal production of cortisol decreases, whereas the negative feedback control on the HPA increases, with a maladaptive overall response to stressing, chronic, and acute stimuli.[2]

HPA Axis in Osteopathy

The very first chapter of *Il ragionamento clinico osteopatico* (Clinical reasoning in osteopathy), by osteopaths Christian Lunghi, Francesca Baroni, and Mariantonietta Alò, focuses on the HPA axis and how it is relevant in osteopathy:

> Osteopaths identify the structures and functions that are overloaded by palpating the alterations of tissue that are attributable to stress and inflammation biomarkers.... These alterations... can involve the hypothalamic-pituitary-adrenal (HPA) axis and/or the sympathetic adrenergic system (SAS).... Adaptation is the main biological mechanism that restores the balance and minimizes the internal effects of stress, and it occurs after the decoding of the environmental demand that the HPA and the SAS convey.... Osteopaths relate the overloaded structures and functions ... to the alterations of tissue mechanics through perceptive palpation.... The tissues react with a generalized state of hypersensitivity, which predisposes the individual to neurological, metabolic, circulatory, and respiratory fatigue and nullifies the ability of the self-regulatory functions to work in connection with the physiological modalities. Endogenous and exogenous environmental stimulations might also foster a local adaptation syndrome, leaving dysfunctional memories impressed in the tissue.[3]

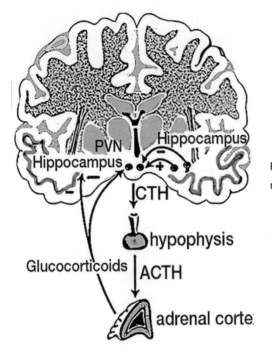

Fig. 19.3. The HPA axis response to stress

HPA Axis in Clinical Psychology

Physicians, psychiatrists, and researchers Mario Guazzelli and Angelo Gemignani, both professors at the University of Pisa, addressed the subject of stress and the stress axis as follows:

> The response to stress can be considered an overall activation of physiological and behavioral reactions initiated by the organism to address stimuli that tend to disturb its homeostatic balance (stressors). The change that the individual must carry out in order to respond to a stressful situation, such as the adaptation to environmental stimuli, is supported by systems with a high level of integration. The adaptive response of these systems is called allostasis. . . . Allostasis is generated by the combined activity of the central and the autonomic nervous systems (CNS and ANS), the hypothalamic-pituitary-adrenal (HPA) axis, the sympathetic system of the adrenal medulla, and the immune/proinflammatory system. . . . Allostasis is a process meant to maintain homeostasis that can produce the so-called "allostatic load" if it lasts excessively, increasing the activity of the mediators on their target cells and provoking phenomena of tissue desensitization and damage. . . . In the long term, the effects of the allostatic load represent tragic consequences for the individual, such as insomnia, mental disorders (e.g., depression and anxiety), and various somatic pathologies that harm the cardiovascular and the respiratory systems in particular. . . . On a functional level, chronic stress is generally associated

with the reduction of the excitability of the hippocampus and the long-term potentiation (LTP) mechanisms, which mainly alter the mnemonic function of the hippocampus. . . . Through the so-called neurogenesis hypothesis, it has been suggested that the physiopathogenic mechanism underlying some mental disorders that are connected with stress (e.g., depression and PTSD) is connected with a loss of neurons and an alteration of the neurogenesis in the hippocampus.[4]

HPA Axis in Chiropractic

To complete our overview of the HPA axis, we are going to refer to the observations of chiropractor and ergonomist Giovanni Chetta:

The union of mind and body, now unanimously recognized thanks to the scientific evidence provided by psychoneuroimmunology, allows emotions, feelings, thoughts, and physiological reactions all to be strictly integrated and to constantly condition each other. In fact, psychological well-being and physical well-being are two unavoidably interconnected aspects. . . . Stress is an adaptive energy. . . . It provokes a physiological reaction in response to the needs caused by external stimuli (stressors), which mobilizes the available resources in order to produce a "specific high-efficiency energy." The biochemical process that releases such energy is a natural reaction that is inevitably repeated in the organism every day, every time it is needed. All of this means that stress evokes increased activity of natural functions that are stimulated by specific hormones, especially adrenaline and noradrenaline, and therefore an intensification of vitality that allows the organism to adapt and react to changing circumstances. . . . What distinguishes positive stress is essentially the degree of uncertainty; stress is positive when it is searched for and provides us with the sensation of controlling our environment, increasing our vitality (eustress); it is negative when it is unsolicited, unpleasant, and followed by uncertainty, discomfort, uneasiness, and similar sensations (distress). . . . The hypothalamic-pituitary-adrenal (HPA) axis seems essential since it is characterized by regular oscillations in stress-free situations, but it is more active when stress occurs. . . . The human organism is like an integrated network that unifies various organs, systems, and apparatuses both on a physical and on a chemical level. All the components of this network recognize certain messages, whether they come from cerebral circuits through emotions and thoughts or from vegetative nervous circuits through the stimuli or feedbacks of organs and systems, from the connective system through mechanical pushes and tensions or from endocrine or immune organs. In brief, between biological, physical, and psychological events there is a two-way connection rather than a cause-effect relation.[5]

THOUGHT-FORM

The concept of thought-form is widely addressed by the studies of theosophist Charles W. Leadbeater—previously mentioned in chapter 16, in our discussion of chakras—and his collaborator, the theosophist and esotericist Annie (Wood) Besant. Anthroposophist Rudolf Steiner also made use of it. We will need it to introduce and understand a particular aspect of the treatment carried out by Facilitators with nonverbal SER.

In an extremely simplistic explanation, the thought-form could be defined as the "energy of thought" (sometimes associated with psychic energy). As such, it might take on either negative/destructive connotations or positive/constructive ones.

The mental energy that is focused into the thought-form can assume a definite and structured dimension, created and fed by thought itself. The thought-form is often referred to as elemental or egregore (derived from the ancient Greek word for "guardian"), even though the latter is mostly used to interpret a collective figuration/action.

After Leadbeater and Besant, other academics grew a cautious interest in this phenomenon—cautious because until the past century it was considered a prerogative of occultism. More recently, thanks mostly to the progress and discoveries of neuroscience and quantum physics, the thought-form's esoteric reputation has been downsized.

As we have seen, the quality of emotions, thoughts, ideas, and intuitions can play an essential—if not determining—role in an individual's well-being or discomfort in the widest connotations of this concept. Let us analyze some definitions of thought-form given by various scholars in their field of expertise.

To begin, we'll hear from psychologists Dario Sepe, Adriana Onorati, and Fortunata Folino:

> The Mental Dimension is the system of thoughts, ideas, convictions, and conceptual and theoretical knowledge that all individuals own. It can be compared to a house built with bricks in which the bricks are the thought-forms, the series of beliefs and convictions that we have built throughout our existence. Thought-forms represent a "reality" in the mind of the individual, and their quality and vibration especially relate to their history, prejudices, beliefs, experiences, and relationships. Most of our thoughts disappear shortly after being born, since they are unconscious, but some of them become actual thought-forms, stable over time because they are constantly retrieved from memory and can affect other individuals on an emotional level. . . . The effect of thought-forms on our lives is evident, based on the principle that "energy follows thought": what we create on a mental level, even if it is unconscious, has an effect on a material level, conditioning our life and that

of the people around us. . . . Any thought is a vibration, which is elevated or raw according to what we think and introduce in the space. . . . Masaru Emoto's studies highlight the ability of water to record the vibrations of an environment, reacting according to the thought or vibration it is exposed to; crystals assume either a symmetrical and harmonious shape or a chaotic and disorganized one depending on the energy around them. Since the human body is largely composed of water, it is easy to image how our words and thoughts can encourage a harmonious disposition of the crystals and, subsequently, an optimization of cellular processes. . . . The importance of introducing in our daily life positive thoughts and vibrations that generate harmony and beauty in our organism is more and more evident. Traditional science confirms as well that "energy does follow thought"![6]

As psychologist, humanist, and scientist Guido Brunetti stresses in his perspective on brain, mind, and consciousness within neuroscience:

The fascination we have toward these three elements is ambiguous . . . they can produce Mozart's *Requiem,* the Sistine Chapel, the Divine Comedy, Beethoven's symphony, the genius of Leonardo, the unique beauty of Raphael's art, but also Auschwitz, Hiroshima, and many other tragedies. . . . The explanation of the mental act as physical act brings us to the core of neuroscience and to the methods of positive sciences (reductionism). New neuroscience carries a radical twist . . . grasping the concept of brain, mind, and consciousness thanks to brain imaging techniques, genetics, and molecular biology. . . . The newest sciences of the mind allow us to start anew. . . . in the unified vision of mind, consciousness, and brain, creating an initial principle that establishes that all normal and abnormal processes, even the most complex such as thought, language, creativity, art, and music, come from cerebral operations. . . . We are animated objects, and therefore our physical bodies are subjected to the laws of physics, but there is also essence—thought, self, spirit, mind, soul—a mental property that is neither visible nor observable, does not comply to physical laws, and does not coincide completely with the body. . . . In its intellectual dimension, the soul transcends the body and, at the same time, "resides in it, as form of the vegetative body," "incarnating" and "embodying" our mental and spiritual acts. This means that thought exists on a plane that is above time, but it incarnates in the temporal dimension when it is rooted in the brain . . . so that finiteness (matter) finds its connection with the infinite, hidden, and undisclosed. The essence is fascinating, upsetting, attractive, and dismaying, in a conception that unites and integrates the neuroscientific vision with a spiritual and metaphysical vision that encompasses all the manifestations of the absoluteness of human spirit.[7]

Theosophist Edoardo Bratina reminds us:

It is commonly believed that when an individual creates a thought, the thought disappears into thin air or stops having any influence on the psychophysical structure of the individual as soon as it is forgotten. On the contrary, each thought has its own life span, which extends in time in proportion to the emotional charge it is given. Its existence per se, even if it is ignored, influences the behavior of the subject, his thinking, emotions, dreams, etc. . . . As Besant and Leadbeater wrote in their work on thought-forms and their effects, "every impulse sent out, either from the mental body or from the astral body of man, immediately clothes itself in a temporary vehicle of this vitalized matter. Such a thought or impulse becomes for the time a kind of living creature, the thought-form being the soul, and the vivified matter the body."[8]

NONVERBAL SOMATOEMOTIONAL RELEASE

We have already seen how to carry out a verbal SER treatment with Therapeutic Imagery and Dialogue, but we should keep in mind that the Facilitator is not always able to verbalize what is occurring during the treatment, and patients are sometimes unable to communicate their emotions verbally. These cases are not very common, but it is necessary to take them into account because Facilitators might have to treat people who speak a language they do not know, who have speech impediments, who are in a vegetative coma, who have cognitive deficits, or who suffer from a disabling form of autism.

Such cases require the Facilitator to make use of nonverbal SER, a treatment in which the dialogue occurs solely between the non-conscious of the patient and that of the Facilitator. It can be implemented when the Facilitator is trained to listen to the patient's body and subtle energy. The latter is the energy that belongs to the particular dimension we call Third Space, where the Higher Self—or Inner Physician, if you prefer—is able to express itself.

It is certainly necessary for the Facilitator to constantly practice and train in the correct therapeutic approach, but the particular space that enables the individual to access the information that is useful for their self-healing, which is the space that the Facilitator has the privilege to access if the patient's non-conscious agrees to it, is the most fascinating and constructive element of SER and does not need any words.

We could continue to describe neural processes, the exchanges of quantum electromagnetism, or the results of various implementations of the imaging technologies in relation to the emotions that are elicited during an SER treatment. We could also spend much more time in the detailed description of this modality of dialogue/

nondialogue. Nonetheless, we firmly believe that knowledge of SER should be experienced rather than told, documented, read, or listened to. It is certainly only in the actual treatment that the individual who receives SER and participates in it is able to experience the melding Dr. Upledger wrote about.

However, we can certainly go through some of the theoretical information that, in addition to the learning, technical, and ethical protocols and practices, is made available to Facilitators in their training to learn how to implement one of the modalities of nonverbal SER.

A Facilitator's objectives in this practice are:

- to stimulate and activate the therapeutic imagery in themselves (in any sensory or imaginative form)
- to provide patients with a healing/restoring imagery and encourage them to associate it with a constructive transformation that can help them solve their problem

Nonverbal SER Technique

This technique is carried out nonverbally until the final stage, when the patient and the Facilitator might share/communicate (if that is possible).

1. Locate the Energy Cyst through the Arcing technique.
2. Nonverbally ask the patient's non-conscious to convey (in a way the patient can easily perceive) a thought-form/sensation/vibration, such as an image, thought, word, sensation, smell, sound, or emotion, that can help you identify the patient's problem and the cause that generated it.
3. Once you have received the feedback of the patient's non-conscious, ask again—still with no verbalization—for a thought-form (image, thought, word, etc.) that belongs to the patient, is easily recognizable, that represents an experience the patient associates with positive/constructive characteristics, and whose constructive energy is equal in intensity to the negative/destructive energy of the trauma. Memorize whatever is transmitted.
4. Communicate the second thought-form (image, thought, word, etc.) to the patient through intention—or verbally, if possible—while sending syntropic/therapeutic energy in the same amount as the entropic/destructive energy that generated and/or is feeding the problem. At the same time, ask the patient to make a simple gesture, one that can be easily repeated in everyday life. The gesture will become a tool that enables the patient to recall the energy of the constructive thought-form or reconnect with their healing space (Higher Self) every time they make it.

Note: If the patient cannot communicate, you will need to associate the constructive thought-form with an action that is easily repeatable in everyday life by the patient's caretakers or people close to them (e.g., folding back their sheets if they're forced into bed).

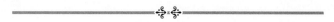

Clinical Observations

One of my students once introduced me to a couple whose daughter, a university student, was in poor health. Her boyfriend had left her some time before, and afterward, with no apparent physiological cause, all her muscles had started to gradually atrophy until she was forced into a wheelchair. Her parents had obviously made sure she underwent a long series of clinical tests and psychiatric assessments, which she had agreed to.

The couple asked me to examine and treat their daughter.

When the girl came to my office, the first thing I did was assess her craniosacral rhythm. I perceived an intense sadness, and I asked her whether she felt discouraged or fatigued. She replied that, even though she was aware of her situation, she wanted to live for her parents and felt her physical conditions were improving.

Nevertheless, her craniosacral rhythm was telling me the exact opposite through the Significance Detector.

At her parents' insistence, I treated her three times a week for three months while she was also being treated with allopathic medicine and seeing a psychiatrist. I implemented all the techniques I knew, but every time I used the Therapeutic Imagery and Dialogue, I felt she did not allow me to contact her non-conscious and kept eluding me (and lying about wanting to live).

Though it was hard to admit, I felt she was strongly feeding the thought of scarcity and consumption, transforming it in a destructive invocation that was taking her to the end of her life as the means of her liberation.

Sometimes, it is hard to respect the free will of others, but in that case the only option I had was to propose to her parents that I treat them to alleviate their suffering and to help them let their daughter go. It was with unbelievable pain, but they understood. Thereafter, I treated them and kept treating her until her last month of life.

CHAPTER 20

CST and SER in Death

Support for the Dying

Nothing in life is to be feared, it is only to be understood. Now is the time to understand more, so that we may fear less.

MARIE CURIE

This chapter introduces concepts that can help the Facilitator address the subject of death. Our attention will focus specifically on both personal perceptions about death and on the work the Facilitator might want to carry out to assist a person who is dealing with it. Let us start with a brief analysis of what could commonly be the perception of death for the living.

The first crucial question we should ask ourselves is, *What exactly is death for the living?*

Essentially, our personal take on the meaning of death might have its roots in our fear of death. Where does this fear come from? What are our experiences of the perception of death?

As was previously observed in this text, for the living, death is an indirect experience that is evoked by the loss that comes with separation, abandonment, or small deaths occurring during our Life Cycle. Again, this means that death does not really exist for the living. It may seem redundant and unnecessary to repeat it over and over, but we are going to see why it is so fundamental.

We know only the fear of death and the energy of the fear of death, which comes from our perception of the interruption of the vital energy continuum in the experiences of our Life Cycle.

The fear of death, then, is the fear of the interruption of our life continuum, which is our energy. The traumatic events and situations we have experienced, and the specific emotions and their energies connected with them, caused us to perceive this interruption. These are the situations that our Cellular Memory registered as loss.

The first perception of this fear could probably be traced back to birth. In fact, birth is the first experience within our Life Cycle in which we experience an interruption of our vital energy continuum (separation from the fetal environment). This experience can sometimes remain connected with destructive emotions if the individual associates the natural physiological separation with a sense of loss and this sense of loss with grief.

Could this be the authentic root of the fear of death? Some people are positive it is. At least it is surely one of the probable causes.

In fact, we tend to associate the sensations connected with our well-being to the perception of stability of our life energy, which allows us to implement strategies of energy management. This perception is connected with our self-confidence, with our confidence to live life as we can and, especially, would like to, and with the perception of our innate human self-transcendence.

THE THERAPIST'S FOCUS WHEN ADDRESSING THE SUBJECT OF DEATH

Taking care of patients in the last phase of their Life Cycle, envisaging the passage from the last known scenario to a completely unknown one, can certainly move a Facilitator to reflect on a similar situation in their own life. Below are the foundational concepts for a correct approach to such work.

Reject the Ego

We have already addressed the Ego, and therefore we should know how fundamental it is for therapists—or anyone else—to LET IT GO and replace it with the self-confidence that is needed to be aware of their own role, abilities, knowledge, and skills.

Empathize

It is also important for Facilitators to always empathize with the patient and never sympathize, as is the same for anyone who wants to offer their best when they are listening to the actual needs of another person. Practicing empathy prevents Facilitators from activating their Ego to solve the patient's problem at any cost. Instead, it allows them to listen to what the patient's Higher Self is really communicating in the dialogue with the non-conscious and to offer the maximum support to the patient's natural physiological process.

Respect Free Will

The job of Facilitators is to make use of their skills, therapeutic abilities, and knowledge to remove all the dysfunctions that inhibit the functions of homeostasis in the patient's organism, letting the patient's free will choose whether to accept spontaneous remission and acquiescence in the transition or to reject them (in the same way all of us should behave to respect other people's free will). Therefore, the Facilitator must do everything it takes to give the patient all the options to address their self-healing—even the chance to refuse it.

Recognize Constructive Opportunities

As we have learned on this path, another crucial point is to stay focused on the chance to face loss, not as a merely negative/destructive element but rather as the factor that initiates the most meaningful mechanisms of transformation and change—that is, as a constructive opportunity.

LOSS AS AN OPPORTUNITY FOR TRANSFORMATION

Facing a scenario of loss could provide Facilitators, as well as anyone else, with two fundamental opportunities:

- to work on themselves, addressing the theme of loss in order to transform it into a constructive opportunity, action, possibility, or change for themselves and others
- to accept others without judgment and with the highest respect, especially those who are going through a scenario of loss, and learn from their actions, emotions, and feelings in one of the most significant, delicate, and pivotal moments of their lives

More than any other situation or scenario, the process that brings another individual to the end of their life offers the Facilitator the ability to acquire knowledge and awareness about the fundamental factor that initiates the transformation process in all living systems. That information provides the Facilitator with confirmation

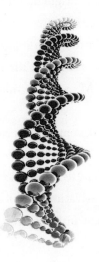

Fig. 20.1. DNA holds genetic information on the end of life.

that we would not know what transformation is if there was no perception of the interruption of the vital energy continuum; it is a phase that is necessary for the change of state.

The Facilitator is thus able to come into contact with one of the most important occurrences in human life, activating Cellular Memory and the memory of the non-conscious and retracing the individual's experiences that emotionally connect that person to the experience of fear due to the presence of entropic energy and the interruption of the vital energy continuum.

We have therefore discovered together that addressing separation, loss, and bereavement also means taking care of some of the highest expressions of human life itself.

It is an Ode to Life that finds a transformative answer in gratefulness and the emotions connected with it.

It is clear that gratefulness itself is the feeling and attitude that has the potential, the qualities, and the ability to eradicate the nourishment of the Ego, and it finds its roots in love, trust, and the joy of living life in every moment and during any occurrence.

One of my students once told me about a dialogue she had witnessed by chance (but chance does not exist, remember?). The dialogue had been between a Catholic priest and a middle-aged woman. The woman was searching for comfort because she was going through the difficult situation of taking care of one of her relatives who was about to die. She looked broken as she described to the priest all the attention and daily care she was offering to her relative, as well as her relative's reactions. Her relative kept talking about the past, the affection they had shared, and their common experiences, even though pain was sometimes blurring her lucidity. Moreover, this person was arranging all her affairs as best she could in order to leave as little chaos as possible after her death.

Assisting someone who is critically ill is generally one of the hardest tasks anyone might have to endure. The woman was extremely fatigued, and she looked worn out as well. When she had finished letting out her thoughts and emotions, the priest had taken her hands and brought them to his heart. While looking her in the eyes, he had called her by her name, smiled, and said, "So much life, my dear! There is so much life in you and what you are telling me!" My student told me that after those words, the woman seemed lighter.

My student had been puzzled, however, and kept asking herself why the priest had said such a thing in a situation so full of pain, loss, and death. She told me that she had understood only much later, when she had to assist one of her parents in the final stage of life. In that situation of suffering, privation, and loss, what had actually lingered longest in her mind was the sense of the wholeness of life she had perceived, rather than her parent's life coming to an end.

SCENARIOS A FACILITATOR MIGHT EXPECT

Here, we will not treat death from a social or anthropological point of view, although that subject might open interesting and culturally enriching discussions. Instead, we will focus on the most common cases for which a Facilitator might be called upon to assist with death:

- a terminally ill patient at a public or private health care facility
- a terminally ill patient being taken care of in their own home
- relatives or friends of a dying person
- someone dying from disease
- someone dying from old age
- someone who has chosen euthanasia or assisted suicide

FEELINGS AND EMOTIONS CONCERNING DEATH AND DYING

We are now going to present you with a selection of citations and observations about subjects concerning the emotionality of death and dying.

Death and the Fear of Death

Some reflections on this subject may be found in a paper written by surgeon, psychotherapist, psychiatrist, and writer Anna Maria Pacilli. In her review of the stance of history's eminent philosophers, we can see the possibility of opening up to a propositional reflection.[1]

Pacilli begins with the Greek philosopher Epicurus (341–270 BCE), who wondered why we think about death and fear it, assuring us that "the most terrifying of fears, death, is nothing to us since so long as we exist death is not present with us, and when death comes, then we no longer exist. Death, then, is of no concern either to the living or to the dead—to the living, death has no existence, and to the dead, no concerns of any kind are possible."[2] What he seems to tell us is that there is no use in fearing death if we cannot really know it.

Blaise Pascal (1623–1662), a French mathematician, physicist, philosopher, and theologian, believed, instead, that even though it is easier to accept death without thinking about it, the greatness of human beings lies in their ability to be aware of their own experience. He wrote, "Man is but a reed, the most feeble thing in nature; but he is a thinking reed. . . . But, if the universe were to crush him, man would still be more noble than that which killed him, because he knows that he dies. . . . All our dignity consists, then, in thought."[3]

German philosopher Martin Heidegger (1889–1976), a major exponent of ontological idealism, encouraged us to give up talking about death, calling it an impersonal dying, not the death of the speaking subject. From this perspective, death is not real for anyone. He claimed that it only makes sense to talk about death through the observation not of death but of the phenomenon of dying, which is certainly painful when it touches those we love. According to Heidegger, human beings mostly consider death to be an uncertain event, one that will occur some day but does not threaten them because it is not yet present. People, he said, do not have the courage to bear the anxiety that would make them face themselves authentically and recognize that death is certain and possible at all times.

On the contrary, Jean-Paul Sartre (1905–1980), the French existentialist philosopher and playwright, believed that human beings find death to be only absurd; it comes from the outside and remains unintelligible since meaning is always realized through the subject, but death erases the subject. . . . Nonetheless, Heidegger regarded death as a life event that must be understood also on an existential level, not only biologically, because it is the ultimate meaning of existence, the "being for death."

Pacilli notes that the laic response to the fear of death seems to be to exorcise it by intensely experiencing pleasures, affections, and desires and trying to make them come true as much as possible. We try to exorcise death because most of us regard death as an event that must be avoided as much as possible, living intensely in the present moment and projecting into the future through more and more projects.

Yet, as German philosopher Max Scheler (1875–1928) tells us, the more we run from death, the closer we get to it; at each instant, the time of the past increases, the present compresses, and the future shortens, bringing death ever closer to our present.

In his 2015 book *Morire di paura* (Dying of fear), Alberto Mazzocchi analyzes the fear of death through the observations of laic and religious physicians, researchers, philosophers, and thinkers of different epochs. He quotes Socrates: "Death is one of two things. Either it is annihilation, and the dead have no consciousness of anything, or, as we are told, it is really a change—a migration of the soul from this place to another."

Mazzocchi continues:

Some say that fear is the main cause for our illnesses. . . . Perhaps this is a bit of an exaggeration, but the modern world certainly seems to be oriented toward the transmission and diffusion of fears of all kinds. . . . We are constantly overwhelmed by the news reports telling us of tragedies and negative events. In a society that makes sure to provide all kinds of certainties, from financial investments to political programs, from working activities to hobbies, we often hear about illness—often not adequately—but no one is eager to talk about death. . . . Death is avoided, as if addressing it will bring bad luck. . . .

Paradoxically, it seems that the progress of modern medicine, emphasized so greatly in media, can do little or nothing against degenerative diseases, the major cause of death in the richest countries. People still die, but with much more fear. The fear of death conditions our entire life, in particular with the appearance of the inevitable "signs of aging," but death can only rarely be foretold. The lady with the scythe, as death is portrayed in ancient paintings and in films of the past century, comes when she wants and usually takes our body in an instant. Why are we afraid then?

Few people had the chance to explore what happens after that fatal moment. They tell us about experiences of light and great peace and serenity. Science has a hard time believing it and regards this experience as hallucinatory mechanisms of suffering brains. We do not know for sure who is right, but I believe we should at least wonder whether it is worth being so afraid of such an inevitable event, preventing ourselves from serenely living life at its fullest.[4]

Stereotypes about Death

Nowadays, Western society is often said to practice the dehumanization of death and dying. That claim is itself a stereotype. In some cases it is true; in others it is not. It is never helpful to generalize.

There are many stereotypes surrounding death, and to analyze them we are going to borrow the point of view of Italian sociologist, scholar, and essayist Marzo Barbagli, who explains them through the perspective of various thinkers in different fields of knowledge, as reviewed in an article by journalist Raffaele Liucci:

> In contemporary times, the latest false myth is the removal of death, which according to several historians, sociologists, philosophers, anthropologists, and psychologists is a prerogative of our society.... The estrangement of death was [said to be] an aspect of the "civilization process," consisting in emotional self-control.... On the contrary, Barbagli believes arguments of this kind are suggestive but refutable through empirical and historical research. His widely multidisciplinary investigation, in which he even draws upon the history of thinking and ideas, is an implicit apology about the risks of nostalgic ahistorical perspectives on the past.... That is not only because in times gone by it was possible to suddenly die on the street, but also because war, famine, and epidemics made it extremely hard to plan and manage one's own death, especially for the poor. Furthermore, dying was generally painful and anything but serene. "For at least three hundred years after the fourth century, an incredible number of people died either in a lazaretto [an institution for people with contagious diseases] or on a carriage that was forcibly taking them there, avoided by family and friends and surrounded by cries and screams of other dying people." Barbagli believes that contemporary society does not hide and fear death more than

it used to in the past; what happened is that the average life span lengthened, family ties loosened, the role of religion was downsized, bacteriology and microbiology revolutionized medical knowledge, big epidemics that used to kill quickly and indiscriminately gave way to long-term chronic and degenerative illnesses. For this reason, the "hospitalization of death," which started at the end of the nineteenth century, has now taken over—though not everywhere—family rituals that used to be adequate in a traditional society that gave to the external manifestations of grief the function of sharing pain, something that is now done through Facebook pages dedicated to friends who have died. The ever-growing diffusion of hospices, palliative care, and biological testaments proves that death was never removed from our horizon but rather recalibrated on the basis of an ethic focused on the reduction of suffering. The control of pain is one of the greatest achievements of modern medicine, despite those who believe that it transforms individuals into insensitive spectators of human decadence (Ivan Illich). . . . We left behind the patronizing model that used to hide death and achieved a medical discipline that privileges the patient's autonomy and right to know. Wittgenstein wrote, "I was in no way shocked when I heard I had cancer, but I was when I heard that one can do something about it, because I had no will to live on." Not all the ill are so seraphic in their reaction to a negative diagnosis, since each death obviously constitutes a unique event. We can try to grasp its general tendencies through demographic statistics, but we have to give up in front of the singularity of each death.[5]

One of the most well-known therapists in Italy to work with all aspects of assistance to the dying is Ange Fey. Fey works with different organizations and institutions to support and educate health care professionals in assisting the dying. He created the Early Declaration of Treatment (DAT in Italian), a form that, in Italy, allows people to state their own will about their final stage of life should anything occur that deprives them of their ability to make a decision.[6] (Other countries have different versions of similar documentation.) An organization for oncological volunteers described Fey's training as a "process meant to help people contact the intimate part of themselves in which they can find the understanding of death and dying, enabling them to recognize and activate their own inner path on various levels. . . . Its purpose is serving as an encounter with life, an experience that never rejects deaths nor discourages the fear of meeting it, through a program full of practical aspects that are articulated within a wide cultural context."[7]

Transformative Chances

Thanatology is a branch of forensic medicine that studies death and the losses it causes, as well as the biological changes that occur during it. In this text, we have already encountered Elisabeth Kübler-Ross's psychothanatology, which introduced the psychological changes surrounding death and dying. We now offer an excerpt of an interview by thanatologist Maria Angela Gelati of philosopher, pedagogic counselor, and writer Laura Campanello.

M.A.G.: Epicurus said, "It is possible to provide security against other ills, but as far as death is concerned, men live in a city without walls."

L.C.: Death, fragility, and precariousness concern all human beings indiscriminately. On the one hand, that is what allows us to share the experience of life and pain; but on the other hand, it's what makes us distance ourselves from those who suffer—leaving them alone!—because in their pain we see what could occur to us, something we cannot escape from and are exposed to exactly because we are human. Never considering such dimension of life often causes us to live life with superficiality and fear, but considering it too much mortifies life and makes it gloomier. Philosophy invites us to give meaning and value to our life because it has a purpose and because what we experience is unique and unrepeatable. . . .

M.A.G.: Can philosophic exercise about death help us act through existential movements that are crucial for human life? How?

L.C.: For sure. That is why I recommend it as a way to live each day as if it were the last and to allow ourselves the right to cry and to grieve. It can help us to better identify our position in life for what it is and find hope, happiness, friendship, and true dialogue.

M.A.G.: To sum it up, it's better to wake up every morning saying, "I'm alive, and it's just the beginning!"

L.C.: Yes, to wake up and realize we are alive, because it's not something to take for granted. To realize that every day is the day to acknowledge what's good; to try to bear what's not and transform it; to consider the condition of our soul and make sure that we search for its authenticity and happiness no matter what; to elevate above our overwhelming routine and observe life from the perspective of the whole, look at ourselves from above, and give due weight to ourselves and to life events. Despite everything, happiness is possible, not only when there is no pain or fatigue.

M.A.G.: What does it mean to take care of people in fragility, fear, and death?

L.C.: It means being there for them; making them feel less alone; helping them weave a weft of meaning made of their personal history and find possible life directions; letting them express their fears, anger, and dismay so that these emotions don't stop their possible transformations. For me, it mostly means doing everyday the philosophical exercise of death and feeling the depth of life, giving it value, and trying to give a chance to those who think they do not have any. I do all of that with respect and the certainty that a spiritual path—either religious or not—is always possible for anyone.[8]

OBSERVATIONS

We have intentionally exempted ourselves from offering a specific arbitrary perspective on the end of life, meaning the transition from the known phases of the Life Cycle to possible unknown ones, underlining the aspect of possibility over any subjective opinion on the subject. We have done so in the respect of any conviction or faith (agnostic, laic, religious, etc.), and at the same time, we have tried to avoid an ethical disquisition about the end of life in cases of assisted voluntary death (euthanasia) by proposing various accounts of researchers, philosophers, physicians, writers, and therapists who address, study, and interpret the phenomenon of death.

What we can add to that is only our perception about the need of the dying and those who assist them to have physical contact with another human being—a perception that, with no intention to be arrogant or conceited, is more of a certainty. The sense of abandonment that many people feel in the final stage of their lives is strongly connected with the absence of a loving and compassionate contact (meant as intimate communion, communication, and sharing transmitted through touch even more than through words), the tactile perception associated with reassuring gestures previously experienced in life (one need only think of the embrace, which is the first contact after birth). That is why techniques such as CST and SER can be of extreme importance in these moments, and not only for their connection to quantum mechanics. Shared care happens also through touch.

THE PHYSIOLOGY OF DEATH IN CST AND SER

When examining the different parts of the system that are most involved in the process of death, we need to bear in mind that every part of the physiological system is important in the holistic perspective of CST and SER. Therefore, when we talk about single functional parts, we must not lose sight of the overall vision of the entire Open-System Human Being.

The energetic framework of the system is essential in the CST and SER approach to the process of the biological conclusion of existence. If the vectors are dysfunctional and not aligned to their axis, the spirit has difficulty coming out of the body. The feet listening station is crucial to introduce us to the profundity of total contact and to verify the treatments, especially when patients are bedridden and intubated.

From the feet station, by patiently listening to the craniosacral rhythm and the entire system, we can observe the realignment of the vector/axis system.

In addition to that realignment, Dr. Upledger indicated some physiological structures to dialogue with, using Therapeutic Imagery and Dialogue, to support those who are approaching the end of their existence. Below, we'll describe those structures with specific reference to aspects that are functional to the subjects we are addressing. Any further detail in this respect can be found in Dr. Upledger's *A Brain Is Born* and *Cell Talk*.

Pons

The pons is known as the "great connector." It is located in the brain stem just beneath the midbrain; therefore, it connects the higher centers of the brain with the entire body through the structures beneath it. Underneath the pons we find the cerebellum, the medulla oblongata, and the spinal cord.

Dr. Upledger tells us that our spirit leaves the body through the pons. When our physical body stops existing, the spirit passes upward through the pons. Moreover, the pons perceives cosmic information and is involved in all vital decisions. It carries out a great work of selection and also has an isolating and/or stabilizing function for the various cerebral subsystems. If necessary, it carries out some of the tasks of the RAS.

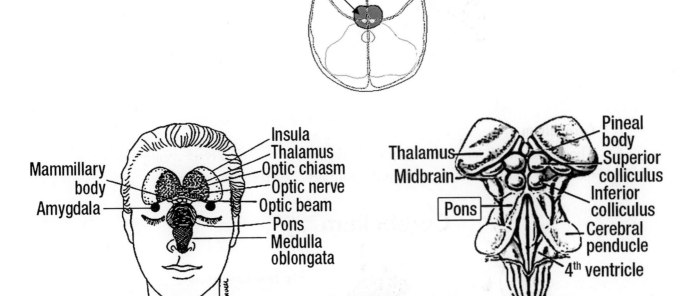

Fig. 20.2. Pons and adjacent anatomical structures

Vagus Nerve

This tenth cranial nerve is influenced by the cerebellum, which sends to it the message to arrest cardiac and respiratory activities, inducing the death process, when it perceives it is the proper moment. When writing about the vagus system and how it is influenced by the cerebellum, Dr. Upledger explained it through the experiences of therapists who reported working with patients who passed away quickly and easily only a few hours after being treated with CST, even though they had been suffering for a long time before that.

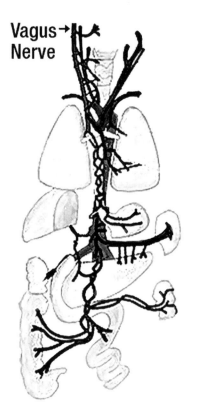

Fig. 20.3. Vagus nerve

Cerebellum

The cerebellum decides when it is time for the body to die and is consequently able to induce the death process, often through its influence on the vagus nerve.

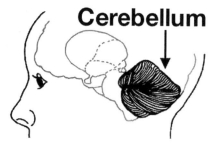

Fig. 20.4. Cerebellum

Center

The center does not receive much attention in anatomy and neurology textbooks. It is located between the two hippocampi, which constitute its base and support. Its structure is pyramidal and its summit is located exactly on the medial line of the head. Anatomically speaking, the center is connected with the hippocampi and the central lobe of the brain (insula).

Most of the center's work is done through energetic connections. It receives spiritual and cosmic energy through the crown chakra (seventh chakra), which is located in the bregma, and sends that energy to wherever it is needed in the organism. Its energetic connection passes through the heart and reaches down to the sacrum. If the vertex of the center is not in the correct position, it receives only part of the incoming energy.

The center works constantly to monitor the Ego, keep us alive and functional, and allow us to relax when it is required in order to heal on a physical, psychoemotional, and spiritual level.

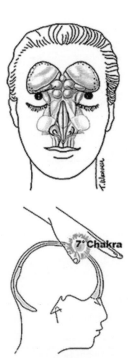

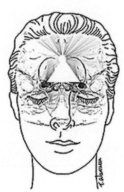

Fig. 20.5. The pons, crown chakra, and center

TWO EXERCISES FOR PERSONAL GROWTH

The exercises for personal growth that we propose are useful to stimulate a subjective focus on what you have read so far. They could surprise you. Facilitators complete these exercises during their training; we encourage you to try them as well, if and when you feel like it. We invite you to write down your impressions, thoughts, and answers about the exercises and what you have learned up to this point.

Personal Growth Exercise 1: What Is Death for the Living?

On the fear of death: What is death for the living? Give at least three brief answers.

1. _____

2. _____

3. _____

On your thoughts about death: What do the words *death*, *separation*, and *loss* mean for you? Summarize your thoughts.

Death_____

Separation _____

Loss _____

On your fear of death: Answer the following questions.

Right now, what are your thoughts and fears about death?

_____

_____

Which scares you more: your death or other people's death? Why?

_____

_____

If you could choose, how would you want to die?

_____

_____

Personal Growth Exercise 2

You have only one last chance to communicate. To whom would you feel the need to write your last message? Write what you have to say to that person in the form of a letter.

_____

_____

_____

_____

_____

_____

You might later find a chance to reflect on what you wrote.

Clinical Observations

I was teaching an advanced CST seminar to a group of ten students. During this seminar, as I coordinated a multi-hands treatment in which four Facilitators were treating one of their fellow students who was in the role of patient, I experienced something very surprising.

The student who was being treated by the others was someone I had known for years. I had been his Instructor on many occasions as he went through the various levels of his core training. To help you understand why I was so surprised, let me tell you a little about him.

Up until that moment, even though he had very positive qualities as a human being, as a student he had perplexed me. Yet there was nothing about his learning path and work as a Facilitator that could be criticized. I will try to make myself clear: I had always considered him to be an extremely honest, polite, sensitive, respectful, attentive, focused, and kind person, so much so that I could define him as a gentleman—and I assure you that this characterization is appropriate.

What perplexed me concerned his SER treatments. Generally, when students are being treated by the others, they are encouraged to express their emotionality with no inhibition. Whereas the other students followed their emotions, this student never seemed to manifest much. His emotionality always looked somehow dormant, or so calm that he never seemed to have any emotional factor to work on. Therefore, I had always thought that when he was in the role of patient, the exercises were inconclusive for him.

I had started to think that he was not benefiting from the treatments he received, and yet he always came to all the SER seminars. I wondered why; as a therapist, he was in attendance to learn a method he would later have to employ with his patients, but it did not make sense to delve further in that subject if he could not understand its beneficial effects. Nonetheless, he was always eager to carry out all the seminar exercises, both as a patient and as a Facilitator.

I started to have personal conversations with him outside of classes, trying to grasp in his words any emotional aspects I might have overlooked. Nothing emerged.

Now, during this advanced seminar, he opened up emotionally with his fellow therapists, and he disclosed a scenario he had never before revealed—and it was not exactly a little thing!

He had experienced fetal death, not his own, but that of his twin sister who had shared their mother's womb with him.

He had basically experienced death even before experiencing birth.

It seems appropriate now to open the subject of vanishing twin syndrome.

Psychosynthetic counselor Chiara Pasin, in an article on the subject, described what a surviving twin experiences when they finally address bereavement and grief:

> With twins, it sometimes happens that one cannot be born, or that they "sacrifice" themselves to let the other live. This causes the surviving twin to live with a constant burden and a sense of guilt that seems not to have a concrete, specific reason to exist. . . . This individual may experience later in life emotional blockages and/or a constant agitation that fades only when they address their prenatal bereavement; until this loss is dealt with, it feels unbearable and unexplainable. . . . Other symptoms of the survivor twin generally include a sense of dismay, perennial incompleteness and lack, a nostalgia about something unknown that at the same time feels like it used to belong to the individual but did not have the chance to be experienced, anger, sadness, guilt, emotional attachments so strong they become actual addictions, and great difficulty in dealing with any kind of abandonment or bereavement. It is as if the survivor could not live fully, as if they were only a half of a whole, or as if they were living for two.[9]

Psychologists Alfred R. and Bettina Austermann's book *Drama in the Womb: The Surviving Twin Syndrome* mentions Belgian physician Dr. Sartenaer, who specialized in prenatal therapy. In his analysis of this work, Umberto Carmignani wrote,

> Sartenaer observed through ultrasound scan that one pregnancy out of eight shows a multiple conception, and sometimes multiple embryos, but only one case out of 70 childbirths involves twins. The death of the other embryos occurs usually by the first trimester of pregnancy; when it does before the fourteenth gestational week, the embryo is completely absorbed by the placenta and integrated in the body of the twin; when it does after, it is possible to see in the placenta a sort of fossilized fetus. Before the [19]80s and the advent of ultrasound methods, a vanishing twin was rarely noticed since the mother does not feel anything unusual on a physical level. However, prenatal psychology found out that the fetus, even in its state of embryo, suffers hugely for such a precocious bereavement, which will become for millions of people the cause of discomfort, sometimes aggressiveness and restlessness, or even a sense of guilt for being alive and/or a death wish. In our work, we realized that many cases of unexplainable suffering or constant difficulties in the relationship with others are connected with the issue of the vanishing twin. In all of those cases, their patients always asked what

was wrong with them, why their relationships were so bad, and/or why their professional life was so awful.[10]

I believe we have now contextualized the scenario I was facing when I was supervising the exercise in which that particular student was being treated.

I do not wish to describe the treatment in detail—it would not be fair since it was not carried out by me but by the Facilitators participating in that seminar. What I will tell you is what my student confided in me, and agreed for me to share, when I asked him to tell me about that experience quite some time later—because some time was necessary for him to process that treatment.

As the conscious person he has always proven to be, he had considered several factors and investigated with his family the results of the treatment. He had dealt with his peculiar prenatal experience in different ways, even asking for help from experts in that field who used the same methods as the professionals I have mentioned before. He had taken an interest in family constellations (which have their foundation in phenomenological and systemic psychology and whose first form of methodological approach was developed in 1980 thanks to Bert Hellinger) and chronogenetics (founded in 2001 by Temogim Schreiber Perotti, Mariane Wetzel, Mario Grilli, and Domenica Nieddu as a technique of psychogenealogy and neurolinguistic planning).

Here I must insert a sidebar.

If a student of mine seeks the answers that are the most adequate to their problem or situation, without stopping at the first therapeutic solution encountered, I always feel proud. I feel like I have contributed (at least partly, I hope) to the reinforcement of the concept of freedom and free will in other people, and it is a concept that I really try to convey as a teacher and Facilitator.

Not only that, I am so convinced that Dr. Upledger's techniques are extremely effective that I feel confident in stating that they are a way to achieve the awareness that every person needs for self-healing. Even though their effect cannot be immediately observed in some cases, CST and SER techniques constitute the foundation for the virtuous and constructive process of self-awareness—and therefore also the encounter/dialogue with the Higher Self.

In fact, I often tell my students and patients that CranioSacral Therapy is not THE therapy but ONE of the therapies. Nonetheless, it was for me the most important therapy I have ever encountered in my professional path, and I hope they can understand it and benefit from it as well, either discovering it now or recognizing its value in the future, in any phase of their Life Cycle.

Anyway, when I asked my student whether he wished to talk to me about his experience, he agreed. First he told me that becoming aware of what had happened at the beginning of his own life brought him some comfort in relation to several emotional issues that he had faced up until that point but could not explain. He was now able to recognize symptoms of vanishing twin syndrome, such as immense loneliness and a sense of guilt for being alive when his twin was not, which made it possible for him to describe his symptoms and deal with them with greater serenity.

After listening to him, I asked him which symptoms he recognized as his own. He replied that he recognized almost all of them since they were all connected with each other. He also added that the important thing was that his sensation of being different had faded, or at least he had accepted it as an unavoidable aspect of being alive. After all, who is really the same as anyone else?

Apart from all of that, he told me that his syndrome is considered a radicalized trauma, and among its distinctive signs is difficulty in choosing a professional sector. He had always been torn between a military career and specialization in manual therapies. He thought the army was his own true choice, whereas it was his twin—who had sacrificed herself to leave him the vital space he needed in order to grow—who was the actual therapist, and it was for that reason she had saved him. It was to honor his twin's soul that he had become a therapist while still pursuing his military career.

Let me disagree on this point. Even considering his syndrome, as his Instructor and colleague I am convinced that his choice of working in the therapeutic field is due mostly to his desire to help others and maybe partly to his need to compensate for not being able to help his twin survive (as the general symptoms of the syndrome indicate).

After the clarifications he gave me, I felt relief from my doubts that he could receive successful SER treatments. I understood that his recalcitrance was connected with his discretion in expressing something intimate concerning another person, his twin sister, and in thinking at the same time that he did not deserve to pour out his emotions in search of relief. As the survivor twin, he deemed himself privileged for having been born. Nonetheless, he had actually benefited from the treatments since he admitted that he had felt each one of them only after some time and gradually, as if he was being reminded of something exactly when he needed it the most.

I hope he will be able to believe and understand that he was born with a bright light, and that might have been a cause of serenity and peace for his twin sister.

⁘ A CST-CENTERED VISION ⁘

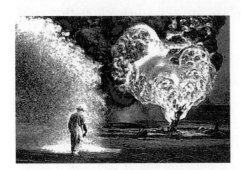

Fig. 20.6. Reproduction of *Kuwait: A Desert on Fire,* by Sebastião Salgado

Commenting on his photograph *Kuwait: A Desert on Fire* (fig. 20.6), Sebastião Salgado said, "Never before or since have I witnessed an unnatural disaster on such a scale. It was like facing the end of the world, a world filled with blackness and death."[11] The photo was taken in Kuwait in 1991, when, in the so-called "black gold war," Iraqi soldiers set more than six hundred oil wells on fire to prevent the U.S. coalition from advancing.

Salgado was traumatized by his experience in Kuwait. Nonetheless, he was able to document everything he observed as a spectator and to offer his insights to those who would see his photographs. In fact, those powerful images succeeded in bringing awareness about that tragedy to the world.

Facilitators, too, witness tragic events, in this case through their patients. Like Salgado, they do not need a specific or personal interpretation; they just need to be impartial witnesses. By relying on their Higher Self, Facilitators can help their patients become aware of their condition—whatever it may be—and find all the tools to deal with it.

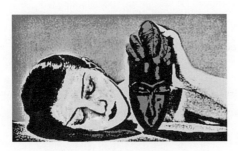

Fig. 20.7. Reproduction of *Black and White,* by Man Ray (aka Emmanuel Radnitzky)

Man Ray, a surrealist photographer, chose the title for *Black and White* (fig. 20.7) to highlight the opposition between the white complexion of the woman and the blackness of the African mask in a game of contrasts. The woman looks like she is absorbed in a dream.

Dreams are an essential element in surrealist art; they represent freedom and transgression, just as in real life they help us overcome mental barriers and censures as well as directly access the unconscious, the essence of our thoughts. The two feminine figures in the photo—the woman and the mask—get closer to each other beyond time and space.

The contrast of black and white is emblematic in the representation of opposites like life and death. In *Black and White,* it is fundamental to note that the two faces are on the same surface, representing the dialogue between differences that must occur on a communal plane. For us, in the dialogue between the scenarios of life and death, everything starts with a question: *What is death for the living?*

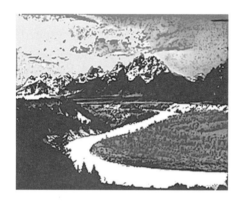

Fig. 20.8. Reproduction of *The Tetons and the Snake River,* by Ansel Adams

Ansel Adams is well-known for his black-and-white photographs of landscapes taken in American national parks. Among his most popular, *The Tetons and Snake River* (fig. 20.8) offers us a breathtaking sight. The sinuous river is highlighted by the play of light resulting from the black and white of the photographic image, giving the impression that in the stillness of the picture, the river is waiting to find its path in the landscape, although the trace it has left over time is very clear. The observer may believe that the river can still choose whether to flow down toward the sea or to climb the mountain, challenging the laws of physics. In the same way, the CST therapist simply listens to the patient, respecting their free will and disregarding any expectation.

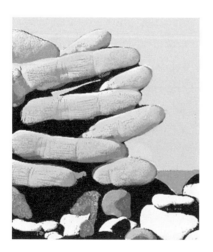

Fig. 20.9. Reproduction of *Nude, Baie des Anges,* by Bill Brandt

Bill Brandt was a British photographer of the twentieth century who became famous for his nocturnal and nude photographs. About his work, he said, "I interfered very little, and the lens produced anatomical images and shapes which my eyes had never observed."

While we observe our patients as they process a stage of their path in the vital energy continuum of their Life Cycle, we may witness physical and emotional phenomena that we never would have observed otherwise. CST provides us with the means (the lens) to exercise this new type of observation. The richness of the images we can obtain through that can allow us to help ourselves as well as our patients. The interweaving of the therapist's experiences and those of the patients during treatments provides the strength that is necessary to defeat fear and face transformational phases.

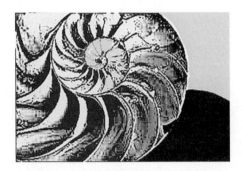

Fig. 20.10. Reproduction of *Shell,* by Edward Weston

To "photograph life" is how Edward Weston himself described the mission he gave to himself. To him, seizing life in any of its forms is the only possible way to be a photographer; that is why he became the representative of realism in photography. He believed a photographer needs to visualize the picture inside himself before taking it.

Similarly, in CST and SER, to see reality, to observe and understand it, and to be aware of the scenarios in which the patient's personal occurrences develop mean to accept seeing the macrocosm in the microcosm. Seizing life means seizing the essence of the particular in a single scenario among the multitude of possible scenarios and translating it in a real and universal language in order to make it intelligible to the patient.

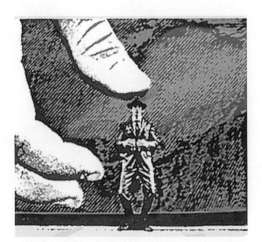

Fig. 20.11. Reproduction of *A Certain Oppression,* by Rodney Smith

Rodney Smith was defined as a minimalist photographer. For him, photography evoked the essence of experience. With *A Certain Oppression* (fig. 20.11), he tells a story about himself through a particular sensation, indicating his transformational epilogue. He described it as the representation of his own sensation, which he concretely visualized as an image of himself turning back and seeing a huge hand behind him that was trying to crush him. What he learned from this, he said, was that if the world itself tries to stop your energy, it is the right time to take a deep breath and use it to trace new paths of light.

We believe there is nothing to add to Rodney Smith's statement. We leave to you the task of reflecting on his vision.

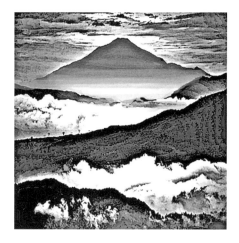

Fig. 20.12. Reproduction of *Tranquility,* by Hengki Koentjoro

Strength, calm, and serenity inviting us to respect nature define the visual representation of the pictures taken by Indonesian artist Hengki Koentjoro. He says that the light he seeks must be bright and contrasting because the right contrast can bring tension and harmony and therefore becomes essential to impart emotion to the image. For Koentjoro, immersing himself in his light and contrasts is a journey into an unknown world whose borders and boundaries he wants to discover. This journey of his certainly excludes any banality and has as its goal the serenity and well-being of the mind.

When we observe *Tranquility* (fig. 20.12), our eyes are drawn to the highest peak in the background, which pierces the clouds as its base "floats" in the light. The peak is the destination and the base is the preparation to ascend. The valleys and the uplands before it inevitably appear surmountable.

In parallel fashion, the Facilitator supports patients by helping their organism face the way to their destination in any of its phases.

Digression

Real generosity toward the future lies in giving all to the present.
                                                            ALBERT CAMUS

The last exercise of personal growth invited you to write a final message to someone you deem worthy of receiving it. If you wrote it, it may mean you never communicated that message to that person.

Ask yourself, *Why have I not told him/her/them?*

The possible reasons can be several, including the effective impossibility of reaching the recipient (though, ask yourself, *Is that really so?*).

However, if the message is important to you and you have the chance to communicate it, then think about it. Do not leave those fragments of life sedentary; they can become a burden in your path, preventing the smooth flow of your vital energy continuum. If you can, try to express what you need to express and do it in the here and now.

If you cannot do it, let it go with your intention and set yourself free on the way toward the next phase of your Life Cycle.

A CST-CENTERED VISION

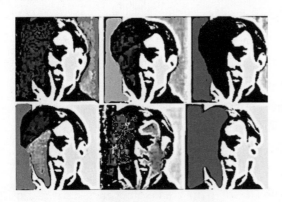

Fig. 20.13. Reproduction of *Self-Portrait,* by Andy Warhol

Ever the unconventional pop artist, Andy Warhol believed art must be consumed as a commercial product. He painted common objects and transformed them into artistic subjects. His multiple portraits with chromatic variations are particularly famous.

When we make choices, we are always ourselves, and yet we are always different. We are recognizable works of art. Can we be as we want to be? We can make it true! We could help ourselves and the people around us by doing so. We can plan it with our intention and modify our attitude in order to transform our actions as we address the test of life.

CHAPTER 21

The Final Treatment

The Origin of Techniques for Death and Transition

A man is completely enveloped by his true nature, which is not divided in two hemispheres to go from one to another as it likes depending on convenience and comfort.

ALDO BUSI, GRAZIE DEL PENSIERO

Even though we need to mention the energetic framework of the human body once again, and we will have the chance to delve into other methods of energetic assessment, we must never forget that the foundation of Dr. Upledger's CranioSacral Therapy and SomatoEmotional Release is knowing, treating, and listening to the human body through the aptonomy of touch, and that no technique or assessment method occurs outside the contact with the patient's body. Though other techniques can be implemented at a close distance from the patient's body when it is strictly necessary, the core cognitive base is anatomical-physiological. Physical contact through noninvasive palpation is the foundation for any assessment (e.g., the assessment of the craniosacral rhythm) and fascial mobilization; this procedure constitutes an integral part of the fundamental requirements of CST and SER treatments.

To support people in the various phases of pain they sometimes have to go through during their Life Cycle as a consequence of the loss of a loved one or a small death, or during a scenario of death and transition, Facilitators must employ the therapeutic gesture in all treatments. It consists of the manual techniques that Facilitators have learned in their professional training and have contributed to their competence, ability, and knowledge of CST and SER, contributing at the same time to their personal growth and specialization in the treatment of patients who had to go through a loss, abandonment, or bereavement.

Obviously, in the protocol of the final treatment that we are going to propose for the process of death and transition, there are specific techniques to employ. The first

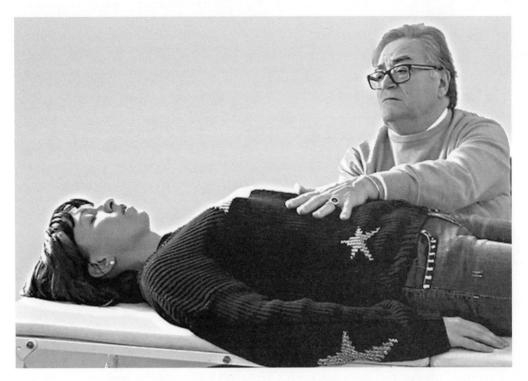

Fig. 21.1. Diego Maggio treating the respiratory diaphragm

is the realignment of the vectors, which we have covered previously, but the vectors have, additionally, another quality that can help our treatment protocol support the loss of losses. Let us see how and why before delving into further assessment methods.

UNITING THE CNS, RAS, LIMBIC SYSTEM, AND THE THREE BRAINS

The Facilitator starts in the preferred position for assessing the layout of the vector/axis system in the organism: at the feet listening station, with their hands on the patient's insteps (in the position of tactile/listening perception).

The Facilitator must work on the realignment of the energetic framework of the vector/axis system to rebalance and harmonize the energetic connection of the Open-System Human Being with the universe, preparing what is necessary for the following work on the other structures of the organism.

The Facilitator checks whether the central vector is aligned with the superior directional pole of the skull, using as a reference the ideal line that unites the first chakra to the seventh (which is located on the bregma). Once the correct alignment of the central vector with its axis is verified or restored, the most adequate cranial vault hold for the case at hand will help the Facilitator focus on the path of the vector from the sixth to the seventh chakra. This is the same energetic reference the

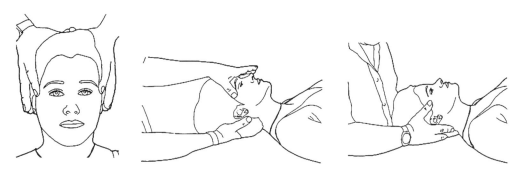

Fig. 21.2. The three cranial vault holds

Facilitator will use to work also with the corpus callosum, which unites the two cerebral hemispheres. In this way, they will connect as well with the central nervous system, the RAS, the limbic system, and the three brains (reptilian brain, mammalian brain, and neocortex).

An Intuitive Analogy

We certainly know that matter is energy and everything is interconnected. We know of the connection between the two cerebral hemispheres through the corpus callosum, which joins them. We know that we will interact with the entire energetic structure of the human body, including the physiological components of the central nervous system.

In this respect, before giving more reasons to explain the importance of the energetic framework of the human body, we would like to focus on what Dr. Upledger wrote on the subject: "The energy particle can easily transform from Nerve Cell to Immune Cell or Hormonal Cell or cell located wherever it decides (exactly: 'decides') to move to. One of the characteristics of consciousness is intelligence; therefore, an energy particle can certainly decide when and where to move."[1]

By acquiring awareness about this connection, which is rooted both on equating matter and energy (matter is energy) and on the ontological aspects of the connection itself, we are able to consider a scenario in which the passage from one known phase to the following unknown phase of the Life Cycle (the loss of losses, or death) occurs.

The treatment that the Facilitator is about to carry out involves first all the vectors and the entire vector/axis system, the two cerebral hemispheres, and the corpus callosum. In order to better understand the importance of this initial target of treatment for this extremely delicate and crucial phase of the Life Cycle, we propose an intuitive analogy found by Dr. Upledger during his eclectic studies, which was quite useful in his research: the correlation between the image of the Shem Ha Meforash ("the Name," meaning the name of God) and the graphical image with which the energetic framework of the human body is usually represented.

Dr. Upledger did not write about this analogy in any of his textbooks, but we are now able to give a written form to what he transmitted to us only orally, thanks to next section, which Facilitator Devid Caressa wrote for us, summarizing a subject on which rabbis and rebbes (the rabbis of Jewish mysticism) have been debating for thousands of years.

A Work of Mind and Body
By Devid Caressa

Devid Caressa is a Facilitator and a masseur with a diploma of CranioSacral Therapy from the Upledger Institute in Italy and a diploma of naturopathy from the Riza Institute of Psychosomatic Medicine in Milan. He comes from a Sephardic family (a Jewish ethnic group originally from North Africa and the Iberian Peninsula); his ancestors were Spanish Jews. At the moment, he is one of the three cantors (hazzan or chazzan, from the singular of the Hebrew word) at the reform synagogue Lev Chadash (whose name literally means "new heart") of Milan. He is also a teacher of kabbalah, the discipline of Jewish mysticism, and was qualified by the schools Chokmat Ha Emet (literally "wisdom of the truth") and Leitel Leitel (an initiatory name used by King Salomon in Proverbs) in Jerusalem and Milan, respectively.

It is extremely interesting how Dr. Upledger saw what had been noticed in the Jewish cultural context a long time ago. Since in Judaism there is the prohibition to depict the Lord graphically, no one had ever compared the Shem Ha Meforash to the human body in such a detailed way.

I must first make a premise, which is that Dr. Upledger came to this analogy while he was reflecting on the image you can see in figure 21.5, which to him could represent the vector/axis system, the energetic framework of the human body. At first it was only an intuition, but then he started searching for the meaning of that image until he deduced that his intuitive vision brought him before a much wider reality, the YodHeiVavHei.

In fact, Genesis 1:27 is explicit that "G-d made man in His own image."

According to Jewish mysticism, YodHeiVavHei has a series of correspondences with anything quadripartite. For example, in physics yod = gravity, superior hei = weak interaction, vav = electromagnetism, inferior hei = strong interaction.

However, let us go back to Dr. Upledger.

I believe that many would agree with me if I claimed that Dr. Upledger can be considered one of the Chasidei Umot Ha Olam ("Just among Nations"). It is a title usually attributed to those who follow in the footsteps of the Lord and cooperate with the Jewish people in the *tikkun olam* (restoration of the world).

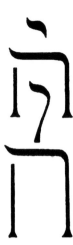

Fig. 21.3. Shem Ha Meforash

According to the Talmud, in all generations there are thirty-six Lamedvavnikim, thirty-six human beings whose conduct determines the destiny of mankind. It is believed that there can be thirty-six among the Jews and thirty-six among the "Gentiles," a term that indicates the non-Jews. Dr. Upledger could be included in this last group of thirty-six, given that his personal writings talk about an "energetic framework" of the human body—how Dr. John used to call it. This energetic framework has a very peculiar appearance, even more for a Jew or someone who speaks Hebrew; in fact, this framework looks exactly the same as one of the names the Jews use to designate the Lord, only written vertically. Of course the Jewish people have known for a long time that the most sacred name of G-d (who is called in various different ways in Judaism) looks like a human figure if written vertically. Anyway, no one had ever dared say before that that same name, the holiest name to call G-d in Judaism, could be the very energetic framework of human body, which gives credit to those who claim that the Lord must be searched for and exists inside ourselves, a complicated matter that is still being debated today among rabbis and rebbes.

The term Y-H-W-H (yod-hei-vav-hei) is employed in writings as the most sacred name of G-d in Judaism, and it is also known as Shem Ha Meforash, "distinctive name," or Havayah or Tetragrammaton.

However, its pronunciation was lost over the centuries; when Jews read this word, they replace it with the term Adonai (literally "my Lord") or Ha Shem (literally "the name").

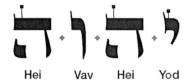

Fig. 21.4. Hebrew is read from right to left, thus Yod Hei Vav Hei

According to Jewish traditions (Mishnà, Sota 7:6), in the time of the first Temple this word could be pronounced only during the celebrations in the Temple. According to the Talmud (Kiddushin 71a, Yoma 40), because of spiritual degradation, in the last period of the Temple only the Cohen Gadol (high priest) knew its correct pronunciation and used it solely on Yom Kippur, the holiest day of the Jewish calendar, and only once he had entered the Qadosh Qadoshim, the Holy of Holies, where no one else could go. The reason for this is that the holy name has extraordinary powers for Jewish mysticism, including the power to heal any illness.

According to Kabbalah, such powers are connected to the fact that this name represents a human figure when the letters are placed vertically and that, since there are different ways of "filling in" the name, one of the four main fillings equals the number 45 [in the Hebrew alphabet, each letter is associated with a number.—*Ed.*], the same number as ADAM, which means literally "human being." The yod represents the head, the first hei represents the arms, the vav stands for the torso, the second hei stands for the legs. This image has been used for centuries in mysticism to meditate, even imagining it inside the body. Moreover, it has different levels of interpretation, but it is interesting to note that Dr. Upledger understood it to be one of the keys for healing the human body!

Jewish mysticism (Zohar) considers the existence of four worlds, which are reflected on the human being: the material world, called Asyiah (represented by the inferior hei of the body); the emotional world, called Yetzirah (the vav); the mental world, called Beri'ah (the superior hei), and the spiritual world, called Atziluth (the Yod).

In Judaism the letter hei is associated with actions on the material plane; it equals the number 5 in the Hebrew alphabet, just like the fingers of each hand that are used to build things and the toes of each foot that are used to move in the world (Asyiah). However, in order to do anything, we must first think about it; therefore, we must pass through the mental world (Beri'ah).

In the middle of the image of the name stands vav, which equals the number 6 and corresponds to the thorax and abdomen. It is interesting to note that traditional Chinese medicine associates the organs of these bodily areas to basic emotions; according to several neuroscientists, there would be exactly six basic emotions (joy, surprise, sadness, fear, disgust, and anger), just like the functional circles of TCM, and each of these emotions would be associated with a specific functional circle. (Dr. Upledger knew well this subject since he was an acupuncturist and developed the SomatoEmotional approach!) Kabbalah talks of the world of Yetzirah.

Above the others, we have the letter yod representing the head. This letter equals the number 10 and represents the entire potential of human beings, corresponding to the spiritual aspect (Atziluth).

They say that if these four worlds are not perfectly aligned, their disharmony could reflect on everything, human beings included.

Well, Dr. Upledger called this image "energetic vectors" and claimed that vectorial misalignments cause an imbalance in the individual. For this reason, Dr. John developed a technique to rebalance this energetic framework, a very important technique because it goes beyond the merely physical aspect, touching upon the energetic parts of the body and giving the therapist an opportunity to restore in the patient's body the primeval balance that is innate in the human matrix. That conception merges with concepts that have been part of Jewish mysticism for centuries.

Jewish mysticism claims that, by chanting repeatedly this name with the formula YoHeVaHe (as taught by Avraham Abulafia, famous mystic of the thirteenth century), the body can be restored from any pain because the voice—which is made of sound waves and biophonons—impacts the body directly and encourages the work of the cells that resound with the name of God, which is the source of all healing.

It is also possible to chant with different tonalities depending on the areas that need to be worked on; just like the Vedanta traditions say about chakras, Judaism has different mantras/divine names that can be chanted with various tonalities, each of which resounds with some of the energetic centers of the body (called *ofanim* in Hebrew). The name Y-H-W-H would include them all.

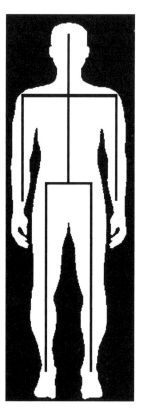

Fig. 21.5. The energetic framework of the human body

It is also important to consider how words are fundamental in Judaism; in Genesis we read, "And G-d said, 'Let there be light" (Gen. 1:3), and throughout all the first chapter this verb ("say") is used every time the narration describes G-d creating the world.

It is for this reason that the greatest Jewish mystics chanted constantly YoHeVaHe as a mantra to connect with the universe through the word and awake that "divine spark" (as it is called, translated from the Hebrew *netzotz*) that lies within us and is able to restore anything.

Chazaq, Dr. Upledger! Thank you for giving all therapists the opportunity to help their patients on all levels, from the physical to the spiritual one, passing through emotions and mind!

✦ ✦ ✦

Another Synergy

Rebbe Rav Menachem Mendel Schneerson (1902–1994), Ukrainian orthodox rabbi, philosopher, mystic, and naturalized American, was the seventh and last rebbe of the Chabad-Lubavitch movement and the Chassidim of the Chabad movement. Today he remains a point of reference for Judaism all over the world because of his knowledge and especially because of his dedication in the search for the *tikkun olam,* the "restoration of the world." In 1978 the U.S. government established Education and Sharing Day in honor of the Rebbe, as he was known, and in 1995 granted him posthumously the Congressional Gold Medal, an honor given only to 130 American citizens from the presidency of Thomas Jefferson to contemporary times.

Many of the teachings of Rebbe Rav Menachem Mendel Schneerson were reported and developed in *Bringing Heaven Down to Earth* and *Wisdom to Heal the World,* two volumes written by Chabad Rabbi Rav Tzvi Freeman. The acknowledgments at the end of *Wisdom to Heal the World* caught our interest since Freeman thanks Rebbe Rav Menachem Mendel Schneerson for encouraging someone to turn to CranioSacral Therapy, defining the latter as "a work of mind and body to heal the soul in collaboration with God."

Dr. Upledger was a Gentile, a non-Jew, and we do not know whether he ever encountered Rebbe Rav Menachem Mendel Schneerson, but we certainly know that synergy exists.

ANTIREDUCTIONISM AND ONTOLOGY

In its philosophical meaning, ontology studies the nature and relations of being, including the higher categories that enable us to give being an order. Depending on the context (philosophical, anthropological, medical, theological, etc.), ontology has been mainly defined as the "phenomenology of being," a branch of metaphysics, the study of phenomena as they are and appear to be, or the group of principles regarding all kinds of knowledge (sensory, psychic, spiritual). Depending on the science, discipline, or school of thought in which it is being employed, ontology also contemplates the concept of Higher Being (God), Absolute, or Higher Principle.

Though these concepts might seem abstract, ontology has been investigated by more concrete scientific fields such as mathematics, modern physics, medicine, and information science (the latter specifically in the context of artificial intelligence).

When we talk about modern physics, especially in this respect, we mean that part of antireductionist physics that studies particles, considering objects not as substances but rather as bundles of properties or collections whose qualities do not depend on a fundamental substratum but on the general properties of the fields. (In physics, a field is a quantity that can be expressed as a function of the location in space and time or, on a relativistic level, in the space-time.)

There is no doubt that in his life as a physician, researcher, and scientist, Dr. Upledger relied on an ontological and antireductionist vision; for this reason, it seems only right to dedicate a part of this chapter to the synthesis of these concepts, which we believe substantiate the details just given by Devid Caressa. Not only that, the concepts of antireductionism and ontology are complementary to the peculiarity of Dr. Upledger's CranioSacral Therapy and SomatoEmotional Release, which are methods that introduce and develop the knowledge of manual techniques in their antireductionist and ontological dimension.

Let us briefly develop the concepts of antireductionism as they relate to biological phenomena. To do so, we cite an article on the subject written by neurologist, iridologist, and homeopath Flavio Gazzola:

> Reductionism claims the reducibility of all biological phenomena to physical-chemical terms. . . . Nonetheless, the advent of quantum physics has demonstrated the inadequacy of classic physics in the explanation of more complex phenomena. . . . Even if we tried to reduce biological systems to a group of chemical elements and physical forces, their functioning would be altered, therefore altering also the outcomes. It is not possible to study the biological principles and the physical-chemical principles on a living being at the same time since the study of one of them excludes the other.
>
> In 1968, M. Polanyi stated that the morphology of living beings transcends the laws of physics and chemistry and is subjected to higher principles, which are additional to those of physics and chemistry. To sum up the situation, we can say that

the antireductionist movement highlights the tendency of reductionist scientists to reduce the complexity of life to a small number of variables in order to be able to study it by employing exclusively physical and chemical principles, thus corrupting the essence of research.[2]

We are now going to see how antireductionism and ontology are closely connected with each other and with neuroscience, as explained in the master's thesis on reductionism and antireductionism written by Federico Zilio, a philosopher specializing in the philosophy of mind, neuroscience, and epistemology. Epistemology is the critical study of nature and the limits of scientific knowledge, with a particular reference to logical structures and scientific methodology; in the past decades, the term has also been increasingly used to more generally designate the theory of knowledge.

Zilio opens the third chapter of his extensive thesis, which analyzes the mind-brain-body problem, by quoting a poem by Emily Dickinson, which we find extremely fitting as well:

I felt a Cleaving in my Mind As if my Brain had split—
I tried to match it—Seam by Seam—But could not make them fit—

As Zilio explains, developments in neuroscience in the twentieth century brought the "mind-body problem" to the attention of both scientists and philosophers. Multidisciplinary research focused on the concept of "embodied cognition" brought an alternative to psychological and philosophical positions such as cognitivism, which left out the body and focused solely on the mind-brain connection. According to this approach,

Cognitive processes—even those of higher level—are intrinsically connected with our bodily structure, sensitivity, and experience; therefore, not only is the body a machine that the mind-brain can direct, but it plays an active role in the determination of cognitive activities.... The mind-brain-body problem cannot be easily labeled as an exclusively epistemological or ontological issue.

Zilio goes on to analyze Northoff's approach, which used methodological cross-functional principles to move between different levels—logical-natural, epistemological-ontological, metaphysical-empirical. He goes on to say,

From here, many examples of dualisms with different degrees of ontological engagement followed.... Mental approaches essentially share one premise, which is that there appear to be phenomena—such as conscious experience—that contain size, weight, shape, and other characteristics that are directly measurable through physical methodologies.... Other perspectives that are essentially dualist but more moderate include "property dualism," which entails the emergence of nonphysical characteristics (thinking in general, consciousness, mental concepts, intentionality, etc.) from a single physical substratum (the brain as an organ); from here we get to the problem of mental causation, meaning a typical example of nonphysical dimension, that is nonetheless useless for the neuroscientific explanation of conscious action.... According to Hart, what can be imagined is also possible, since imagination is to the knowledge of nonactual possibilities what perception is to the knowledge of actuality. Therefore, there would be a direct inference between imagination, conceivability, and possibility.... Mental approaches of this kind ... are founded on the existence of external reality as actuality and try to retrieve from this ontological assumption "something different" that the physical world cannot explain.[3]

We now return to the analysis of scientist and humanist Guido Brunetti, whom we previously encountered in chapter 19, and his overview on the connections between the concept of soul and neuroscience.

We are considering the existence of two ontological principles ... an immaterial one, the "soul," and a material one, the body and the brain. This conception is called "metaphysical dualism" since it envisions the human body as a dual substance made of soul—autonomous and immortal principle of all things, according to Pythagoras—and body. Conscious mind and body are two distinct worlds. The distinction between soul and body as the two dimensions of man is traditional to most cultures, religions, and philosophical currents. Today, since the notion of soul got lost, we usually talk about the mind-body dualism (the mind-body problem) and mind-brain (the mind-brain problem). This dualism is defined as "the problem of problems." Therefore, the term *dualism* indicates the theory claiming the existence of two dimensions of the human body, one that is corporeal and another that is incorporeal and traditionally defined as soul, spirit, mind, breath, pneuma, consciousness, psyche, reason, or intellect. ... The new science of the brain is based on the concept that brain and mind are not two distinct realities (dualism) but rather identical realities (monism). ... Neuroscientists are convinced that mind and consciousness can therefore be investigated experimentally....

The soul, as Brunetti points out, is still taboo in the reductionist neuroscientific equation. It tries to reduce the soul to a function of the brain—"a combination of neural connections, a group of cerebral functions." However, Brunetti goes on to draw connections between the worlds of science and spirit, of brain and soul, to show their unity rather than their dichotomy not only through philosophy but through measurable research.

> Science is an activity of the spirit. To divide these two worlds creates an artificial and unsustainable dichotomy. . . . We have results coming from neuroscience itself, notable scientists (biologists, physicists, mathematicians, evolutionists, geneticists), philosophers, and writers. In fact, recent neuroscientific research clarified that our brain has an innate ability to "build" beliefs and the concepts of sacredness, transcendence, and God. These are biological and therefore "measurable" properties (Gazzaniga). Then, brain imaging experiments indicated that in the brain there is a "divine center" and a "deep moral spark that is universal, common to all humankind" (Green). There is evidence, going from Einstein (who talked of a superior mind that reveals itself in the world of experience) to Darwin (who mentioned laws impressed on matter by the Creator) to Nobel Prize winners Eccles and Sperry (who claimed that the mind is a noncorporeal reality that is not reducible to neurological events) to Popper (who defined man as a spiritual being). . . . We started from the soul, through the neurons, the body, the brain, the mind, and the consciousness to land again on the marvelous coasts of spirit (noùs) or soul.[4]

OBSERVATIONS

The soul becomes a taboo. This statement, taken from Brunetti's article above, brings to mind a question I was asked by an elderly patient during a treatment, which directed me toward the resolution of her problem.

The woman had asked me to assist her beloved brother—whom she had always defined as a "man of science"—during the final phase of his life and to treat her after his death.

From the moment her brother received the diagnosis of a terminal illness, the woman had started to suffer from sudden panic attacks, which occurred more frequently when she went out of her house. The panic attacks decreased in frequency and intensity for a short period after each treatment and became sudden and frequent again after some time. This situation went on until the patient, during an SER treatment, told me, "You know, neither my brother nor I believed in the existence of a soul or an afterlife . . . so . . . I mean . . . I was wondering . . . maybe he was afraid of . . . death?"

HORROR VACUI

"Nature abhors a vacuum," said Aristotle, synthesizing the nature of *horror vacui* (literally "terror of the void"). In fact, in nature absolute void does not exist, or at least it was never demonstrable, though for a long time many schools of thought (e.g., atomist philosophy) claimed that the existence of the void is an ontological principle that is unavoidable in the existence of entities. Absolute void is not obtainable in a laboratory and cannot be observed in nature, but it was hypothesized that a part of intergalactic space is constituted of almost complete void, with the exception of some gravitational and electromagnetic fields.

Let us go hear now from philosopher Francesca De Fanis, discussing the concept of *horror vacui*:

> This Latin expression is used in different fields, from philosophy to psychology and art. The first formulation of this concept is attributed to Aristotle in his studies on physics. After proving that each place exists in relation to the bodies it contains, the Greek philosopher stated that a void is not necessary to explain movement, in opposition to the theories of atomists. Moreover, he claimed that postulating its existence means transforming it into a place, which represents a contradiction. . . . Even today [the concept] fascinates us and gives birth to various speculations. What is the key to its "popularity"? Why has humankind wondered about it from ancient Greece to today's Generation Y? The answer is extremely simple: the terror of the void is something that deeply characterizes us, and it always has. In psychology, the Aristotelian horror vacui takes on the technical name of kenophobia, often connected with agoraphobia . . . , the anxiety felt in open or unfamiliar spaces that do not allow us to control the situation. However, the fear of the void is maybe not only a characteristic of pathological conditions. Each of us experiences uncertainty, fragility, and the sense of abandonment. We all have at least once seen our own certainties waver, said goodbye to a friend or a partner, or given up on something we consider essential. More importantly, we all have had to confront ourselves; this is maybe the real challenge of every human being.[5]

Finally, let us turn to theologian Vito Mancuso on the subject of interior silence and the experience of the spirit:

> Horror vacui, a concept of ancient physics that is a little outdated in modern sciences of nature, remains a valid principle in the context of philosophy. In this perspective, it is connected with the fear of boredom and the constant search for entertainment as a way out and diversion meant to win against this fear. Our inner

energy is always projected toward the outside, so if there is no external support, it breaks down, perceives the void, and feels like dying. That is the reason why there is an immense difficulty in creating silence. It seems like it can be done only if we win against the fear of the void, which is so close to the sense of nothingness and death, and most importantly, only if we have an internal support tied to the need of relation we host and, essentially, are. . . .

For the common consciousness, silence recalls death because it has a strict connection with the great silence it represents. Learning to be silent means learning to die, and it is not surprising that the objective of philosophy and spiritual life is exactly that. Vedas, Upanishads, Buddha, the Tao Te Ching, Plato, Epicurus, Stoicism, Qoelet, and later on Montaigne, Spinoza, Wittgenstein, and Weil all teach that the apex of human knowledge consists in learning to die, which means not being afraid of death. . . . In the Canticle of the Sun, Francis of Assisi talks about death as a sister and praises the Lord for it: "Praised be You, my Lord, / through our Sister Bodily Death, / from whom no living man can escape." . . . The list could go on and on. . . . Learning to die does not mean making every day a funeral; on the contrary, it means defying all fears and making every day the purest experience of joy, which is very different from worldly happiness. This joy is simplicity, detachment, and lightheartedness.[6]

INTRODUCTION TO TREATMENT TECHNIQUES

Horror . . . fear . . . trauma . . . grief . . . major transitions . . . reorganization of our very being . . .

The main consequences on a physiological level for these are the modification or blockage of the craniosacral rhythm, the modification or absence of breathing, the modification or stiffening of the fascial system.

We have seen that fears and the like can be determined by different factors and take on different proportions. We can therefore imagine in proportion the more or less intense reactions that occur in our organism when faced with the stress of changes, from the smallest and most common ones in our daily lives to the most difficult ones faced throughout our existence.

How can CranioSacral Therapy intervene to stem the damage these reactions cause in our body? Below we will begin to consider some of the techniques that are used in the treatment protocol to facilitate the transition between one phase of the life cycle and another. Let us try to immerse ourselves in the practice, starting from how to evaluate and deal with the first symptoms of fear and progressing to understand all the practical work the Facilitator can offer to help us transition when faced with the trauma of fear, absence of separation, and loss at the end of life.

Releasing the Respiratory Diaphragm and Thoracic Inlet

Copyright 1987, 2020 Upledger Publishing. All rights reserved.

What follows is an excerpt from the study guide written by Dr. Upledger for all first-level students of CranioSacral Therapy (CS1 Seminar).

Listening to the Craniosacral Rhythm: Palpation

The respiratory pulse is produced by the movement of the rib cage and the diaphragm as they assist in the constant filling and emptying of the lungs during breathing. It is conveniently palpated almost anywhere on the anterior chest surface.

Once you have become familiar with the respiratory pulse at the chest, move your hands to another station. Just like the cardiac pulse, the respiratory pulse can be palpated almost anywhere on the body. This is not the ordinary way of palpating the respiratory pulse, but it can be done.

Some suggested locations for palpating the respiratory pulse are:

- abdomen
- anterior thigh or calf
- ankles
- shoulders

As you palpate the respiratory pulse in these different areas, ask yourself how the tissue underneath your hands is moving in response to the respiratory pulse. Is it rotating, expanding and contracting, or moving up and down? Allow the answer to come through your hands.

The cardiac pulse can be felt in every location you palpated a respiratory pulse—and vice versa.

Now, add the following steps to your palpation:

1. Select an area and palpate the cardiac pulse.
2. Without moving your hands, palpate the respiratory pulse.
3. Move back and forth between palpation of both pulses without moving your hands.
4. Superimpose the palpation of one pulse on the other so that you are experiencing both cardiac and respiratory pulses at the same time.
5. What new information comes from this experience of palpating?

The craniosacral rhythm, like the cardiac and respiratory pulse, can be felt throughout the body. Also like the other pulses, the craniosacral rhythm has a distinctive character at different locations in the body. You will learn to use palpation of the craniosacral rhythm as a means of monitoring the function of the craniosacral system. The craniosacral rhythm will tell you where the system is operating normally and abnormally. It will also indicate the success of your therapeutic efforts to reestablish normal function. Learning to palpate the craniosacral rhythm is the foundation of successful CranioSacral Therapy.

The craniosacral rhythm is reflected throughout the body. However, the actual movement at various body locations differs slightly.

Therapeutic Pulse

The therapeutic pulse is a phenomenon that we have observed on many occasions when the subject's body is in the process of self-correction. It may occur anywhere on or in the body under treatment. The amplitude of the therapeutic pulse seems to increase from near zero until it comes into the conscious awareness of the therapist. It is not the cardiac pulse, although it seems almost the same when you first experience it. The high-amplitude therapeutic pulse may last seconds or minutes. Its presence seems to indicate that something good is occurring. After the self-correction is complete, the therapeutic pulse diminishes in amplitude until it becomes imperceptible. It is my policy not to change whatever I am doing while the therapeutic pulse is perceptible.

Respiratory Diaphragm Release

Core Intent: To mobilize the tissues and structures at the respiratory diaphragm

Posterior Hand Placement: Transverse under T12–L1

Anterior Hand Placement: Contacting the ribs borders/xiphoid process

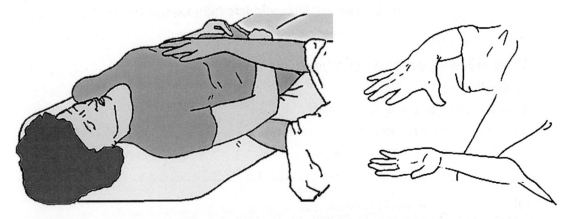

Fig. 21.6. Hand placement for the respiratory diaphragm release

Technique for Respiratory Diaphragm Release

1. Find landmarks.
2. Lighten to 0 grams.
3. Blend/meld.
4. Add 1 gram at a time to engage the tissues.
5. Follow in the direction of ease (not allowing any repeating patterns) until tissue release signs are felt.

Thoracic Inlet Release

Core Intent: To mobilize the tissues and structures at the thoracic inlet

Posterior Hand Placement: Transverse under C7–T1

Anterior Hand Placement: Thumb and second finger contacting sternoclavicular joints and clavicles

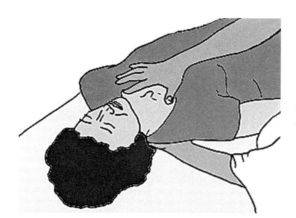

Fig. 21.7. Hand placement for the thoracic inlet release

Technique for Thoracic Inlet Release

1. Find landmarks.
2. Lighten to 0 grams.
3. Blend/meld.
4. Add 1 gram at a time to engage the tissues.
5. Follow in the direction of ease (not allowing any repeating patterns) until tissue release signs are felt.

Objectives for Respiratory Diaphragm and Thoracic Inlet Release

A Facilitator's objectives with these techniques are:

- to develop an appreciation of the total-body fascial system and its transverse diaphragms
- to develop experience and confidence in the perception of tissue release and therapeutic pulse
- to be able to obtain tissue release in the pelvic diaphragm
- to be able to obtain tissue release in the respiratory diaphragm
- to be able to obtain tissue release at the thoracic inlet
- to be able to obtain tissue release at and relating to the hyoid
- to gain a working knowledge of the anatomy of the pelvic diaphragm, respiratory diaphragm, thoracic inlet, and hyoid

The respiratory diaphragm, pelvic diaphragm, thoracic inlet, and hyoid are considered the four diaphragms. Any abnormal contraction of the diaphragms may produce a "drag" on the craniosacral system as evaluated from the head or the feet. It is therefore suggested that the participant evaluate the quality of the craniosacral system's activity from both the head and the sacrum before and after releasing each of the four diaphragms.

This chapter only directly addresses the respiratory diaphragm and thoracic inlet but the pelvic diaphragm is treated the same way (i.e. the technique is the same). The treatment of the hyoid bone differs. As noted, to treat the indicated diaphragms it is necessary to develop an appreciation of the total-body fascial system and its transverse diaphragms. Though we only discuss two of the diaphrams in detail here, you must consider that each part of the body is always closely related to other parts and structures. It must not be forgotten that in CST the body is always seen as a unit and therefore it is inevitable that to treat a single part you must necessarily involve other parts during the treatment.

This exercise will begin to give you an appreciation of the impact upon the craniosacral system function produced by diaphragmatic restriction.

Fascial Release of Intracranial Structures
Copyright 1987, 2020 Upledger Publishing. All rights reserved.

What follows is an excerpt from the study guide written by Dr. Upledger for all first-level students of CranioSacral Therapy (CS1 Seminar).

First Vault Hold
Core Intent: To assess mobility and restrictions of the cranial bones (and relating membranes), primarily from a medial-lateral perspective

Hand Placement: Hands on the lateral aspect of the cranium making light, with fingers spread, conforming contact

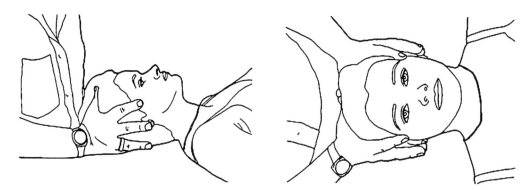

Fig. 21.8. First vault hold

Technique: Evaluate the craniosacral rhythm (CSR) using this hand placement on the medial-lateral aspect of the cranium.

Clinical Observations: To evaluate/gain information about the CSR as it is reflected in the lateral bones of the cranium

Second Vault Hold

Core Intent: To assess mobility and restrictions of the cranial bones (and relating membranes), primarily from an anterior-posterior perspective, as well as to focus on the cranial floor

Hand Placement: One hand "cups" the occiput, while the thumb and fifth finger of the other hand make contact with the greater wings of the sphenoid.

Technique: Evaluate the CSR using this hand placement on the anterior-posterior aspect of the cranium.

Clinical Observations: To evaluate/gain information about the CSR as it is reflected in the anterior-posterior bones of the cranium.

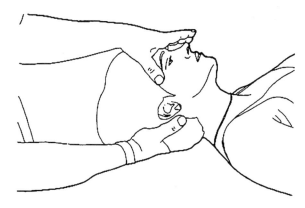

Fig. 21.9. Second vault hold

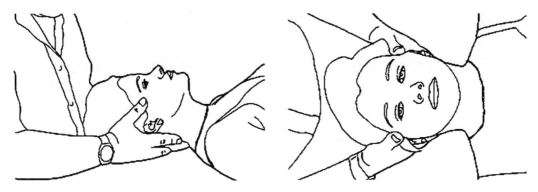

Fig. 21.10. Third vault hold

Third Vault Hold

Core Intent: To assess mobility and restrictions of the cranial bones (and relating membranes), with primary focus on the occiput and sphenoid

Hand Placement: Both hands "cup" the occiput, with the thumbs extending laterally and anteriorly to the greater wings of the sphenoid.

Technique: Evaluate the CSR using this hand placement on the occiput, sphenoid, and temporal bones.

Clinical Observations: To evaluate/gain information about the CSR as it is reflected in the occiput and sphenoid.

OBSERVATIONS

All therapists will have to address in their professional careers the skepticism of some of their patients toward them or the therapy they employ. That can influence therapists in the treatment, making them lose their self-confidence and their confidence in the techniques they use.

In this respect, I must say that I received one of the best gifts in a the seminar taught by Dr. Upledger at the workshop "The Brain Speaks," which I attended as a student.

Dr. Upledger chose to create this specific course to help Facilitators understand the various parts of the brain, their physiological functions, and their reactions to stimuli generated by emotions. He treated these subjects by characterizing all anatomical elements with a specific role, a specific task, their own difficulties, and their sensitivity toward the influences they may be subjected to by other elements (organs and systems) or external factors (e.g., sensory stimuli), as if each element were a participant in the life of a family unit that represents the entire organism.

Therefore, there I was, considering the two cerebral hemispheres and the corpus callosum.

We have seen that the left hemisphere is identified as the analytical aspect, and the right hemisphere as intuitive. The analytical element (the logical, rational, and skeptical member of the family) tries to prevail over the intuitive one (the extroverted, open, curious, and confident member of the same family) and block it because it is too abstract.

In this family, the corpus callosum is the mediator, the trustworthy person who evaluates any information and situation, not per se but in the specific context in which it developed and considering how it could evolve to be useful and support the well-being of all members of the family.

Suddenly, all this information translated for me into an idea, and this idea developed into a practice that could be employed in treatments. Therefore, when patients seem to be somewhat skeptical , the first thing I do is connect through touch with the two hemispheres and ask the left hemisphere to allow me to carry out the treatment and judge what happens only after the treatment itself. At the same time, I ask the right hemisphere not to overexcite emotional manifestations and the corpus callosum to leave all other elements to manifest their need through the hemispheres, thus giving me all the necessary information to accomplish the objective of the patient's best homeostatic condition and well-being.

When I do this, I immediately sense that the patient lets go of tension, and their facial expression often changes as well since the muscles relax and the entire organism is open to accept the treatment.

Once I accomplish this initial objective, I can continue in the most important part of the treatment by aligning the vectors and passing through the three brains (MacLean's reptilian brain, limbic system, and neocortex).

Since I started putting this technique into action, I have also started encouraging my students to verify the validity of the technique by practicing it among themselves, during seminars, knowing it will be useful to them later, in their practice, when they need to face the skepticism of recalcitrant people who stiffen and squint their eyes when they are asked to lie down on the therapy table to be treated.

Clinical Observations

A woman came to my office telling me she had been suffering from a "heavy head" for months. That symptom was causing her issues in facing any everyday situation, bringing her to a state of depression. She had already undergone clinical tests, and they fortunately had not revealed anything anomalous, but they had also proved to be useless in the identification of the cause of her discomfort and in the indication of a possible way to address and solve the situation.

When we were going through her anamnesis, the woman told me that the sensation of heaviness became drastically stronger when atmospheric pressure changed and even more when she was at a different altitude. She noticed it because she had tried to stay at her mountain chalet. She had bought it with her husband some years before to make it a vacation house, but it had always remained unused until the renovation of some months before.

In fact, she had hoped very much to spend some time in that chalet, which she could finally renovate according to her taste. Yet every time she went up there, in the mountains, the sensation of heaviness in her head became so acute that she had to give up on her stay and go back down to the city.

For a Facilitator, an issue in the head always represents something deep that could also turn out to be inscrutable. We do not know all the functions of the brain yet, but we know that there are myriad connections in each of its parts. We always wonder what we will find out when we start to assess the patient. Will we face something that goes beyond what we expect and know? Into what universe will we be transported? And how could we orient ourselves to manage all of that?

I started with the basics, trying to find any tension in the membranes. Almost immediately, I perceived that the vector placed on the central axis was bringing me toward the cerebellum. I focused on that direction and, at a certain point, perceived that the energy flow of the vector was blocked in the area of the cerebellum.

I continued to listen, focusing on that position. In the meantime, while I was wondering what to do, I had the intuition to dialogue with the cerebellum, which, in that moment, I was in contact with and was blocking me.

Nothing happens without a reason. I had just recently attended Dr. Upledger's "The Brain Speaks" seminar. There could have been no better occasion to put into practice what I had just learned than the situation I was addressing.

That is when I dialogued with the cerebellum for the first time.

I informed the patient that I would ask her some questions, and she would have to answer as if she were the mediator of a third party, without really rationally thinking about the question I was asking and without trying to make sense of the answer she would come up with. She only needed to report the first thing she immediately thought of.

I explained to her that her voice needed to be the channel through which her internal organs could inform me of what I wanted to know about them.

It may seem weird, but in situations that would normally seem absurd to anyone, patients are much more cooperative than any therapist may think. I believe that when patients are in contact with their non-conscious, they can distinctly perceive whether what they are asked is actually useful to improve their well-being or can only bring further physical, mental, and emotional discomfort.

I started my dialogue with the cerebellum, where the energy path of the vector indicated an obstruction. Through my targeted questions and the patient's words, the cerebellum thanked me for my interest and told me that it was actually responsible for the woman's symptom. It was its task to express that symptom, but the cerebellum was not its direct cause.

I asked if it knew what the cause was or what other part, organ, or system was responsible. I perceived that my attention was moved toward the cerebellar tentorium.

I tried to focus and proceeded with that surreal dialogue. I asked the cerebellum why I was drawn toward the tentorium. The answer was that the cerebellum was being subjected to heavy pressure because of the tentorium, which was almost modifying its anatomical position under the influence of atmospheric pressure and its downward compression.

Since this situation was not acknowledged in any way, the cerebellum created a perceptible sensation of heaviness to provide a symptom that could be noticed, initiating a search for the cause of and relief for the discomfort .

Since at that point I was completely immersed in that dialogue and had realized that it was the most natural thing in the world (more for the patient than for me), I needed to go on with that investigation. I decided to ask the tentorium what the cause of that anatomical displacement was. To my surprise, the answer I got was that it was due to the weight gain of the third ventricle, which was absorbing and withholding a deep sadness and melancholy, becoming the seat for those emotions.

Therefore, it was those emotions that had caused all the disorders connected with the changes of atmospheric pressure and altitude.

In that moment, the patient expressed her emotionality by starting to cry. I asked her whether she wanted to stop, but she said she did not and encouraged me to go on, even though she was still crying.

I had on my hands a cerebellum irritated by the tentorium, which, without respect but also without guilt, was sliding down on it under the weight of the third ventricle, burdened with sadness and melancholy. Once I acknowledged this situation, I had no suggestions or intuitions on how to continue.

I decided to extend my dialogue to other parts—even addressing the components of the central nervous system—in search of an ally or any kind of help. I thought of the corpus callosum and, as soon as I did, it started participating. The patient started to speak again and told me she had the impression that the right part of her head was divided from the left part.

I asked the corpus callosum whether the patient's sensation could be attributable to the sadness and melancholy and whether it could do something to get rid of it. The corpus callosum replied that, in order to release sadness and melancholy from the third ventricle, it would act as a bridge between the two cerebral hemispheres.

At that point the patient was extremely tired and I decided to stop, telling her we could analyze the subject in the two following sessions if she decided to address it again. To be honest, I did not know whether the patient would actually come back. Though I knew Dr. Upledger generally employed these techniques, I was so astounded by the modality with which I had carried out that treatment that it was hard for me to believe that someone who was not a Facilitator or did not study anything about those complementary techniques could accept it.

However, the patient did come back and even asked to go on with the treatments, booking a series of biweekly appointments.

I treated her for three months more, working on the emergence of the emotions of sadness and melancholy through the Therapeutic Imagery and Dialogue and the cerebral hemispheres, which started to cooperate with each other and continued to do so, sharing information through the corpus callosum, which was acting as a mediator between the analytical part and the artistic part in order to solve the situation.

In short, what emerged was that she had bought that mountain chalet with her husband before he got sick and died prematurely. They had never used the chalet because it needed to be renovated completely, and their dream was to use the sum her husband was going to receive upon retirement to restore it and be able to spend their summer vacations there and invite their friends over.

Unfortunately, things went differently, and my patient ended up restoring and using it by herself. Deep inside her, even though she could use her creativity and taste to make it her own, she still saw that chalet as the dream of two people, not just one, and now when she stayed there she could not stop thinking that the dream was not her own anymore.

The rational part of the patient said that the chalet was now useless because its maintenance could be expensive for just one person and it had lost its initial objective. The creative part said that the beauty of the landscape surrounding the chalet was the reason why it had been bought, and this was something that could not be ignored but needed to be enjoyed in every season.

During the treatments, it emerged that among the patient's resources was quite a lot of creativity (the artistic part). What she actually needed was a way to transform the objective of that chalet, both creatively and functionally, without abandoning that resource. It was emotionally important for her to do so without removing the memory of the original objective.

Ultimately, she needed to transform that dream—which was currently bringing her the energy of loss and bereavement—into a new situation that could enable her to accept and express a restoring energy through a new objective that was open to change and life.

Anyway, all of this had to come from her . . . and without heaviness.

If you ever pass by Sappada, a very pleasant place among the Italian Dolomites, you will find an enchanting bed-and-breakfast chalet, where a smiling and energetic lady will provide you with an amusing and relaxing stay in well-furnished rooms and with an organic homemade breakfast. If you see her climbing up mountain paths, or even just look at her, you will know that she enjoys perfect health.

❧ A CST-CENTERED VISION ❧

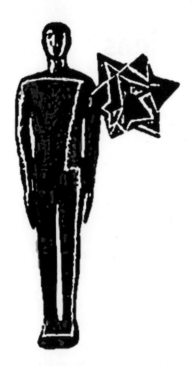

Fig. 21.11. Reproduction of *Zenith*, by Mimmo Paladino (the original features a horse; here, we substitute the human figure)

Domenico "Mimmo" Paladino is a leading artist in the Transavanguardia movement. He is known worldwide for his bronze totem sculptures. Paladino says, "The truth of things lies in the truth of images that refer only to themselves and consequently don't lie about their own nature. . . . Art is always an investigation on language; it's never a matter of surface per se or a visceral expression of poetic attitudes."[7]

In astronomy, the zenith is the apex. For a Facilitator, the zenith is the investigation through the language of the non-conscious, which manifests itself in order to be recognized and acknowledged in any way it can. That is how the Facilitator contacts the truth of things and what was decided by the patient's Higher Self for their own good.

CHAPTER 22

Therapeutic Vibrations
Harmonizing Energy Flow with Sound Frequencies

Everything in the universe is . . . is . . . is made of one element, which is a note, a single note. Atoms are really vibrations, you know, which are extensions of THE BIG NOTE. Everything's one note.

FRANK ZAPPA

Listening to the vibrations produced by sounds and perceived by the organism on various levels is part of the training to learn how to perceive reality through sensory experiences. By using our senses without stopping at the objective or apparent interpretation of the sensations we perceive, and by connecting the cerebral hemispheres, we can use the stimuli we perceive through them in ways that are different from those we are used to.

We have already encountered in the text some definitions of vibration. We've looked at the oscillation produced by entropic energy vibrations in the Energy Cyst; at cellular, electromagnetic, and mechanical vibrations; at the vibration of the universe, of the chakras, of an environment or thought; and more. In this chapter, we will address sound vibrations in particular in order to better understand the effects of these vibrations on our organism and to learn to employ this knowledge to achieve possible therapeutic objectives.

When we talk about sound or sound vibrations, we must first consider that voice is a sound. It has its own vibration, which changes from person to person, and it identifies an individual just as a fingerprint would. One of its functions/manifestations is to express the emotions of the individual. It is also a means to induce the manifestation of the listener's emotion, since it impacts different perceptive and cognitive levels. You only need to think about the satisfaction of hearing someone reply in a reassuring or enthusiastic tone, "Sounds good!"

Let us think of the implications and potential that can be expressed through

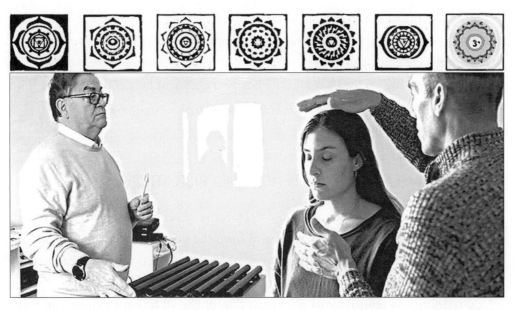

Fig. 22.1. Assessment of energy vortex frequencies and reharmonization

different tones of voice, as Devid Caressa excellently underscored in the previous chapter.

One of the foundations of SomatoEmotional Release is the technique of Therapeutic Imagery and Dialogue. Through it, the Facilitator connects with the Higher Self and addresses the patient's non-conscious, which replies by giving a voice to the Inner Physician. (We encountered an example of this process in the clinical observation in the previous chapter.)

If we let the energy of sound flow, words vibrate far beyond their communicative meaning, as it is commonly considered. For this reason, it becomes important to understand sound, know its potential, and know how to use it on all levels.

For example, the Facilitator can use sound vibrations not only in Therapeutic Imagery and Dialogue but also as a method of assessment and reharmonization of the patient's organism in combination with SER techniques. As noted previously, it is essential for a Facilitator to train in the correct attitude for listening to the patient. Since the main means through which this listening occurs is touch (the Facilitator's hands), we could say that vibrational perception can be simultaneously tactile and auditory for CST and SER practitioners.

I will always remember something Dr. Upledger said when, in 2010, I brought a group of my students to Upledger Institute International in Florida to participate in a course where I was the co-Instructor with him. On that occasion, Dr. Upledger treated all students, and I was his assistant and co-therapist in the multi-hands treatments. I also served as the interpreter for those who did not speak English. During the treatments, Dr. John often exchanged some words with me about the techniques he was employing or some opinions about their results. At a certain point, he noticed that some of the students who were carrying out treatments on the therapy tables next to him were getting distracted and listening to what he was saying.

Without moving his hands from the body of the student he was treating, Dr. John said to the other students, "Instead of listening to what I say, look at my hands; they know what they are doing."

ENERGY VORTEXES AND VIBRATIONS

As we all know, from a two-dimensional perspective, a pebble dropped in water produces concentric circular waves that expand from the point where the pebble fell in.

Similarly, but from a three-dimensional perspective, Energy Cysts create energy vortexes, each of them with a specific size, direction, speed, and intensity.

By training our sensitivity to the perception of the vibration field, we can learn to locate an Energy Cyst through a vibrational dissonance.

The Arcing technique and the numerous methods to assess and listen to the organism allow the Facilitator to perceive/detect Energy Cysts and especially the nature of their vibration. The Facilitator's hands can perceive the fascial modifications occurring in the patient's organism and, through the various methods of assessment, also the release of energy as Energy Cysts are dissipated. Evidently, the listening method also depends on the therapist's perception of the signs received from the Inner Physician of the patient. (Several people experience visualizations during the treatments; others experience bodily sensations or memories about tastes, smells, or sounds.)

In order to accomplish their job and empathize with the patient, Facilitators sometimes might have to use a nonverbal or an unconventional language. One of these unconventional languages and its respective techniques is based on sensory integration, which involves the five senses. One of the languages Facilitators can use in this case is sound, which may not necessarily be their voice.

Imagine Energy Cysts as physical points in our organism, located in correspondence with an energy channel (e.g., a meridian of traditional Chinese medicine) or in one of the organs of our physical body (liver, spleen, etc.). The energy vortexes created by Energy Cysts might spread in the organism, from the inside toward the external surface of the body, expanding from the point of origin, which is the Energy Cyst itself. They could be compared to the movement of chakras, which is fairly similar.

If we think of this movement, we could compare it visually to the propagation of a wave, which could lead us to draw a parallel with the diffusion diagram of electromagnetic and sound waves (we will see the scientific explanation of these phenomena later on).

These vortexes of Energy Cysts interfere with the normal energy flow (which is detectable also with the main meridians of TCM, as we have previously seen). The vortexes have their own movement, amplitude, and intensity and various frequencies. Their vibration creates a dissonance in relation to the normal vibrational energy of the physiological organ involved.

A Facilitator can detect that dissonance or disharmony in their assessment of the patient. By employing the language of sound, the Facilitator will also be able to contact the patient's non-conscious through musical instruments used as antagonists and harmonizers for the distorted vibration fed by the energy vortexes.

SOUND AS A UNIVERSAL LANGUAGE

Starting from the assumption that one of the methods to identify Energy Cysts is the harmonic dissonance generated by the entropic energy of the Energy Cysts themselves, we must imagine that this type of energy might be perceived as a cacophony of some notes, each of which is at the same time connected with various organs and physiological systems of our body, or as a single note with a distorted sound that is associated with one specific organ and produces an altered resonance in relation to the general harmony of the entire organism.

Let us briefly remind you that the hearing impaired perceive sound through its vibrations/waves or through its first impact on an epidermal level.

Therefore, during treatments and more specifically during the assessment of the organs, the patient might gladly accept the sound of some musical notes (which means there is probably no anomaly or dysfunction in the organ connected with those specific notes) and feel annoyance or discomfort toward the sound of others (which means there might be a dysfunction in the organ connected with them).

In this respect, I would like to quote some excerpts from the chapter "Music and Tissue Consciousness" in Dr. Upledger's book *Cell Talk*. Before you read it, I want to add that this passage initiated the research on therapeutic developments of sound in CST and SER, a research that brought me to put this assessment and treatment method among the other SER techniques I propose in this text.

Dr. Upledger was also a musician and particularly fond of jazz. He notes, "As a musician, I became aware at a very early age that certain parts of my body would resonate to certain notes." He then goes on to describe a meeting with some of his friends, including a musician and a friend who suffered from back pain, on which occasion they experimented with sound.

> We all reclined on the floor and paid attention to which notes felt good and which did not. It became clear that a single note might give me pain but relieve a pain that one of the others had. All of us had our own best and worst notes. . . .

> I would try to help him [the friend with back pain] find which notes were best for his back. I could do this by palpating the changes in muscle tension in the affected areas as the cellist played different notes. . . .
>
> We have found that when we find the note to which the tissue in question resonates, we can then entice it to follow the cello into simple melodic lines. As this progresses, we can feel increased relaxation, vitality, and energy flow in the tissue. It seems to be very effective therapeutically.
>
> I am somewhat convinced that individual organs, muscles, and nerves not only have their own consciousness energies, but also have their own musical likes and dislikes. Our director of intensive treatment programs, a physical therapist, and I are both piano players. Both of us usually heard the same melody line in our consciousness that is appropriate for a given tissue once the note of initial resonance is found. Could this be the tissue consciousness letting us know the melodic lines that would be therapeutic?. . . .
>
> All of these experiences, and many more, have led me to believe that matter is dense energy, that energy is very thin matter, and that every stage of density or thinness between the two exists. I also believe that things are in a constant state of density flux between the two extremes. I also have a visceral knowing that all things have a consciousness and that the energy fields of this infinite number of consciousnesses are constantly blending and interacting. Therefore, the feelings that you experience at any time, or the ideas that enter your head, may be due to the effects of the changing consciousness energy fields, either in your close proximity or at a distance. . . . Since all fields are constantly interacting, the consciousness energy that you project has an effect, diluted though it may be, on distant consciousness energy fields, and perhaps a more powerful effect upon the closer fields.[1]

Therefore, once we establish a scale of notes/vibrations produced by an instrument in order to use it as a parameter/indicator/ideal systemic model (as a litmus test), sound can be used to identify physiological anomalies and as a resonance element to reharmonize the entire organ/physiological system through the correct sound/vibration. Note that the correct tones we refer to are produced by a musical instrument that a CST and SER therapist might use during treatments. This instrument must be tuned on the 432 Hz grid.

432 HERTZ VERSUS 440 HERTZ

To explain the choice of relying on the 432 Hz grid (Hz = hertz, a unit of frequency equal to one cycle per second; grid = sound frequency range), we cite once more Dr. Upledger's *Cell Talk:*

Harmonization with the Sound Frequencies and the Notes of the Chakras
– another mode of perception –

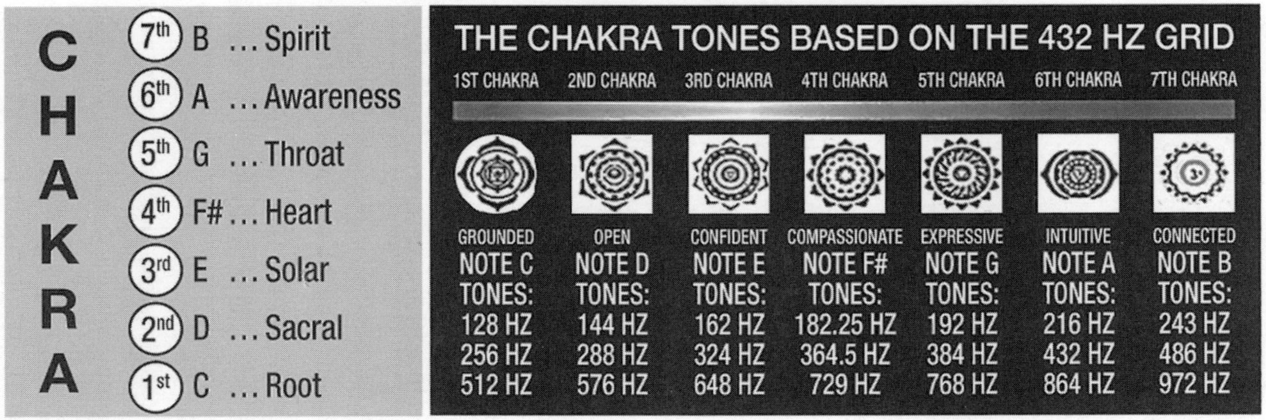

C — 7th — B ... Spirit
H — 6th — A ... Awareness
A — 5th — G ... Throat
K — 4th — F# ... Heart
R — 3rd — E ... Solar
A — 2nd — D ... Sacral
— 1st — C ... Root

THE CHAKRA TONES BASED ON THE 432 HZ GRID

	1ST CHAKRA	2ND CHAKRA	3RD CHAKRA	4TH CHAKRA	5TH CHAKRA	6TH CHAKRA	7TH CHAKRA
	GROUNDED	OPEN	CONFIDENT	COMPASSIONATE	EXPRESSIVE	INTUITIVE	CONNECTED
	NOTE C	NOTE D	NOTE E	NOTE F#	NOTE G	NOTE A	NOTE B
TONES:	128 HZ	144 HZ	162 HZ	182.25 HZ	192 HZ	216 HZ	243 HZ
	256 HZ	288 HZ	324 HZ	364.5 HZ	384 HZ	432 HZ	486 HZ
	512 HZ	576 HZ	648 HZ	729 HZ	768 HZ	864 HZ	972 HZ

Chakra	Name	Main landmark	Color	Note	Hz
1st	Root	perineum/pubis/coccyx	red	C	256
2nd	Sacral/Sexual	intraumbilical	orange	D	288
3rd	Solar plexus	area of the umbilicus/solar plexus	yellow	E	324
4th	Heart	halfway between spinal chord and heart	green	F#	364,5
5th	Throat	in the center of the throat	blue	G	384
6th	Third eye	on the glabella	indigo	A	432
7th	Crown	coronal suture/bregma	violet/golden	B	486

Fig. 22.2. Chakra landmarks and musical notes based on the 432 hertz grid

It did not take long to discover that an open-string G relaxed his muscles and relieved his pain. It also became apparent that concert A 440, the note the orchestra routinely tuned up to, caused his back muscles to contract and produce discomfort.[2]

Unfortunately, most musical pieces of our age vibrate at incoherent frequencies of 440 Hz. In fact, the note A, which is currently used by all orchestras to tune the instruments, is set on 440 Hz, and the same goes for 99 percent of music produced by record companies, spread through media, listened to through phonographic players such as CD and DVD players, or found online.

The official formalization of the tuning method set on 440 Hz dates back to 1939, when Nazi minister of propaganda Joseph Goebbels imposed the 440 Hz tuning fork, causing protests from most musicians. Twenty-five thousand French musicians voted against this decision in a referendum that was completely ignored. Goebbels, during the Nazi regime, imposed his choice on all musicians based on research on sound carried out by Nazi scientists. These scientists claimed that 440 Hz music influences the masses negatively, making them highly excitable and easier to manipulate. It is only recently that the world of musicians started to go back to other frequencies, including the 432 Hz grid. (There are various interpretations concerning the historical and chronological aspects of this matter. Nonetheless, thanks to an original document kept at the Music Conservatory of Milan, we can say that well-known composer Giuseppe Verdi supported the 432 Hz in 1884.)

In the past decades, several bands, including Pink Floyd, Rolling Stones, Tool, The Renegades, and Archangel, experimented with 432 hertz intonation, but most bands unfortunately still conform to the 440 Hz standard requirements.

Even science, and more specifically physics, is starting to promote studies and research about the effects of vibrational resonance on organic and inorganic bodies. In fact, contemporary science now claims that the universe *is* vibrational energy.

The vibrational rhythm of any body (either organic or inorganic) is called resonance. According to scientific definitions, sound is nothing but "the vibration of an elastic body transmitted to a surrounding medium (air, water, etc.) and propagated as a wave through periodic molecular condensation and rarefaction, vibrating in sympathy not only with same note instruments but also with the multiples and submultiples of its frequency."[3]

Recent research established that if we apply this principle on a cellular level, 432 Hz music might have the property of coding cells harmoniously, thus promoting the production of whole proteins in the organism. Moreover, what is commonly called "genetic wave"—which is the vibrational frequency that allows hypercommunication between human beings—is tuned to 432 Hz harmonic waves.

On the contrary, if we bring this concept even further, 440 Hz frequency blocks our species, inducing us to perceive evolutionary separation and limitation, producing damage and stress and provoking negative behaviors and emotional instability.

What we can gather from all this is that if the universe has what we could define as a beat (pulse), and if this beat normally vibrates at 432 Hz in nature, there may be a correlation between sound, harmony, human emotions, and so on.

VIBRATIONS: A MULTIDISCIPLINARY REVIEW

The following paragraphs elaborating on vibrations are taken from various authors and experts in different disciplines. They integrate briefly what has been written so far on the subject before we delve into it in detail. See the references at the back of the book for more information.

Music Therapy and Cosmology

In this context, sound is also meant as a vibratory phenomenon that has an intrinsic energetic power able to influence the physiological and biological activity of the individual. We thus enter fields of study and experimentation that consider vibratory phenomena, sound, and music as a subject of investigation (e.g., music therapy) both on an anthropological and on a medical level. . . . These observations take us into a dimension that widens the normal way of considering the sound phenomenon, expands its borders, and sometimes brings us back to ancient cosmologies that regard the origin of the universe as an auditory phenomenon (in analogy to that, we nowadays call it "Big Bang"). In fact, when the genesis of the world is described with sufficient scientific precision, in the decisive moment of the event an auditory element intervenes.[4]

Quantum Medicine

Quantum medicine (QM) is similar to other forms of vibrational and energetic medicine since its objective is to determine the imbalances in the "subtle" electromagnetic fields and to correct or reactivate biological communication when it is affected by irreversible metabolic or structural alterations and disorders. In the field of QM, any physical or emotional discomfort can be defined as a disorder within the bioelectromagnetic-informational field. QM therapies are meant to correct energetic disorders in order to activate both body and mind and encourage them to develop self-healing processes. . . . It is necessary to note that "quantum medicine" relates theoretically to quantum biophysics, but it often makes use of tools of investigation that instead of acting on energy quanta, such as the biophotons of light and the biophonons of sound, is based on the classic concept of electromagnetic resonance between vibrations of coinciding frequencies, such as acoustic vibrations.[5]

Acoustics and Acoustic Signaling

Many applications of acoustics and acoustic signal processing deem it essential to understand how sound is perceived by human beings. Sound can currently be measured accurately thanks to sophisticated equipment, and the acoustic stimulus connected with it is composed by pressure waves that propagate through air. . . . Nonetheless, the process through which these waves are received and converted into thoughts inside our brains must not be overlooked. Sound is a continuous analogical signal that can theoretically carry infinite information since there are an infinite number of carrier frequencies, each with information about amplitude and intensity.[6]

PHONONS AND BIOPHONONS

It is necessary to explore quantum physics and talk about the particles called phonons and biophonons. Let us start by synthesizing a few concepts and quoting some relevant texts before delving into the details of the subjects we need the most. See the references at the back of the book for more information.

As a paper produced by the department of geology at the University of Turin notes:

Sound diffuses through phonons, quantum particles associated with the vibrational waves of solids and analogous to the photons of electromagnetic waves. . . . In physics, phonons are energy quanta associated with elastic waves, just like photons, but in this case the waves are electromagnetic waves. That means the energy quanta are to vibrational mechanics what photons are to radiant electromagnetic energy. . . . From the equations that describe vibrational dynamics taking into account the translational invariance of crystals, we can obtain the equations associated with independent harmonic oscillators, which all have an energetic spectrum once they are quantized.[7]

In its definition of a phonon, the Treccani online encyclopedia tells us:

In physics the phonon is a quasiparticle constituted by a normal quantized mode of vibration of an elastic means. Phonons intervene in various phenomena of energetic exchange between atoms of solids . . . [and] between atoms of crystals and radiations.[8]

To sum up, phonons can modify through their vibrations the heat capacity of solids and subsequently their structure—like what happens with water crystals. In this respect, we must mention the studies of Japanese researcher and essayist Masaru Emoto on the modification/transformation of water crystals in relation to sound

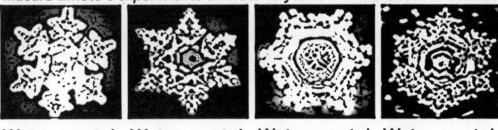

Fig. 22.3. Experiments on water crystals with the vibrations of sounds

vibrations—and therefore also the human voice—which highlighted the effect of sound vibrations on the organism. (Keep in mind that the human organism is, on average, 70 percent liquid, including the cerebrospinal fluid.)

Returning to the University of Turin's geology department, we read:

> The energy of the vibration of a crystal depends on the number of existing phonons for each frequency; such number depends on the temperature of the crystal and is regulated by a precise statistical law that determines the number of phonons for each frequency at different temperatures. . . . This law, called the "Bose-Einstein distribution," regulates all particles analogous to phonons, like photons and other elementary particles that constitute matter, such as electrons, protons, etc.[9]

With their movement, phonons influence the movement of atoms; therefore, the frequency of phonons in solids influences the vibratory frequency of atoms. For each quantity related to the fundamental frequency, there is a series of energetic levels. Nonetheless, unlike what happens in molecules, the vibration propagates through the cells with a wave vector. Therefore, at the normal mode, a quasiparticle (phonon) can be associated to a sound quantum.

CYMATICS

Cymatics is the scientific field that studies the shapes produced by waves, which means the shapes produced by vibratory, auditory, or electromagnetic frequencies. We are now going to provide a brief overview of the subject, constructed of analyses and commentary from a range of authoritative sources. See the references at the back of the book for more information.

According to ancient Indian texts derived from the oral Vedic tradition, Nada Brahma is the divine sound that originated the material, mental, psychic, and intellectual universe—in short, creation. Derived from Sanskrit and known among Hindus and Buddhists as the sound of creation, the Om or Aum corresponds to the Word (Logos) of the Bible cited in the Gospel of John ("In the beginning was the Word").

> The primordial, creating vibration is acknowledged in several religions and ancient civilizations. According to the esotericism of ancient Egypt, the universe was created by the sound that the deity Thot produced at the beginning of times, a cosmic cry articulated in seven musical notes that would have originated the various deified realities such as the Earth, destiny, the day, the night, and so on. . . . The traditions of Aboriginal Australians mention the rumbling sound that gave birth to an evolutionary process with specific syllables and musical notes; its first concretizations were the stars and constellations, then human beings. Even Druidic tradition contemplates an initial condition of existence from which a vibration emerged; it was an undulatory phenomenon of huge power that propagated in all directions, creating everything that exists.[10]

Ultimately, how do vibrations (meaning sound vibrations) actually work? And how can we verify their actual effect on matter? We can begin with the work of German physicist Ernst Florens Friedrich Chladni, who, in the eighteenth century, made it possible for the first time to visualize the vibrations caused by sound. Chladni set up a series of glass plates, covered them with a fine layer of sand, and then "played" the plates with a violin bow. The sand moved, shifting away from the areas of greatest vibration, eventually forming unique patterns (still today called Chladni figures). Such figures find their explanation in classical physics while opening the way to research by drawing parallels between the phenomena of cymatics and undulatory formation in quantum mechanics and the phenomena that gives birth to the so-called fractal structures.[11]

> Hans Jenny, who studied Ernst Chladni's theories, believed that a subtle power allows sound to structure matter through the morphogenic effect of sound waves. The name "cymatics" was coined by Hans Jenny himself from the Greek word *kymatika* (κυματικά), which means "study of the waves" (from κῦμα = "wave").
>
> He noted that if he poured some powder of lycopodium on a membrane, it responded to the sound vibrations of a vocalization such as "Om" by generating a circle with a point in the middle, the symbol ancient Indian peoples actually used as a graphic representation of the "Om" or Aum. In the sixth century BC, Pythagoras had already claimed that "the geometry of shapes is solidified music."[12]

Some Chladni figures

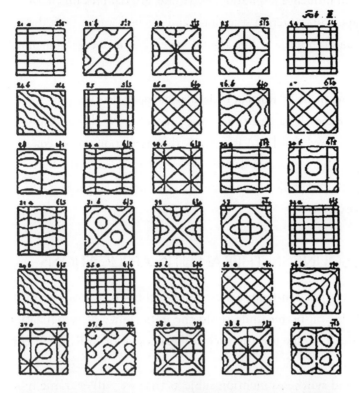

Fig. 22.4. Chladni figures, formed by the vibrations of sound

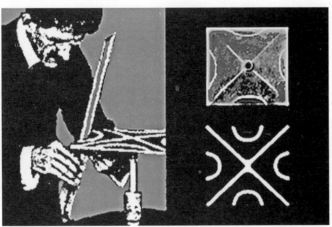

Fig. 22.5. Hans Jenny's experiments in cymatics

According to Dr. Victor Beasley of the University of the Trees research group every cell has a magnetic field that combines with the field of adjacent similar cells, thereby giving rise to the magnetic field of a particular system within the human body.[13]

The vibrations of atoms create a resonance and aggregate in cells with similar atoms. If these notes of inner resonance happen to be off-key for some reason, sickness might ensue. We can "tune" our body again with meditation and music. That is how we can reestablish order in the organism. It has been extensively proven that sounds have the ability to influence respiration, heart rate, arterial pressure, muscular tension, skin temperature, internal secretions, and cerebral waves. Even the sounds that human beings cannot hear (ultrasound waves) can influence human beings on a deep level.[14]

The sensational discoveries made by Russian molecular biologist Petr Garyaev are not very well-known, yet they have an extraordinary meaning. With some colleagues, Garyaev has discovered that DNA is not only the foundation for the construction of our body; it also serves as a deposit for memory. What is the most striking is that the genetic code follows the same rules of human language, even for what concerns musicality.[15]

INTRODUCING SOUND IN THERAPEUTIC APPLICATIONS

The following concepts, extrapolated from articles and authors in various contexts and fields, are meant to help you better understand the importance of verbalization within the technique of the Therapeutic Imagery and Dialogue of SER, given that voice is sound and vibration.

Some of these quotes and syntheses mention subjects that we will examine more in depth later. In the meantime, if you want to consult the sources and read the complete texts, see the references at the back of the book.

Cognitive Science

Meaningful interdisciplinary research carried out by the association Vocal Sound of Lugano, Switzerland, in the fields of physics, medicine, and music on the subject of "human response to sound and vibration," led to a new way of experiencing information. Physicist Fritjof Capra defined it as a "new way to access cognitive science through sound." In the cognitive approach, human beings can recognize that they are always in syntony with the profound nature of reality, where there is an alignment of different levels of frequency that express different levels of existence. The process through which implicit information aligns with the intuitive human antenna can be recognized as an alignment with the frequencies of the vibrational field surrounding us, which constitutes the origin and true nature of reality. . . .

In fact, one of the most interesting characteristics of the process . . . is that the emission of pure vocal frequencies has an extraordinary energetically balancing effect on the organism. . . . These pure frequencies are recordable in processes in which listening and understanding are predominant.[16]

Bioenergetics

Information can rebalance the bioenergetical frame of an organism through the pure frequencies emitted by the sound of voice. The voice itself does not choose a technique to emit sound or the sound itself, but it is oriented and "plays itself," whereas the consciousness of the voice is aligned with the organism that receives the sound. After such process, the bioenergetic rebalance of the organism is measurable.[17]

Epigenetics

"Epigenetics" is the scientific field that studies heritable modifications of the expression of genes that do not alter the sequence of DNA (especially in the context of cellular hereditary phenomena). The "epigenetic quality of health" manifests itself by releasing life energy information through the flow of biophotons and biophonons that goes from quantum vibratory levels to the basic state of balance.[18]

Psychoacoustics

It is crucial to note that what we hear is not only a physiological consequence connected with the anatomy of our ears, but it also entails psychological and emotional implications. . . . These considerations come from the study of subjective human perception of sounds, and especially the study of the psychology of acoustic perception, a branch of psychophysics called "psychoacoustics." . . . The domain of psychoacoustics can be subdivided in two different fields of observation: (a) the ability of hearing to evaluate the physical characteristics of sounds; (b) the ability of hearing to distinguish their variations. For both perspectives, it is fundamental to consider the concept of "threshold," a term that in biology and psychology generically designates the minimum intensity of stimulation that is necessary for a certain biological or psychological response to occur. . . . In order to obtain easily quantifiable outcomes, psychoacoustic research predominantly uses pure sounds, called tones, as well as specifically calibrated noises such as white noise.[19]

Psychophysics

In psychophysics, when the focus is to determine the difference between perceptible and nonperceptible stimuli, we use the term "absolute threshold"; on the contrary, when we want to determine the minimum measurable variation, we talk about "differential threshold." Nonetheless, the percentile ratio between the absolute value of the variation and the intensity of the initial stimulus is more meaningful than the absolute value of the variation by itself. In fact, as Weber's law states, a stimulus must be increased following a constant fraction of its value in order for the difference to be perceivable.[20]

Chakras

In the practice of yoga, if a chakra is not "tuned" and does not vibrate harmoniously, it is possible to tune it again with a process of sympathetic vibration. Harmonious vibrations with the correct frequency access directly the rotation field of chakras and are able to bring their vibratory sequence to the proper frequency in order for them to work effectively as transducers for the energy coming from the universal field of energy that is required by the organs and glands associated with the chakras.[21]

VIBRATIONAL ENERGY OF THE 432 HZ GRID IN CST AND SER

When we speak of therapeutic vibrations in CST and SER, we are not referring to a vibrational therapy set on the frequencies produced by mechanical vibrations (although in physiotherapy, for example, ultrasounds and vibrating platforms with high-frequency mechanical vibrations are used for rehabilitative purposes).

In the context of CST and SER, sound vibrations serve as detectors and conductors that allow us to understand how energetic phenomena manifest on a vibrational scale (e.g., sound). The therapist who consciously recognizes them in the human body will be able to use them and convey them into the rehabilitative action of CST and SER.

By internalizing the correct sound vibration corresponding to the organ or physiological system involved in the vibrational field of the Energy Cyst—with its negative/destructive vortex—and then sending it to the patient's body as a therapeutic harmonization (like a litmus test or a systemic model with a therapeutic index), we can correct the dissonance coming from the dysfunctional organ or the Energy Cyst itself.

In this case, sound vibrations constitute a further method to orient the Facilitator in the perception, assessment, and dissipation of Energy Cysts. One of the simplest methods is to produce and/or perceive the vibrations of the sounds that are associated with major and secondary chakras.

All Facilitators can train their perception of the correct vibrations associated with each organ or system of the human body, relating it to the specific, peculiar, and subjective vibration of the patient's organism, in order to recognize the dissonances (created by the entropic energy of the Energy Cyst) and proceed with the reharmonization of the entire system by sending the correct vibration. The sound vibration might be produced with an instrument or with the voice, with a single note, a melody, a mantra, a prayer, and so on, depending on what the patient's nonconscious and the Facilitator's Higher Self indicate.

The correct vibration is a therapeutic vibration that is antagonistic to the dissonance.

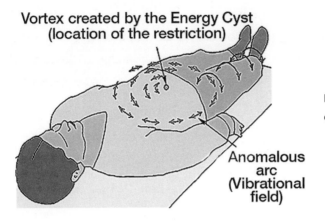

Fig. 22.6. Vortex of movement of Energy Cyst

Technique: Therapeutic Vibrations

This technique enables us to work with the vibrations that correspond to the pure sound of musical notes produced through a musical instrument (tuned on the scale of the 432 Hz grid). Remember that each note coincides with a specific vibration, a specific major chakra and its secondary (or lower) chakras, and the anatomical parts (physiological organs and systems) associated with them.

A Facilitator's objectives in this practice are:

- to propose an assessment made through the tactile perception of any vibrational dissonances that might correspond to one or more chakras
- to harmonize the entropic and dysfunctional energy detected through the dissonance by sending the syntropic energy of the correct vibration through touch in order to rebalance the energy flow in the organs and physiological systems, harmonizing at the same time the emotions connected with them and the chakras involved
- to adopt sound vibrations as an additional method to perceive, assess, and dissipate Energy Cysts

Perceiving Vibrations and Harmonizing Energy

This exercise offers one of the simplest methods to train our perception of the vibrations produced by the sounds (notes) associated with the various major and/or secondary chakras.

1. Internalize the correct sound vibration for each note of the musical scale from C to B.
2. Place one hand on the first chakra and the other hand underneath it. Listen to the vibration of the first chakra, corresponding to note C. Reproduce inside yourself the corresponding note/vibration.

3. Take a ten-second break, and then move on to next chakra. Continue in this manner through each of the major (or secondary) chakras, perceiving their vibrations, proceeding from the first to the seventh (corresponding to the note B). Take a ten-second break between one chakra and the next. If you detect dissonance/disharmony—an antagonistic vibration opposing the correct vibration you are sending—in any chakra, make note of it.

4. Identify the physiological part involved and, consequently, the emotion connected and associated with the chakras in which you detected dissonance.

5. Place your hands on the physiological part you identified (either directly on it or on the respective distal point) and let your hands be drawn toward the most intense vibration perceived until you find the energy vortex (the center of the restriction/Energy Cyst/active lesion).

6. Once you have identified the center of the vortex, use intention to send the correct internalized note (vibration), and wait for the dissonant vibration to harmonize into a neutral phase. By sending the correct vibration until you perceive no dissonance, you are carrying out a therapeutic harmonization (systemic model with a therapeutic index).

7. If necessary, repeat the exercise (from step 2) for a second assessment.

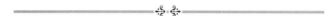

OBSERVATIONS

My following observations report an occurrence that anticipated a clinical diagnosis during one of Dr. Upledger's CST Sensory Integrations workshops.

At the beginning of the first day of the workshop, Instructor Rebecca Flowers welcomed the students to the classroom with a piece of music. In that moment, I considered it simply a light-hearted and cheerful introduction to put the students at ease. I would find out later that this particular piece of music was based on the rhythm of the vibrational frequencies of a regular heartbeat.

After the music ended, when the lesson was about to begin, one of the students told Rebecca that the music had upset and unsettled him. With as much tact as possible, she replied that one possible reason for his emotional response could be the presence of a dysfunction in his organism.

Rebecca's answer impressed me; I knew she would never dare to guess something like that if there were no solid foundation for her assumption. Nevertheless, it sounded a bit over the top, and I decided to set it aside as just an excuse to introduce one of the subjects of the sensory integrations workshop.

Months later, the student who had shared his sense of unsettlement about that piece of music called me and informed me that he had cancer. Not only that, the cancer was probably already developing when he had attended the workshop, even though he was unaware of it at the time. (He received his diagnosis only later, after his physician suggested a CAT scan to investigate a series of anomalous symptoms.)

Had the vibrational frequency of the heartbeat caused him to feel upset just by chance?

I DO NOT BELIEVE IN COINCIDENCE! I believe his organism was already manifesting an antagonism to the correct frequency (vibration).

Now the student has mostly regained his health. He fought the cancer with both conventional and CST and SER treatments and has long overcome the critical stage.

Clinical Observations

During a trip in the United States, I spent some time with my friend Dr. Fabio Burigana at the home of another friend, Ramona Sierra, who is a Facilitator as well. While we were staying at her place, we organized an excursion to the Great Salt Lake in Utah.

As a Native American, Ramona often used a drum to connect with the energies of the Earth when she is out in nature. That day, she brought a drum and some eagle feathers for Fabio and me, and we started to play and move the feathers as we walked.

In the distance, a buffalo appeared (it is not uncommon in that area), and Ramona suggested we get closer to it while playing the drum and sending a message to it with our intention. The message was that we were just passing by. We did not want to invade its space but just wanted to get closer to admire it.

Drawing from the practices of her ancestors, Ramona suggested that I modulate the sound of the drum with this message so that the buffalo could understand it.

I must say that being so close to a buffalo in person is impressive. At some point, I also had some doubts about its ability to understand our intentions.

I trusted Ramona. I knew she used this technique to tame wild horses, and it was not the first time she had approached a buffalo. Notwithstanding, I was new to this experience, and it was hard not to feel scared, which made it hard to focus on the message I was sending to the buffalo because I was too concerned about how I could escape if it proved to be necessary. Ramona understood what I was thinking, so she kept kindly encouraging me to continue to focus and play the drum.

There were some stalls as the buffalo looked at us, and we looked back at it, and it looked back at us. Then, with great joy, I noticed that it was bending its front legs. Immediately after, our buffalo lay down and started to carelessly roll on the ground, as if we were not there.

After that experience I bought some handmade drums, each of which produces a different type of sound and comes from a place that has a significant meaning.

I begin with this long premise so that what follows will be easier to understand. On that note, let us go back to my work as a Facilitator and my clinical experiences.

A ten-year-old boy was once brought to my office by his parents. He had autism, and his parents wanted me to treat him since they had read some articles about Dr. Upledger's positive outcomes using CST and SER in the treatment of autistic children.

The boy was not able to stay still and kept spinning around anything he saw in my office and walking in very quick circles around the perimeter of the room. It was not possible to make him lie down on the therapy table or sit on a chair (it was not even a hypothesis in my mind), but it was hard even just to get him to stop moving.

I certainly could not run after him.

I had accepted the invitation to treat him after a long conversation on the phone with his parents, but I was starting to regret my decision because it looked like I was just making those good people waste their time.

Then, I do not know why, I thought about the buffalo. I took one of the drums hanging on the wall (I had bought it in Utah, and it was painted with an image of a buffalo and some feathers) and sat in the middle of the circle the boy was tracing counterclockwise in the room. I started to play the drum like I had done in Utah.

Animals and children have a wonderful subtle energy and do not like intrusiveness. Therefore, I just played the drum following a rhythm similar to a human heartbeat. I sat there for more than ten minutes playing the drum.

The boy's parents, who were sitting in front of my desk, were now looking at me quite puzzled. As had happened with the buffalo, I started to wonder whether my actions were wise. I was about to give up on my strategy and get up when the boy stopped, came closer to me, and started to listen. He took the beater from my hand and started to play the drum, which I was holding with the other hand. I am not able to describe my joy in that moment!

I realized that the buffalo I had trusted in Utah, after all my doubts, had helped me.

The boy's parents cried with happiness. They had never seen their son focus on or listen to something and interact in such a way. I was told they bought a drum and the boy started to play it regularly.

The boy was also under the care of the therapists at a specialized center for autistic children. These therapists informed the parents that since that first encounter with me and the drum, their son had started to be more sociable and to interact more with strangers, always in his own way, of course.

❧ A CST-CENTERED VISION ❧

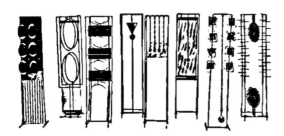

Fig. 22.7. Sketches of sculptures by Fausto Melotti from his Harmony and Counterpoints series

Fausto Melottie, born at the very beginning of the twentieth century, creates extremely light steel sculptures that are pervaded with irony and a surreal aura. After his musical studies, he decided to become a sculptor and started applying musical rules to his art; the compositions he creates evoke a harmony of variations, intervals, and legatos. His works are the plastic representation of a musical rhythm. They appear fragile and fluctuating but have solid metaphysical roots.

Melotti's artworks bring out the incorporeal (music) in matter (sculpture as a musical, artistic, and expressive instrument). He actually got a degree in theology, and music is, after all, the natural expression of spirituality. It is one of the highest artistic expressions of humankind and a powerful universal means of communication that both causes and is caused by emotion. It is able to make all the cells of our organism vibrate in harmony. Music is a versatile coefficient, adaptable to any structural foundation.

CHAPTER 23

Form of the Third Space
Visualizing the Perception

Science may set limits to knowledge, but should not set limits to imagination.

BERTRAND RUSSELL

As we continue our learning path, deepening the conceptual elements and the technical bases that are necessary to prepare for the treatment of patients in the last known phase of transformation of their Life Cycle, we want to underline once again the objective of the treatment itself.

The aim of this energetic work is to facilitate the passage between various phases of patients' Life Cycles through the optimization of all the systems, meant to give them as many possibilities and as much comfort as possible and allow them to follow what their Higher Self has predisposed for their own good.

This treatment is indicated as a way to allow a person's vital energy continuum to flow when there is a blockage during any passage from one phase of the Life Cycle to the next. It is equally useful in the facilitation of the transformative passage from the last known phase to the unknown, helping the Open-System Human Being in the transition. In his books, Dr. Upledger reports the work of Facilitators who were able to ease the phases of the dying process, alleviating the physical and emotional suffering of that passage.

In chapter 25, when we examine the seven-step treatment protocol, we must keep in mind that our objective during the treatment is to make contact with the space where we can meet the Higher Self, where everything takes place, and where we are, were, and will be. It is the Third Space, where everything transforms and where we can interact with everything around us, with all information and scenarios, and with all that apparently starts and ends. The seven steps of the protocol comprise seven techniques that we have already encountered in this text.

In addition, we are going to consider an additional step, represented by the space where the therapeutic gesture takes place (assessment, treatment, and reassessment), which becomes an integral and meaningful part of the treatment, fundamental for the execution of the seven techniques.

This eighth point (and it is not only by chance that number 8 is also the infinity symbol, a line that continues with no interruptions and does not start nor end) will be considered exclusively as the space where we want the therapeutic action to take place, the space where all systems are universally connected, and where transformation happens. That is the space we have already defined as Third Space, where the patient and the Facilitator meet the Higher Self.

Before properly analyzing the technical part, which is the foundation for the experiential phase of perceptive visualization of the Third Space, let us go through some elements that constitute the conceptual and theoretical structure behind the technique itself. We have already mentioned them, but so far we have not explored them sufficiently. We are talking about fractals and the toroid, in the context of the toroidal magnetic field.

FRACTALS: MATHEMATICS AND GEOMETRY IN MEDICINE AND BIOLOGY

Why do we mention the fractals? It might seem strange, but in 2018 the Italian Ministry of Health included fractals as part of the medical entrance exam. It goes without saying that this caused many difficulties to the applicants.

We are in the scope of mathematics, which, we remind you, means science, knowledge, or learning (from the Greek word μάθημα, *máthema*), a subject we should be investigating, as well as physiology, anatomy, chemistry, and physics. As you know, mathematics is the field that includes the study of the quantities and sizes of substances in the physical world, space, and the structures and calculations (cognitive mental processes) also applied to statistics. The latter has similarly become a subject of study for many professionals in the field of health and wellness (physiotherapists, osteopaths, physicians, etc.).

A fractal is a geometric concept, a shape characterized by dimensions that are not integers and by the property of reproducing the initial figure in all scales. This very basic explanation indicates that the fractal process is connected also with phenomena that concern sciences such as medicine and biology.

Since we have already mentioned fractals in this text, it is only right to give you a better definition of what they are and to explain their connection with medicine, biology, natural sciences, and physics since all these disciplines play a key role for Facilitators throughout their professional practice. They are as functional as anatomy and physiology to the knowledge that is needed to practice CST and SER.

"Thought-form" as "Third Space"

Our Thought-form can also be our Third Space, the representation of the universal energy that is connected with the love nourishment that feeds the universe with which the universe feeds us.

Inside of it, all the data you send will be processed, and transformation from entropic energy to syntropic energy will take place, so that you can receive the syntropic energy and send it to the patient through your hands.

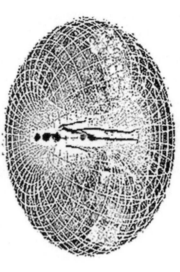

Thought-form as Toroid
(magnetic field of the human being)

Projection of the "thought-form" as therapeutic space of healing
(imaginative visualization)

Fig. 23.1. Thought-form as Third Space

What, then, are fractals, other than a geometric expression? Let us go through some definitions laid out by experts in the field.

The term *fractal* derives from the Latin *fractus,* from the verb *frangere* ("to break into pieces" or "to crush"). As we have seen, it designates specific geometrical figures that can correspond to numbers that are not integers but fractions. Therefore, they can be, for example, "intermediary between one-dimensional figures (lines) and two-dimensional figures (surfaces). They are usually defined through recursive procedures and enjoy specific scalar properties, because of which representations in different scales of the same fractal object share some structural similarities. In other words, if the size of a portion of the object is increased with a proper scalar factor, the structural characteristics of this portion are the same as those of the object that maintains the initial size."[1]

In her all-round perspective on mathematics as applied to natural phenomena and structures and to the entire cosmos, Rosa Mistretta defines fractals in the very title of the article we are going to cite: "Cosmic Spiral: The Golden Ratio of the Universe." She writes:

> One famous aphorism by Galileo Galilei states that "the book of nature is written in the language of mathematics," thus claiming that the harmony of the world manifests itself in shapes and numbers. . . .
>
> By observing nature, we can find expressions of elegance and harmony. The common trait that defines attractive objects is a series of rigorous and unequivocal forces that comply with specific mathematical laws. . . .
>
> Obviously, it is not possible to define a process without taking into account the intuition, experience, and sensitivity of the observer. These are fundamental qualities to find in any kind of relation in a research method. A new way of interpreting nature can thus be actualized . . . in the acceptance of the obedience of the Earth and the sky to the same laws, in the regularity of structures between macrocosm and microcosm; these are necessary and logical premises to discover, for example,

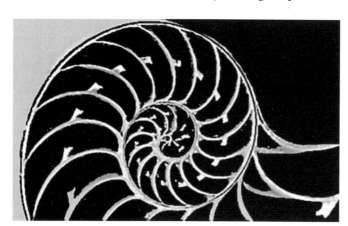

Fig. 23.2. Fractal forms in the nautilus

that the essentiality of the line that creates a spiral represents some types of galaxies, but it also has the characteristics of the vortexes of the Earth.

The spiral . . . is an omnipresent structure. It is one of the most common geometrical shapes in nature, and we can find it everywhere, from sunflowers to the horns of some animals, from the motion of cyclones to the molecule of DNA, from shells to galaxies. . . .

A simple ratio creates the proportions of spiral shapes, proving that even the spiral branches of the Milky Way and other galaxies are connected with constant and orderly phenomena that are attributable to precise patterns. The golden ratio is the mathematical expression of beauty in nature. . . . In a progression of divine proportions, any part is the microcosm, or the minuscule model, of the whole. From the infinitely small to the infinitely big, everything seems to be regulated by mathematical perfections, precise predefined calculations applied to all things, from small snails living in the woods to immense spiral galaxies that contain billions of stars.[2]

Gabriele Angelo Losa, mathematician and biologist, widely described this subject in his article "Fractal Geometry in Biology":

In order to understand and measure natural objects and complex shapes, we had to wait for fractal geometry, conceived and developed by Benoît Mandelbrot (1924–2010). The title of his famous article published in 1967 on "Science, How Long Is the Coast of Britain?" at first provoked some giggles and then became a cause for reflection for several mathematicians and scientists. . . . The answer to the question the title asks was surprising: the length of the coast depends on the resolving power of the ruler or scale employed. Since the analyzed systems are irregular and fractal, the smaller the measuring scale employed is, the bigger the quantity of the measured parameter will be, because there are more portions and details of the whole that can be adequately recognized and evaluated.

Another relevant principle of fractal geometry concerns the unlimited iteration of a part to constitute the object in its entirety, ensuring at the same time a similar shape on any scale. The complex figures obtained through iteration reflect reality, since they are "almost the general rule in nature, in particular in its most visible aspects," so that "clouds are not spheres, mountains are not cones, the outline of a coast is not a circle, barks are not smooth, the lightning does not travel in a straight line." . . . We need to admit that the predominant cultural and scientific attitude in the scientific community remains Euclidean. . . . Biological forms and complex structures and the biochemical mechanisms and physiopathological events they entail are still investigated as if they were Euclidean, deterministic objects, which are

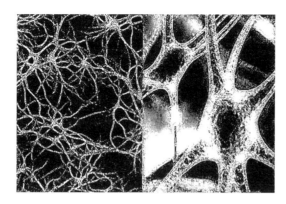

Fig. 23.3. Fractal structures in neuronal ramifications

quite approximate and therefore rarely found in nature. This essentially means that the dimensional, morphological, and functional peculiarities of natural elements that develop according to the "power law" or "scaling law" are still being underestimated. . . . Mandelbrot did deduce anatomical and metabolic complexity, rather than describe it. After observing the convolutions of the folds of human brain and the labyrinthine network of the neural cells in the cerebellum, he postulated a geometrical organization that was not Euclidean, even though he recognized that "the notion that neurons are fractals was still a conjecture."[3]

Doctor Pasquale Venuti wrote the following:

Living organisms are oscillatory, not linear, or better yet, they are nonlinear systems manifesting complex oscillatory behaviors in certain environmental conditions.

A nonlinear system does not comply with the principle that states that the sum of two or more stimulations equals the sum of the responses to each of the stimulations taken singularly. In other words, when the intensity of a cause increases, the intensity of the response does not necessarily do the same. An example of the consequence of nonlinearity is constituted by sudden and catastrophic phenomena such as the collateral effects to a medication, or a sudden cardiac death, etc. Sudden cardiac death allows us to notice that, even in a system in which all the subparts (in this case, the heart cells) work normally, an alteration in the mechanisms that connect them might cause catastrophic effects. . . . This encouraged the development of a new interpretative paradigm in the field of biological sciences. In fact, chaos and the other nonlinear theories show that in a wide range of conditions, highly deterministic and linear processes are quite frail in the preservation of health, while chaotic systems can function effectively in several different conditions, thus providing both adaptability and flexibility. This functional plasticity enables the system to deal with the unpredictability and variability of the environment, providing dynamic adaptability instead of homeostasis, which is more precise but weaker. . . . The nonstationarity and nonlinearity of the signals generated by living organisms threaten the traditional mechanistic approaches, based on homeostasis and conventional biostatic methods. The theory of deterministic chaos allows us to find better explanations. The concept of fractal, described by Benoît Mandelbrot in 1975, refers to irregular geometric objects displaying self-similarity. Fractal shapes are all the geometric shapes that do not belong to Euclidean geometry (lines, planes, surfaces) and are composed of subunits (and sub-subunits, etc.), each of which is similar to the entire object. . . . This property, called self-similarity, is applicable to all dimensional scales. Many non-Euclidean structures of nature are fractal, like for example the branches of a tree, coasts, and the surface of mountains. Even the geometry of many anatomical structures is fractal, like in the case of the arterial and venous systems, the tracheobronchial tree, neural branches, the internal surface of the intestine, the His-Purkinje system, etc. . . . Vortexes are fractal objects . . . ; their global aspect is always recognizable, but it is never the same. . . . A spatial or temporal irregularity could obviously be originated either by randomness or by chaos. The difference between a random phenomenon and a chaotic phenomenon lies in the degrees of freedom involved. In a random system there are infinite degrees of freedom, which generate a random behavior, whereas in a chaotic system the degrees of freedom are finite. . . . The opportunity to register in a continuous way different physiological variables allowed some revolutionary observations to be made. . . . The characteristic irregularity of a healthy individual is the foundation for their adaptability; it is as if the irregularity were an indication of the ability of the organism to react in different ways. If we look at it from this perspective, illness might consist in a modification of one or more parameters of the system that induces the replacement of an irregular behavior with a regular one. The state of illness can therefore be considered as a loss of complexity of the system.[4]

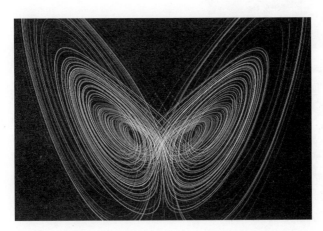

Fig. 23.4. Butterfly-shaped fractal structures

Doctor Giorgio Bianciardi, director of the Italian Center of Bioenergetics, describes fractals as follows:

> Fractal geometry is nothing more than the geometry of chaos, that branch of physics in which the determinism of Galilean science and its ability to make predictions dissolve. The famous butterfly of Edward Lorenz's mathematical model, ideated in the [19]60s, the first mathematical object of the physics of chaos, has a fractal structure. [Edward Norton Lorenz is also remembered for the article that asked, "Does the flap of a butterfly's wings in Brazil set off a tornado in Texas?," which led to the concept of "butterfly effect."—*Ed.*]. . . . More precisely, when there is a passage from regularity (for example, the slow laminar flow of a fluid) to chaos (in our example, the flow surpassing a certain limit speed and starting to whirl), complex, irregular, and "homothetic" structures appear in the frontier line; these are fractal structures. . . . In the field of the study of life, the concept of fractal has strong consequences. There cannot be a sufficient amount of genetic information to describe the shape of a tree's entire foliage or the disposition of the fifty thousand billions of cells that constitute the human being, not to mention the distribution of the million billion intraneural connections of the human brain. Nonetheless, Mandelbrot proved that with around ten lines of program it is possible to obtain a figure, the set of Mandelbrot, which has an incredible complexity. . . . If we look at a microscopic photograph of a portion of the dendritic branch of a neuron, we may be confused about the degree of enlargement of the picture

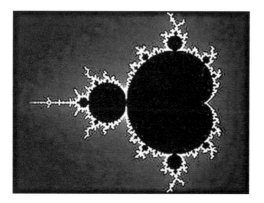

Fig. 23.5. Mandelbrot set

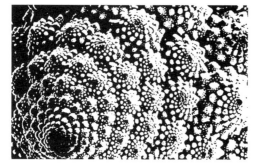

Fig. 23.6. Fractals in the organic structure of a plant

since the ramification of the nerve cell remains extremely similar even when we change the scale. . . . When we get to the single cell, the fractal structure dissolves, maybe reappearing with a different fractal dimension in the subcellular structure. Chaotic dynamics and fractal structure cause us to change the concepts of order and complexity in living beings. . . . The concepts of healthy and unhealthy organism change. The appearance of strong regularities in the fluctuations of the electrocardiogram indicates a bad prognosis for an unhealthy heart. . . . The conventional medical interpretation that considers illness and old age as the results of the exhaustion of a deterministic, orderly, and regular system must be completely revised since order and regularity are actually connected with illness.[5]

Psychologists Ulisse Di Corpo and Antonella Vannini discuss the relationship between fractals and syntropy:

A consequence of introducing attractors (syntropy) in chaotic systems is the creation of complex—but orderly—figures known as fractals, as Mandelbrot showed. . . . The quantity of fractal structures in the human body is extraordinary. Some examples: coronary veins and arteries have fractal ramifications. The main vessels divide into smaller ones, which further divide into even smaller ones. Moreover, these fractal structures would play a key role in the mechanism of contraction and in the conduction of excitatory electrical stimuli; the spectrum analysis of cardiac frequency shows that the normal heartbeat is characterized by a wide chaotic spectrum. Even neural structures are similar to fractals: if we observe them in an enlarged image, we will notice asymmetrical branches (dendrites) connected with the cellular bodies; with a further enlargement we can see smaller branches coming from the bigger ones and dividing in even smaller ones, and so on. The respiratory passages of the lungs are similar to fractals as well. . . . These observations bring us to the hypothesis that the organization and development of living systems (tissues, nervous system, etc.) might be led by a series of attractors, exactly like in fractal geometry.[6]

TOROID: THE TOROIDAL MAGNETIC FIELD AS ENERGETIC SPACE

We previously defined the toroid in the context of the balanced energetic flow of sustainable systems. Now we will examine it both as a magnetic field within quantum biology and as the space where the expression, containment, exchange, and expansion of subtle energy can occur. This will get us closer to the perceptive vision of our Third Space.

Let us then examine the toroidal magnetic field of the heart from the perspective of professor Paolo Manzelli to help us understand the possible energetic space we could need to enter in CST and SER.

An article he wrote 2018 for Eduscuola entitled "Biologia quantica: biofotoni e biofononi" (quantum biology: biophotons and biophonons), highlights that in quantum biology the heart is not considered only as a blood pump but as a much more complex system equipped with its own neurons correlated with a network of receptors afferent to the central brain, the enteric brain, and all parts of the body that are supplied by blood. In addition to this, it must be considered that the heart is responsible for the production of oxytocin and dopamine, the hormones responsible for managing stress. The functioning of the heart begins and is visible and measurable by the electrocardiogram well before the brain is formed in the fetus. Even when it is first formed, the heart creates a powerful electromagnetic field, which is approximately sixty times larger than that generated by the brain waves recorded by the electroencephalogram.

Manzelli explains:

Following the audible heartbeat, the "toroidal magnetic field" takes on a double structure (external and internal) that resounds interactively with a synergistic and coherent rhythm that harmonizes the magnetic component of the body with the overall nonlocal magnetism (the magnetism of the Earth, the sun, the stars) coming from the environment. . . . Sound phonons, unlike light photons, are sound quanta that oscillate at very low frequencies, propagate at long distances, and diffuse sound and color within the electromagnetic toroid. . . . In light of these considerations on the innovations brought by quantum biology, it is possible to highlight the equivalences between quantum biology and the scientificity of the knowledge based on "vital energy and subtle bodies" (considered in the practices of yoga, shiatsu, acupuncture, pranotherapy, laser therapy, . . . and other self-healing systems).[7]

Physicist Nassim Haramein is known for his "theory of everything," formulated after twenty years of study and research in various fields and disciplines, such as physics, cosmology, biology, philosophy, history, and anthropology of ancient civilizations. Here is a brief explanation of the part of his theory that concerns the toroidal field:

Nassim Haramein's "theory of everything" is based on the idea that we are all immersed in a sea of fundamental energy, which is the source for the physical world. . . . This energy would be the void or space surrounding us. Nonetheless, the word "void" is not used in the usual meaning of the term since this space would be

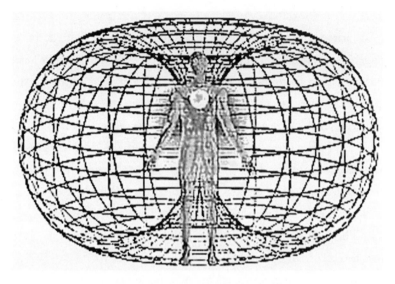

Fig. 23.7. Toroidal magnetic field

literally full of an extraordinary energy that connects everything and carries a huge amount of information. . . . One of the expressions of the universe is the double toroid, visible in the atmosphere of the Earth . . . [and surrounding] other celestial bodies, such as the stars and the galaxies. One of the main characteristics of the toroid is that it has a peculiarity in its center, an immobile balancing point. This central point would connect all the existing systems with the underlying Unified Field. It would be a holographic reality in which every entity informs the entire cosmos of its own local existence through the Unified Field. When the energy moves in this "point zero," geometry is reduced to the minimum quantity of vectors to have absolute balance and stability. . . . One of Haramein's best-known statements is "To be a good scientist you must think with your heart, because that's where the information comes first." The electromagnetic field of the heart would have a toroidal shape as well; through the flow of such field, information would be sent to the brain and all the body. The energy toroid would flow from the heart to the top of the cranium, then downward to the pineal gland, through our nervous system and then back to the heart. All of this would be constantly connected with the universe. . . . There would be an infinite potential inside us. . . . It would be enough to interiorize the senses into the point zero to access the infinite wisdom inside of ourselves.[8]

Writer Claudia Palmas describes the toroid as follows:

Energy flows from one end, circulates around the center, and comes out from the opposite side. It is balanced, self-regulated, and always intact. You can see it everywhere, in atoms, cells, seeds, flowers, trees, . . . galaxies, and even the entire cosmos. Scientist and philosopher Arthur Young explained that the toroid is the only energetic or dynamic model able to support itself, and that it is made of the same substance that surrounds it, like a tornado, a ring of smoke in the air, or a whirlpool. Evolution means development, and what does the universe develop? Self-organized systems that are therefore visible with all scales. It is a system able to organize itself. In nature, we find these self-organizing forms everywhere. . . . The universe has manifested in all its scales a single project, the developments of tori. . . . Galaxies have a toroidal shape in which "white holes" release energy, whereas "black holes" suck it inside themselves. The entire universe has the shape of a toroid. The geometrical shape used to describe the self-reflecting nature of the universe is the torus. The toroid allows energy vortexes to flow outward only to come back inside. That is how the energy of a toroid keeps regenerating itself and, at the same time, expands and self-reflects.[9]

AN INTRODUCTION TO THE THIRD SPACE: PERCEPTIVE REALIZATION AS A RESOURCE

Our perception should start with visualization. In order to allow that, we are going to expand our horizon, train our vision, let our right hemisphere influence us, and focus on what we can perceive through the visualization of a shape in order to give shape to our perceptions.

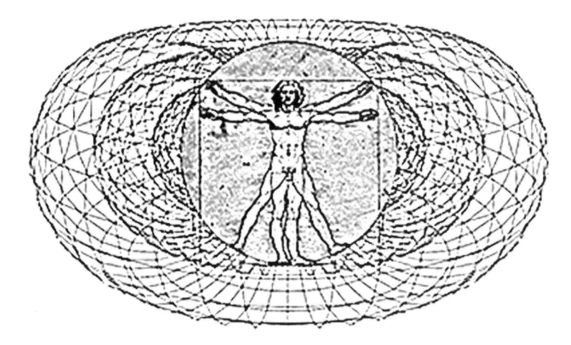

Fig. 23.8. Toroidal magnetic field of da Vinci's *Vitruvian Man*

An example of connection between art and science that can help us in this exercise can be found in the work of Leonardo da Vinci, as mathematician-biologist Gabriele Angelo Losa, whom we encountered in the context of fractals, explains:

> Leonardo's approach to complexity mainly consists in the visualization and description of phenomena. Using an adequate and reproducible methodology is the indispensable and ineludible condition to examine any phenomenon, a method even Leonardo employed. In fact, in his treaty on painting, . . . he explicitly wrote that it was his intention to start from experience, and then to proceed by using reason to prove "why that experience had to occur as it did."[10]

THIRD SPACE AS THOUGHT-FORM

For this phase of the treatment, polarity and the chakras are crucial once again but in combination with the visualization of the Third Space—this time meant as an aspect of the thought-form in which transformation takes place.

We have already mentioned thought-forms; we now need to synthesize the aspects of this subject that can be preparatory to the treatment by drawing on quantum physics again.

Quantum physics (or quantum mechanics) shows that, on an atomic level, thought is a form of energy that is vibratory or undulatory in nature. A thought-form can be compared to an energy accumulator ready either to discharge or to get even more charged when it runs out of energy depending on the vibrations with which it is supplied. Sometimes the thought-form is also called elemental or artificial elemental.

Cellular biologist Bruce Lipton—whom we encountered previously when talking about polarity—excellently explained this from a quantum biological perspective in an interview he gave to the magazine *Altrogiornale*.

As Lipton told interviewer Alessandro Silva, life goes on thanks to the ability to maintain its balance in a constantly evolving and dynamic environment. The energy potentials of environment and spirit are directed inside the body, influencing it, whereas the physical responses of the body create at the same time energy fields that go back to the environment. Instead of responding passively to all the signals coming from the environment, we can become aware of those signals. Through a process of selection, we can use either the subconscious mind to automatically respond to signals or the conscious mind to generate responses that are different from those that were programmed by the subconscious.

From a functional point of view, the human mind looks like a "membrane that allows the spirit to interface with the physical body." In this interface, our mind possesses the awareness that comes from the combination of an external spiritual-environmental source and the life experiences gathered during our physical existence. While the energetic potentials of the environment and the spirit go from the outside to the inside to control the body, the physical responses of the body simultaneously generate energetic fields that go from the inside to the outside environment. That is why we can identify an external environmental energy and a behavioral energy that comes from the body. These energies are tightly connected with each other; when the mind creates a response in the body, this response generates an energy potential that goes back to the environment where the stimulus came from. If we record and integrate the responses over time (just like our cerebellum does) through a device located inside the system, that device will become the database of all information that our mind uses, a "functional interface between physical and nonphysical states of our existence."

The cells of the body respond to both conscious and unconscious minds, and this is how disharmony can enter our lives. If the conscious mind is healthy, for example, and the subconscious mind (which is programmed with acquired perceptions) agrees with it, then, for a matter of coherence, we are healthy. However, if there is discordance between these minds, then the more active of the two will have control over how the body behaves. For instance, the conscious mind can be kept busy with positive thoughts. However, if the subconscious mind is programmed with self-harming thoughts, the destructive behavior of these thoughts will affect the actions taken by the conscious mind, nullifying any positive experience registered. If our doctor tells us that we have a terminal disease and we agree with his perception, then this perception might take control over our biology. Therefore, if we were not sick before, after hearing this opinion we might be on the way to terminal disease.

That, Lipton concludes, is why we need to decide what truth we are going to use to control our own biology and, consequently, our life. If we get stuck in behavioral clichés that we acquired during our development, then these clichés will become the main conductors of our system.[11]

BEFORE THE TREATMENT

Before starting a treatment (through palpation or intention), imagine that the Facilitator's assistant in the treatment is not a colleague but a thought-form. To make it easier, we are now going to identify this thought-form with a sphere that will be present during the treatment and interact with the Facilitator and the patient, playing the role of "functional interface between physical and nonphysical states of our existence," as Bruce Lipton said.

The sphere we are asking you to perceive and visualize will serve as the "membrane that allows the spirit to interface with the physical body" (again in Lipton's

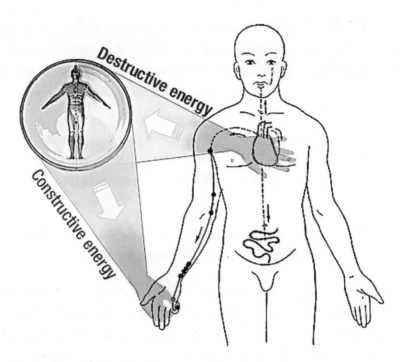

Fig. 23.9. Emptying and filling: transformation of destructive energy into constructive energy

words). The Facilitator will send to it all the information received from the patient's non-conscious and will take from there all the answers coming from the Higher Self on the patient's behalf.

Each person can visualize this sphere in their own way, but we might imagine it as having, for example:

- a vibrant or pulsing nature
- the appearance of a golden light
- the consistency of honey
- a fragrant smell
- a perceptible sound made of the vibrations of the tonality of the note A (which is used to tune all instruments)

Otherwise, we might identify the thought-form with the space of the energetic field of the toroid (or a mandala, or a space that through its imaginative/intuitive/perceptive visualization allows us to store all the information), a space of connection with the Higher Self and the universal energy used to visualize and describe (just like Leonardo da Vinci) beyond all subjectivism.

This will be your thought-form, where you can project the representation (visualization) of the therapeutic space where transformation takes place: the

Third Space (see fig. 3.1, page 24, and fig. 23.1, page 383). It is meant to be the representation of the universal energy, connected with the nourishment of love that fosters the universe and through which the universe nourishes us. Inside it, all the data you send are processed and the transformation from entropic energy to syntropic energy can occur.

Such energy, which is full of information, will be channeled in the process of therapeutic facilitation, transmitted through the Facilitator to the patient with the aptonomic touch (noninvasive palpation) to benefit the patient.

PRACTICING AN INTERACTIVE VISUALIZATION: VECTORS AND THE THIRD SPACE

For this practice, we will start the treatment from the feet station, placing our hands on each of the patient's insteps or soles, at the level of the first chakra (lower/secondary). It is preferable for the patient to be lying down on their back. From this position, we can visually trace the axis of the central vector, starting from the first chakra and proceeding up to the seventh.

Afterward, we carry on with the visualization of the other vectors, mapping the entire vector/axis system with the help of the landmarks of the secondary chakras. If the patient's position does not allow us to place our hands on their body, we may use the intention at a close distance both for the visualization and the rest of the treatment.

Once we have visualized the vectors, we can project (with our intention) the image of the vector/axis system on our "screen" (the Third Space), make the assessment, and establish what corrections are needed in order to realign the vectors. We must then act accordingly, bringing the vectors back to their correct position in relation to their axis. This will facilitate the energy flow in the organism and foster its directionality:

- It starts from the root (first chakra).
- It passes through the heart chakra (fourth chakra).
- It aligns with the energy of vision (sixth chakra).
- It finally connects with universal energy (seventh chakra).

We can follow the last segment of the ascending line (from the sixth to the seventh chakra) through the corpus callosum to reach the bregma (seventh chakra) and channel the universal energy (connection with the Higher Self).

Our objective is to help the patient's organism reach the maximum homeostasis (reestablishing the flow of the vital energy continuum) in order to facilitate every stage of the transformation in any phase or passage of the Life Cycle.

Realigning Vectors Using the Third Space

1. Follow the basic technique to align the vector/axis system, as described beginning on page 244.
2. Without taking your hands off the patient's body, create a thought-form (e.g., a sphere, a toroid, a mandala) and project on it the map of the vector/axis system, as if it were an interactive screen, in order to:

- see/project the image of the vectors (vector/axis system)
- send the entropic energy that is coming out and the information received by the patient's non-conscious
- receive information (through the connection with the Higher Self inside the Third Space) to realign the vector/axis system permanently

3. Still keeping your hands in the initial position, transfer to the patient the information you received in the form of syntropic energy in order to facilitate the transformation from the entropic/disorganized/destructive energy to a new layout of the energetic framework meant to improve and maintain the patient's homeostasis during the process of transition from the current phase of the Life Cycle to the next.

Note: This visualization technique (thought-form) can prove to be especially useful when the patient is in a position that does not allow the correct position of the Facilitator's hands on the body (for example, if the patient is in a fetal position) or the visualization of major and secondary chakras to map the vectors/axes directly on the body.

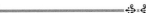

Clinical Observations

A twelve-year-old boy came to my office with his mother. He was suffering from a functional deficiency his family doctor diagnosed as paraplegia. He used a walker to ambulate, and at night he was able to get only a few hours of sleep since he was in a constant state of alert.

This lack of sleep was the dysfunction that was most worrisome to his mother because, on top of the other physical issues, the boy was developing an extremely asocial character, probably due to fatigue. According to his mother, instead of interacting with his schoolmates, he tended to isolate himself and had developed aggressive and destructive intentions toward them.

To be honest, what his mother actually told me was, "He thinks about killing his schoolmates."

Obviously, at that point the boy had been seeing various specialized therapists, each with a specific competence to help his different issues. Nonetheless, his mother had decided to bring him to me since she had been treated with CranioSacral Therapy by a student of mine and found it to be really beneficial for stress management.

First I asked her how her pregnancy with the boy had been. I could not find anything in her description that might point to a cause for the boy's suffering; there was no stress or trauma that might have altered the mother and fetus's RAS and thus triggered a series of anomalies in the fetus.

She added that the delivery had been long, difficult, and very painful, so much so that in that moment she had thought she would prefer to die, even though that meant not seeing her son being born.

As I was listening to the woman and observing her in that difficult and delicate explanation, I noted a tendency to assume a purposely cold and detached attitude, sometimes showing rejection toward what she was talking about. That certainly did not make the dialogue easier, but it made me think that her son had developed his almost misanthropic attitude as a consequence of imprinting with his mother.

She also made me clearly understand that she was in my office because she expected me to perform a miracle on her son, and if I could not do that, she would immediately consider me a charlatan. It was not an easy situation.

Though I commonly begin treatment with Arcing, in this case I did not. Instead I directly started to work on the boy's RAS with the techniques of Direction of Energy through the cranial vault hold. I focused my intentional attention—if I may call it that—on the insertions of the trigeminal nerve, which are connected with the RAS.

Still with the same intention, I brought the image of the therapeutic gesture connected with the patient's organism inside the therapeutic space, my Third Space.

I cannot say what happened next; I just know that I opened my eyes again a few minutes before the time of the session ended.

None of us said much about the session, but the boy's mother booked another appointment for her son.

I was a little shocked, since I could not figure out what happened exactly. I only knew that it felt as if I had fallen asleep, but before starting the treatment I was neither tired nor bored, so I could not explain why it felt like I had dozed off.

When they came back for the following appointment, the boy's mother entered my office saying that she did not see any change in her son. And yet she was there again with him.

Once the boy was on the therapy table, I instinctively repeated the same gestures I had done during the previous session. I used the cranial vault hold and the Direction of Energy on the RAS, connecting through my intention with the roots of the trigeminal nerve. Then I proceeded with the therapeutic gesture in the perceptive visualization of the Third Space.

Exactly like the first time, I inexplicably found myself opening my eyes again just before the session ended.

This time, the boy's mother looked outraged. She told me she had no intention of bringing her son back to me because all I did was sleep!

Before answering, I waited a moment, looking at the boy, who was waking up and had clearly slept with me during both sessions. I asked him how he was feeling.

"I'm okay, thanks," he answered. "I feel very relaxed."

I then addressed his mother and said, "Didn't you say that your son is tense and doesn't sleep much? It certainly doesn't look like that during the treatments."

She had to face the obvious and booked another appointment, though she looked unhappy about having to admit she was wrong.

At the next treatment, after I assumed the usual position, the boy looked at me and said, "Mr. Maggio, let's see who falls asleep first!" and he smiled and closed his eyes. On that occasion, relying on the voice of the Higher Self in my therapeutic space, I somehow went into an alpha state to propose a synergistic connection that could be useful to the boy.

At the end of the session, his mother told me that, though she was not pleased by the "absolute lack of any kind of conventionality" of my technique and my use of unattested and indemonstrable methods, my intervention proved to be effective for her son, who had started to look less tense, sleep more, and soften his attitude in social relationships.

The treatments continued on a weekly basis for more or less six months. The time we spent meeting in what by now was "our" Third Space became gradually shorter, and we did not need the alpha state anymore. I could finally work on the boy to release the restrictions of his intracranial membranes. I focused more on the limbic system—the seat of emotions—and released the Energy Cyst I found.

This story has a happy ending. The boy's mother apologized for the way she had judged me, explaining that she could not conceive a manual therapy carried out without apparent physical work. Despite that, she was extremely happy with the results and told me that the specialized doctors who were taking care of her son were happy as well.

After six months, his ambulation had improved; he had started sleeping eight hours a night again; and he socialized with his schoolmates without thinking about killing them. In fact, he even made a friend.

One of the courses I periodically organize in Italy for my students and fellow Facilitators is called Clinical Applications. This course takes place in a clinical setting with the collaboration of the doctors and staff of the hosting facility, which can be either a public or a private health facility.

During these courses, in accordance with the doctors in charge of the wards involved, I normally propose particular cases that are not likely to be encountered and treated in the everyday work of a Facilitator. I make this choice both to improve each Facilitator's competencies, skills, and knowledge and to bring the aptonomic touch of Dr. Upledger's CST and SER to people who would normally not have the chance to reach a private clinic or office and get to know it or be treated with it.

For some years I found it important to suggest to my students that they work inside wards hosting long-stay patients with serious disabilities, especially patients in a vegetative coma. In this work I also involve patients' families in order to widen the scope in which the benefits of the therapy can occur and to give a new awareness to people who need to take care of ill relatives with which any possibility of interaction seems to have ceased, even before biological death.

In this context, I have generally obtained outcomes that looked minimal at first but were actually huge from a human and therapeutic point of view. It is essential for the Facilitator to be aware of that. In these cases, we often cannot rely on words; there is no placebo effect induced by external stimuli and there are no external stimuli other than the Facilitator's hands and the work with CST and SER techniques.

It is a way of colliding with realities in which there is no big result, but minimal variations can be valued as improvements of the balance of the biological systems that are suffering.

I can assure you, though, that what happens during this type of treatment is a life school for any Facilitator, starting from the foundation of Dr. Upledger's therapy: letting go of the Ego, training the correct attitude, respecting individual free will, and making the difficult choice of empathizing without sympathizing within the Facilitator/patient relationship. It may seem unbelievable, but this happens especially with people who seemingly do not express any emotion that could be useful for building a personal relationship or complicity; they will never thank with words or their eyes those who take care of them, and they will never manifest externally the emotions that each of us could connect with our own life experience. Yet, as that priest told the woman who was taking care of her ill sister (from chapter 20), there is "so much life!" in these people.

Before describing a particular treatment that took place during one of the Clinical Applications courses in Italy, I must make a fundamental clarification.

It is not always easy to find doctors and medical directors who are willing to make their facility and staff available to this kind of initiative or to welcome professionals who do not belong to medical associations. Those who do so usually have an open mind, have no interest in any financial gain, and care only about the possible benefits their patients might experience, but they are so rare that I began to think they are enlightened people. But they do exist, and the actualization of these projects often becomes possible when they themselves experience Upledger CranioSacral Therapy and SomatoEmotional Release through one or more treatments or they attend Upledger Institute International courses as part of their professional continuing education and then bring this knowledge to the health facility where they work.

In Italy, the first person who believed in this project was Dr. Paolo Fusaro, geriatrician and head of the coma ward in a residence for the elderly in Padua. He allowed us to treat the coma patients in his ward. After Bryan, the patient I had met with Dr. Upledger in Ireland many years before, this was only my second experience working with coma patients.

After Dr. Fusaro, with whom I became friends, one of my students, Paola Nobili, introduced Upledger Italia into a health facility in Trieste, where she works as a physiotherapist. With her enthusiasm and passion for her work, she helped me bring CST and SER to the attention of the director of the residence and to Dr. Patrizia Sfreddo, the head of the ward for patients with serious disabilities and in comas. It is thanks to them that I can now describe to you this clinical case and the treatment that was carried out.

During the course, three of the Facilitators worked on the patient. Under my supervision, taking breaks when the medical staff needed to do their work in the ward, they made assessments and treated him for four consecutive days. The man's wife was always there during the treatments, and I encouraged her to interact with the Facilitators by placing her hand on her husband in order to be in constant contact with him during treatment, following the instructions of the group conductor.

A lot of work was done, not only on a physiological level but also on a verbal level. In fact, the Facilitators talked to the man the whole time, as if they were having a conversation and he was replying to their questions through the perceptions they had, while they were employing different techniques of assessment (Significance Detector, Arcing, assessment of the vector/axis system).

One of the Facilitators used the Still Point technique for the whole treatment, while another carried out the dural tube traction and the third one dissipated the Energy Cysts.

During the last treatment, after evaluating the excellent work of the team of Facilitators, I intervened with the technique of energetic emptying and filling through the heart meridian. I emptied the meridian from the residual entropic energy with one hand placed on the heart (with a five-gram pressure) and sent syntropic energy from the distal point of the meridian (the little finger of the right hand) to fill the meridian energetically. In the meantime, I asked his wife to place her hand on his left hand.

When I was about to complete the technique, the patient moved his hand and rolled his palm up, taking his wife's hand into his. We realized what was happening mostly because of the start his wife gave.

When we completed that last part of the treatment, his wife told us what the staff had already informed us of: Ten years before, the man had gone out on his scooter to buy cigarettes and was involved in an accident. The ambulance arrived almost immediately, but he was already in a coma and never regained consciousness.

What we did not know before was that since that moment, even though she kept assisting him daily, she felt her hope of seeing him wake up fading more and more. However, she lived in an entirely irrational state of waiting for his return home with his scooter.

She knew perfectly well that her husband's gesture did not mean he was about to wake up completely, but the feeling she had when it happened was that of hearing him finally come back home, as she confessed to us.

That same day, the last day of Clinical Applications, since all the treatments were completed, we recorded some video footage to report the work that had been done. We also asked the relatives who witnessed the treatments what they thought about those days with us and about the treatments we carried out. When we filmed the wife of the coma patient, she said, "Today, for the first time in so long, he showed his affection and took my hand."

I believe you can imagine how much all of us were touched by that. At last we could allow ourselves to be sympathetic as well as empathic (the treatments were over).

It is essential to consider that, for the relatives or the people taking care of patients in a vegetative coma, even the smallest sign that allows them to have some kind of communication is crucial, especially on an emotional level.

For those who assist their loved ones in these circumstances, the perception of normality is that of living in grief, even though they are at the bedside of a living human being. This happens because they feel like their loved one is in another dimension; therefore, it is not possible to contact them in any way apart from observing and touching their inert body.

On the contrary, when communication is finally made possible in any form, the sensation of grief dissolves and these people perceive again the vital energy continuum of the other person. A new phase of the Life Cycle starts for both, obviously a very different one, but equally intense.

CranioSacral Therapy and SomatoEmotional Release can facilitate this communication.

A CST-CENTERED VISION

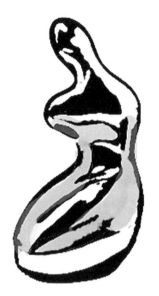

Fig. 23.10. Reproduction of *Demeter,* by Jean Arp

Painter, sculptor, and poet Jean Arp is known all over the world for his sculptures, which feature essential shapes and volumes and smooth surfaces. His creativity is connected with the spiritual essence of reality, beyond the concrete forms through which it manifests itself, an essence we often do not grasp because our perception is used to moving only within the world of concrete forms and sometimes loses the ability to go beyond material reality.

Like Arp, Facilitators can use the imaginative form (thought-form) to shape their work, transforming perception beyond the world of concrete form into reality by manifesting the image of the non-conscious. To do so, they have only to use the gift of perception they were given, just as humans have made use of the gifts of the physical world, such as, in Greek mythology, the gift of grain from the goddess Demeter (a subject of Arp's work; see fig. 23.10).

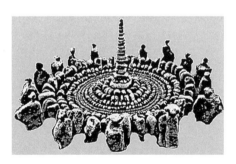

Fig. 23.11. Reproduction of a mandala created by James Brunt

James Brunt is a British "land artist." He creates his artworks in natural landscapes using only the elements nature gives him (rocks, for example). He places materials in the shape of spirals and concentric circles, similar to mandalas, and then lets nature take them back (fig. 23.11).

In Buddhist tradition, the mandala is a symbol that represents the cosmos, in which everything representing the Power of the World has a circular shape. Carl Jung studied mandalas and defined them as an orderly outline that in some measure "is superimposed on the psychic chaos so that each content falls into place and the weltering confusion is held together by the protective circle."[12] In his view, the mandala is the Self, the personality in its entirety, which is harmonious if everything goes well. In Eastern philosophy, the mandala is used as a means to meditate and help individuals set their spirit free, purify their souls, and enter into communion with the positive forces of the cosmos.

CHAPTER 24

Mind-Body-Spirit Continuum

Our Request to the Universe

If the doors of perception were cleansed, every thing would appear to man as it is: infinite.

WILLIAM BLAKE

In his book *Cell Talk: Transmitting Mind into DNA*, Dr. Upledger wrote the following:

> I strongly suspect that all information is energy. Every concept and piece of data to which we are privy has a specifically designed signature in the sea of energy in which each of us is constantly bathing. This sea of energy bathes every cell in our bodies. It knows no boundaries. The energy permeates every nook and cranny, and the same energy is in every particle of our bodies.
>
> So let's assume information is energy and energy is consciousness. Once we allow ourselves to recognize and accept these possibilities/probabilities/facts, we become privy to all of the information or knowledge in the universe on the level of conscious awareness. If it all came into our awareness at once, however, we would be overwhelmed. Rather, it's available to conscious awareness upon request. We just need to learn how to make those requests so that they may be honored.[1]

CONSCIOUSNESS OF THE UNIVERSE

Massimo Teodorani, astrophysicist, researcher, and science communicator, writes about subjects such as entanglement and neurodynamics, offering his observations on synchronicity, the consciousness of the universe, and spirit. The following excerpts are taken from the interview he gave to Anna Biason, writer, poet, and independent researcher.

Quantum physics enters the study of the brain and therefore the generation of conscious processes. . . . The hypothesis that is gaining more and more strength and credibility in the academic world claims that conscious processes are due to "tubulins," proteins located in the microtubules, which are fundamental components of the brain because of their regulating action on the connections between synapses. . . . The process essentially takes place in two phases. During the first phase there is an "unconscious moment" that corresponds with the quantum superimposition of all 109 states of the tubulins in the microtubules. The second phase consists of an actual "conscious moment," consisting in the collapse of the wave function that was keeping together in a single quantum state the complex global entanglement that unites the cerebral microtubules; this phase is also called "orchestrated objective reduction." . . . From this perspective, the brain would be nothing but a carrier able to manifest a consciousness that is actually located "elsewhere." . . .

The quantum model of consciousness that is now definitely taking over the old brain model . . . clarifies that it is not possible in any way to have moments of consciousness if it cannot be explained through a physical carrier with properties of quantum coherence, like the brain and the microtubules. . . . According to this scientific view, the consciousness factor and its functioning absolutely need a physical carrier to be explained . . .

That is the reason why the physical world, as we meant it, exists: to allow the spirit, the consciousness, and the soul to develop, enabling what is actually just a nonphysical database (the spirit, the consciousness, and the soul) . . .

At present, there are no theoretical models able to explain rigorously and coherently a possible interaction between the spirit (or mind, or consciousness) and matter. Quantum potential appears to be linked to matter, but it does not offer any explanation (for now, at least) about how the spirit itself can influence matter directly. . . . There are respectable researchers, such as Dr. Dean Radin, who believe that the influence of the observer (and therefore their mind) on the potential "mental source" of the phenomena works exactly like the classic phenomenon of interference in physics, which can be either destructive or constructive. . . .

After all, there are very interesting studies on quantum electrodynamic coherence like those carried out by physicist Emilio del Giudice (recently passed away) that show that biological matter, and specifically the water it contains, cannot hold out without a "control room" that manages it. This would be a sort of "information field" whose task is not to transport energy but rather to transport information synchronically to all particles. . . . What is the soul exactly, then? We still do not know, but we could deduce it quite easily. . . . This soul is not a physical object, but rather an "information object," which means pure information. . . . Since life without conscience (and therefore without moral and spiritual values) would not make sense in the organization of the universe, it is only logical to think that the soul inside a body must ideally serve also as a sort of "flight recorder" able to register all intellectual and emotional experiences. . . . Science—and physics in particular—is "exploration." Since it represents the main "cognitive gate" of humankind, it lies on a neutral territory, which is critical, healthily skeptical, and objective and strictly rejects any conceit, but also any gratuitous, catatonic, and uncritical form of skepticism.[2]

EXPERIENCING SPIRIT BY CONSCIOUSLY LISTENING TO REALITY

Vito Mancuso, the theologian we encountered in previous chapters, offers another point of view on consciousness, in this case meaning observing and listening to reality.

In the Book of Proverbs (17:27) we can read, "The one who has knowledge uses words with restraint, and whoever has understanding is even-tempered." . . . The mature spiritual dimension relies on the ability to listen in silence to much more than spoken words. Simone Weil identifies the highest spiritual virtue with attention, the prosoché of Stoicism. In order to pay attention, we need to know how to be silent. First, inside ourselves. . . . In all great spiritual traditions, the wise man is the one who does not talk much and is consequently able to listen more. Listening enables him to remember, rethink, and reflect, connecting the multiple contradictory messages of life with each other. This processing of information to find an overall meaning is the highest ability of reasoning. . . .

That is why the degree of maturity of a person is connected with the ability to be silent and listen, which is the only way to see things as they are, understand them, and grow. . . .

If we are able to be silent, we can see the world not in moralistic terms but in physical terms, and we can observe human things as natural phenomena. . . . What do we understand about the world when we interpret it like this? . . . I believe there is an interior way that has three levels with a spiritual hierarchy, which I am going to briefly describe. The first level coincides with the perception of the vanity of the world. The mind that is freed by the silence sees the world and the things most people run after as completely worthless, as deceits and traps. That is the moment of maximum detachment from the world; the liberation from its idols coincides with the detachment from the world as it is. . . . The second level, which is born when the soul acquires maturity, starts the path of reconciliation with the world, which is now understood not as pure negativity but as encompassing also good things. The world emerges as a contradiction, or more precisely as an antinomy. . . . The third and final level in the way of the soul starts when, by continuing to be silent and working on ourselves, we access a more profound level of reality, now seen as a whole in which everything is unified and good. That is what contemporary physics teaches us when it states that all material phenomena are only the energy that constitutes them: everything is energy. . . .

Maybe we now understand what a spiritual experience is; it is not to exit life but rather to understand the profound and true logic of life. The highest spiritual experience coincides with the understanding that everything is energy, which means that everything is spirit, since the Greek term for spirit—pneuma—indicates the igneous breath that creates fire, the perfect representation of energy and its vital heat. To make a spiritual experience means to touch the heart of life. . . .[3]

AN EXPERIENTIAL PERSPECTIVE ON CONSCIOUSNESS

We would like to remember one of the individuals who was able to transmit the concept of unity and harmony of mind, body, and spirit through his own life: journalist and writer Tiziano Terzani (1938–2004), who was awarded several national and international literary prizes and for whom the Premio Terzani per l'Umanizzazione della Medicina (Terzani Prize for the Humanization of Medicine) was named. We are going to do it neither through a synthesis of his biography nor through the citation of paragraphs taken from an interview with or an article about him. Instead, we offer here the most meaningful passages from his books (among the best known are *Letters against the War, A Fortune-Teller Told Me, One More Ride on the Merry-Go-Round,* and *The End Is My Beginning*) in terms of their relevance within the subjects we are examining in this book.* Some of them are his own words; others are the words of figures that appear in the books. All of the Italian books are listed in the bibliography.

> The desire to be complete is shared by all human beings of all continents and all times. It is a universal problem. The solution is universal as well. . . . Without problems, there would be no joy. Problems are the motivation for spiritual research. If you didn't feel miserable and limited, you would not wonder what to do. Human beings become adults and mature through conflict.

> The human mind is behind all human problems, but it also holds their solutions. The mind is a hidden treasure we step on everyday without realizing how much it is worth. We need to own it and dominate it by training to do everything consciously, instead of letting ourselves be distracted.

---

*All the quotions are translated by the translator of this book from the original Italian versions by T. Terzani.—*Ed.*

The world is like this; not an illusion, but something that helps us deal with the universe and recognize that it is supported by Consciousness, that Reality, or Wholeness, or Self everything belongs to. Therefore, all things—hell, heaven, happiness, sadness, joy, the entire world—are inside ourselves.

We look at the world and it appears to us to be divided in parts; we think we are one of those parts ourselves, but the truth is that the universe is a single independent whole and not the sum of its parts. Its parts reflect the whole, but it is absurd to think that reality could be reduced to its parts.

Let it be clear: I don't heal, I take care of. The healer is something that we all have inside ourselves.

Our body has a self-healing system. It just needs to be activated. It needs a stimulus, the faith in a saint, prayers . . .

True knowledge comes not from books, but from experience. The best way to understand reality is through feelings and intuition, not through intellect. Intellect is limited.

The solution of human problems cannot come from reason, because reason is the cause for most of those problems.

Believing exclusively in science cuts us Westerners out from an interesting stock of knowledge. . . . Science is an important tool of knowledge. Our mistake is to believe it is the only one.

When you have a problem, stop. Stop. Stop. Listen to it and try to find the answer inside yourself. It is there. Inside yourself there is something that holds you together and helps you. There is a little voice. Listen to it.

What is outside is also inside, but what is not inside is nowhere else.

Everything that is born shall die; everything that dies shall be reborn. Only the Self, the pure consciousness that has never been born and stays outside of time, remains.

The death of everything that is born is certain, the birth of everything that dies is certain. This is inevitable, and you have no reason to suffer.

Don't ask for perfect health, it would be greedy. Make pain your own medicine, and do not expect a way without obstacles. Without that fire, your light would die out. Use a storm to set yourself free.

What scares us so much about death? What makes us afraid, what petrifies us about it, is the idea that everything we are attached to will disappear in that moment. First, the body. We made an obsession out of our body.

Once we accepted that pain fades, too, like everything else, the biggest step had been taken.

Everything begins and ends in our minds. Mind and body are not two separate entities, like Descartes believed. That was a huge mistake, and we are still suffering its consequences. Mind and body are integrated and the mind controls matter. There is no doubt about that.

Human beings need to acquire a new awareness about themselves, their existence in the world, and their relationship with other human beings and with other living beings. This awareness must find a new spiritual component to balance the obsessive materialism of our time. Only then will it be possible to hope for a new and sustainable global civilization.

Who am I? It is all about asking the question, realizing that I am not my body, I am not what I do, I am not what I own, I am not my relationships, I am neither my thoughts nor my experiences, and I am not even that "I" we care about so much. The answer is not made of words. It is the silent immersion of the I into the Self.

Healing ourselves does not mean swallowing a pill every six hours. It means to purify our mind and use it to support the healing process. . . . It means to move toward a correct lifestyle. Healing means preventing illness by living a life in which our body is in harmony and our mind is at peace.

Anger, fear, hatred, or jealousy contribute to bad health, whereas other emotions like charity, compassion, joy, or laughter contribute to feeling well.

. . . harmony, stability in the realization of the Self. That is true health for us.

There are no shortcuts to show. Sacred books, masters, gurus, and religions are useful, but they are useful like the elevators that bring us upstairs and spare us the stairs. The last part of our path, those little steps to access the roof, from which we can see the world and lie down on it or become a cloud, that last part must be done on foot and by ourselves.

Our concept of death is wrong. We connect it too much with fear, pain, darkness, blackness; it is exactly the opposite of what happens in nature, in which the sun dies every day in a joyous explosion of light, in which the plants die in the fall while they are at their best, so full of colors. We should maybe tell ourselves—just like the Teduray do—that we die only when we have decided it, or we should consider death—just like the Tibetans—not as the opposite of life, but simply as the other side of birth, a door that is the entry when it is seen from one side and the exit from the other.

Life is like this: it is everything and the opposite of everything; it is wonderful and it is cruel. That is because life is also death, and there is no pleasure without pain, there is no happiness without suffering.

This is not an apology to evil or suffering. It is an invitation to look at the world from a different point of view, without thinking only in terms of what we like or don't like. After all, if life were a bed of roses, would it be a blessing or a curse? Maybe it would be a curse, because if you live without ever wondering why you live, you waste a great opportunity. And only pain pushes you to ask yourself this question.

OBSERVATIONS

In a specific moment of our Life Cycle, I believe that all of us—in our different ways, beyond any faith, belief, or religion—became conscious of what it means to enter the spiritual dimension, or at least got close to it.

Some of us have probably considered it the experience of an intimate transcendent connection, the product of meditation or prayer, a spontaneous and unexpected perception, an intuition, or the acquisition of awareness about past experiences. Others, like myself, have experienced it thanks to their encounter with inviduals who live (or lived) every day with the consciousness of life and its spiritual dimension.

In all these cases, we came into contact with information or messages that were perceived, channeled, and brought to awareness through our mind, although they had already been assimilated by all the cells of our body, so much so that we could not consciously deny them afterward.

Here are some of the encounters that brought me a message in the form of personal and specific information that was useful (or even necessary) to improve my vital energy continuum and my life itself.

Patrick Francis

His birth name is Paddy McMahon. He wrote the book series *The Grand Design*. He is Irish, from County Clare. I met him through Mary Kennedy O'Brian—the same person who introduced me to Dr. Upledger. By reading Patrick Francis's books and then meeting him in person, I perceived spirituality for the first time, or at least the spiritual aspect of physical events of life. It was he who led me to understand the potential of SER. In reviews of his books, we can read, "His objective is to connect the spiritual realm with the earthly one and give comfort to the living, helping them win the fear of death and revealing at the same time curious aspects of the new existence. Physical death is not the end but the beginning." Also, "Sooner or later questions like 'Who/what am I?', 'Where do I come from?', 'How can I find meaning in my life?', 'How can I reduce the pain of self-realization?', or 'What will happen to me when I die?' start to come up for all of us, sometimes tormenting us. The books written by Patrick Francis explore life in all its aspects both in the physical and the spiritual world. Moreover, they explain how we came to inhabit physical bodies and what happens when we die; and they provide us with facts, concepts, and suggestions meant to help us find more happiness and satisfaction in our life expression with the collaboration of our guides/guardian angels, if we want to."[4]

The Spirit Guide

After meeting Patrick Francis, I had a peculiar experience during an SER treatment I was carrying out on a woman who defined herself as a *curandera*. She felt that the end of her life was near. In that treatment, I came into contact with her spirit guide, which in SER is another form of contact with the non-conscious, in this case that of the patient. It is expressed through a form of being that was radically different from matter and contained all kinds of manifestation of reality. Everything happened during the Therapeutic Imagery and Dialogue. The spirit guide of the curandera said his name was Demetrio Falareo, he had lived in Greece in 300 BCE, and he had joined the peripatetic school of Plato's followers; through him, I was able to meet the "Seven Sages." They guaranteed that the woman's life was not at its end and that I could reassure her about that. Was it madness? No, or at least I do not think so.

Carl Jung would simply describe the experience as active imagination (and we can find a description of his spirit guide in his autobiography *Memories, Dreams, Reflections*).

Charlie

The day before the treatment on the curandera, I actually encountered my own spirit guide. I was in Florida to learn the first level of SomatoEmotional Release (which is the third core level of CranioSacral Therapy). The course Instructor was Dr. Upledger. During the third day of the seminar, as the protocol indicated, we started to learn the technique of Therapeutic Imagery and Dialogue. In the afternoon of that day, during the practical part, the students treated each other to employ what they had learned during the lecture of that morning. My colleague, who was about to act as Facilitator and treat me as her patient, asked me whether I believed in guardian angels. I told her I did not, but she was not satisfied with that answer and kept asking me about any possible other version of that concept she knew: spiritual guides, angelic spirits, et cetera. Honestly, she was so insistent that I remember at one point I was ready to ask her, "What part of 'no' do you not understand?"

I held back because I did not want to be rude, and at a certain point I finally gave in and told her I might have a spirit guide too. Her face lit up. Though I was assuming that the conversation had finally come to an end and I could relax and receive the treatment, she then asked me the name of my spirit guide. Imagine that! I had said I had a spirit guide out of mere kindness and now I also had to think of a name! I told her the first name I could think of, "Charlie," hoping the issue would be closed for good, and then I lay down on the therapy table.

But no, it was not over. Instead of starting to treat me, she stayed where she was and said, "Weird." I gave up. I sat up on the table and asked her, "Why weird?" She proceeded to tell me that, as she was listening to Dr. Upledger's lecture that morning, a name came to her mind, and she wrote it down in her study guide. I was convinced that this endless dialogue would mean that our actual SER session would last only five minutes or so, but I asked her, "Oh, yeah? And what name was it?"

Willing to share her thought with me, she opened her study guide to the page for Therapeutic Imagery and Dialogue and made me read the name she had written, preceding a question mark: "Charlie?"

That is how I encountered my spirit guide. Charlie stayed with me during my whole first treatment of SER and also for much more time after that. During the courses I taught as an SER Instructor, I used to have the room prepared with a chair for Charlie behind me.

St. Giuseppe Moscati

Several years later, I was in Naples to teach at a seminar, and I went to visit some of the churches of the city. I entered the church of Gesù Nuovo, dedicated to the physician Saint Giuseppe Moscati. I was particularly impressed by the statue of the saint, in which he was represented wearing his scrubs, keeping his hand on the forehead of a patient, and raising the other hand to the sky. That night, I dreamed the funerals of the saint.

I decided to investigate his life. I went back to the church, where there was a small shop with his books, and I bought them. I will always remember a sentence I read in one of those texts, which I sometimes quote to my students in the classroom. It could be translated as follows: "Pain must be treated not as a spasm or a muscular contraction, but as the cry of a soul that solicits another brother, the physician, to rush to the patient with the passion of a kind of love that is called charity."

I remember when I read that, I felt heat inside my chest, and I remained there in reflection for an indefinite time.

St. Francis of Paola

Another spiritual figure I have "met" in my life is Saint Francis of Paola (1416–1507). He was a hermit of the Franciscan Order who later founded the Order of Minims. My first contact with him occurred when I went to Paola in the Italian region of Calabria, where I wanted to visit the church and monastery that were built to accommodate Saint Francis and his order. That day, the church and monastery were unfortunately closed to the public.

Some months later I was in Turin to teach a seminar and, as always, I started my church tour. I entered the first church on my way. I thought I was alone, but the sacristan approached me as I was admiring the architecture of that place. He greeted me, and I took the chance to ask him for some information about that church. He told me that it was dedicated to Saint Francis of Paola.

A little surprised, I told him about my attempt to visit the church in the saint's hometown. It was maybe for this reason that the sacristan was eager to provide me with all the material he could find about the saint's life. He told me Saint Francis of Paola was called "the herbalist" by his contemporaries. He was given this nickname because he used to perform healings during which he went into a trance and, as soon as he woke up again, he gave a medicinal herb to the person he had healed, recommending they use it. The sacristan told me that the herb was not useful for its healing properties, but the person's will to take it every day and get better would result in the reconnection with God, who would operate his healing through the saint.

All of this made me think about the work of Facilitators, who treat their patients only to bring them to the awareness that is necessary for their own self-healing. Until their realization, the patients often do not know that they allow the Facilitator to channel into them what is needed for their good, or that by doing so they open up to something that transcends mere physicality.

St. Nicholas

Not long ago, I myself experienced self-healing in a moment in which I was extremely vulnerable because I was going through the fear of disease. Because of that, I was overly focused on any perceptible signal from my organism. In that period, I did not have any desire to socialize or allow any external stimulus to distract me. I had just received the diagnosis of prostatitis, detected through some clinical tests. I wanted to rest and go through some more clinical tests in order to start a treatment protocol, but I had previously taken some work commitments that led me to momentarily postpone the issue and travel to Bari, a city I had never been to.

In moments of discomfort or illness, it is easy to have a different perception of reality and its priorities. Once I arrived in Bari, my body was asking for some rest, but I decided to go on as if everything was completely normal in order not to think about the pain (which was not an easy task at that point). I decided to visit at least one church and chose the church of Saint Nicholas, the patron saint of the city. Once inside the building, instead of looking around as I usually do, I decided to sit down near the remains of Saint Nicholas, which are kept inside. While I was reflecting on the figure of that saint, who embraced both the Orthodox and the Catholic Church because of his origins, I noticed that next to the relics of the saint were some small bottles of manna on display for those who wanted to buy them.

The manna of Saint Nicholas is a particularly pure liquid that constantly gathers in the saint's tomb and is collected once a year and bottled to be preserved. Believers attribute thaumaturgical qualities to that fluid.

I decided to leave an offering, took a bottle of manna, and brought it with me to the hotel. That night, I put it next to my bed. It goes without saying that I was hoping for the thaumaturgical effects of that liquid to work, and I started to project my thoughts into healing until they became a prayer; at that point I fell asleep. I had awful nightmares all night; I kept waking up and falling asleep again, but I was not able to escape sleep enough to force myself to get up and push away the nightmares and the sense of anxiety they were causing me.

When I definitively woke up in the morning, I could perceive a sense of void in my mind. I remained where I was for a long time, without even feeling the pain caused by the prostatitis. I was immersed in a foreign dimension that was pleasant and reassuring, as if I were floating in a warm and comfortable liquid.

I got up thinking about facing the traces of blood in my urine, a symptom I was experiencing in that period. I started to get ready to go out. I was not feeling pain, and I noticed that the most obvious symptoms of prostatitis were not showing up that morning. In the following days, I did not experience any other symptom.

Once I came back home after that work trip, the first thing I did was go to the analysis lab to repeat the clinical test I had already done, which had been already scheduled. After I got the results, I was told that they were completely normal and that there was no trace of a prostatitis in my organism anymore.

To me, that proved the truth of what I always say to my patients about having faith in what they do. In Bari, I had desperately wanted to believe I could be healed.

Since then, I had been even more convinced that our mind, body, and spirit are able to find the synergy that can make them One and make that One connect with the Whole. This is the vision I propose to my patients during the treatments to facilitate their self-healing path.

ART OF TREATMENT

As soon as Facilitators acquire the correct vision thanks to the training of the correct attitude in the treatments, they become able to see that the work on patients is the work on themselves, which is what allows them to be fully aware about their life.

The objective implied by CST and SER treatments is to consciously live all the actions we carry out in everyday life. Being aware of what we do every day is a form of art, in addition to destroying the barriers that divide and section life into separate and contrasting spaces, times, and phases.

Art is the expression of the consciousness of existing in space, time, and the life energy (vital energy continuum) of the universe as a part of everything that surrounds us. It is one of the highest expressions of life. It does not ignore polarities but integrates them. It is able to channel the essence of the reality of mind, body, and spirit in one single aware gesture (holistic vision).

We like to think that, just like Dr. Upledger transformed his knowledge into an art of treatment with CST and SER and made his message accessible to everyone, many other enlightened minds (and expert hands) shared Dr. Upledger's thought-form, although with different methods and in different scenarios/times/spaces/places. Each of these minds discovered the holistic vision and found out that being in life means harmoniously integrating all of the parts that constitute life.

Here are some examples:

> *Science is no more than an investigation of a miracle we can never explain, and art is an interpretation of that miracle.*
>
> RAY BRADBURY
> AND THE MOON BE STILL AS BRIGHT, 1948

> *He who works with his hands is a laborer. He who works with his hands and his head is a craftsman. He who works with his hands and his head and his heart is an artist.*
>
> LOUIS NIZER
> BETWEEN YOU AND ME, 1948

> *Art is science. It cannot be improvised and it does not settle for banal and superficial approximations, but it requires hard and systematic work.*
>
> LEONARDO DA VINCI
> IL CODICE ATLANTICO DELLA BIBLIOTECA AMBROSIANA DI MILANO,
> (2006 TRANSLATION)

> *CranioSacral Therapy is both a highly intuitive art form and a highly scientific modality.*
>
> JOHN E. UPLEDGER

PREPARING FOR THE SEVEN-STEP TREATMENT

Before carrying out any type of treatment, Facilitators must mainly ask to be able to support patients as much as possible for their sake and in the full respect of their will. This is even more necessary when our patients are going through the delicate phase of dying, the passage from a known place in their life to the unknown.

As Facilitators, we should be the first to prepare to accept with deep gratitude the person we are going to treat and to honor that person for giving us the opportunity to support them in this phase of life. Our emotions in this approach should be focused on the fullness of life represented by the person in front of us, since we were given the gift of being the spectators and participants in this phase of life, the moment of maximum remission.

We are facing the transformation of life. We must be aware that in front of us is not a person in dysfunction but rather an individual who is in the moment of both greatest need and greatest offering. In this person we can find everything we have learned so far and also the experience we still need to learn.

We are facing an extreme polarity: extreme fear and extreme love!

The Facilitator's hands are now touching the fragility of the five petals of a primrose and, at the same time, the richness and complexity of the thousand petals of a chrysanthemum.

When preparing for the final treatment, the correct approach focuses on the following:

10 Fundamental Principles for the Final Treatment

1. Focus on listening, rootedness, and breath (self-focus).
2. Invoke the energetic phase of the relationship: palpation, the electromagnetic field, Arcing.
3. CST is a support to the Life Cycle in every aspect, including in the process of dying or for an irreversible vegetative state.
4. Dissipate entropic energy to relieve the mind of trauma.
5. Employ the therapeutic position and intention.
6. Practice being there, listening, and unconditional love; avoid judgment.
7. Give dignity and respect of/in death.
8. Help the patient and their loved ones in transforming the approach toward loss.
9. In the dying process, in the phase of remission, focus on gratitude beyond forgiveness.
10. Remember: Gratitude in the therapist's heart transforms loss.

Clinical Observations

I had been treating a patient suffering from tinnitus for a long time, and I could not solve his problem in any way. I had treated him using various techniques on his temporal bones and masticatory apparatus, and I had worked on his fifth diaphragm and intracranial membranes. And nothing. No improvements. The more he lost faith in my care, the more I lost my inspirations in the treatments.

During one of the sessions, as I was thinking I was about to give up, the patient suddenly told me that he saw the apparition of a purple light. I could not believe it! A glimmer of hope at last.

It goes without saying that when I asked him what the meaning of that purple light could be and he answered that he had no idea, I thought it was the final sign of closure. What I had believed might be an opening that could give a twist to the treatments proved to be just another closed door.

I decided to make one last attempt. I visualized a sheltered space that surrounded the patient and me and had the appearance of a golden sphere. I then projected that sphere in front of me to make myself a spectator of what was happening.

It worked. I could see the treatment as if it were an image projected on a three-dimensional screen. I focused on the image of the patient and filled the sphere with purple light, concentrating on his sixth chakra (pineal gland). From there, I accessed the structures of the center, the insula, and the pituitary gland. The sphere started vibrating, and the vibration indicated buzzing, a sort of unpleasant cacophony.

We could say I was "in his tinnitus." I was astonished.

The louder the buzz became, the more the sphere seemed to vibrate. At the same time, I felt the need to give harmony to that noise. How? It was imperative to tune that orchestra of off-key sound vibrations. I knew I had to give it a try. The worst thing that could happen, I thought, would be that my patient's growing lack of faith in my abilities would be confirmed.

Therefore, I asked the patient if he was comfortable enough to vocalize an A note for me. To my surprise, the patient looked like he was indeed willing to cooperate, for the first time, and he vocalized the A note.

After various attempts at reproducing the harmonic scale to get to a more coherent A (which was hard for him because he tended to follow the ringing he was hearing in his ears), he succeeded in reproducing a perfect A. He was so satisfied with himself that he almost did not want to stop.

In the meantime, the sphere had stabilized and did not vibrate anymore. As I was encouraging the patient to go on with his vocalization, I let my hands be guided by the vibration of the note, moving to the greater wings of the sphenoid bone, while I was focusing again on the pineal gland (hypophysis).

I had come into contact with that specific part of the body, and I took this opportunity to dialogue with it. It told me that it was losing its sense of direction because of the patient's stressful rhythm of life. It was lost in time and space and was not finding north anymore.

I asked the patient whether he was under pressure for any reason and whether stress was getting him away from his objectives. He confirmed that he was undergoing a wearying period of intense stress at work and that this had serious consequences on his family dynamics as well.

We then finally started the dialogue.

He told me he had lost his way in life, or at least what he believed was his way, and this had created a lack of direction in his path. He could not find his place, purpose, or ideal destination in life. He could not focus on any project unless it was short term. He saw no way out and felt as if he had been "thrown off the right way."

I told him that sometimes we need to search for a wider space in which to project our problems in order to redefine and downsize them. Sometimes, if we really think about it, our problems are much smaller than we think they are. We need to put them in a different dimension, outside the box of our everyday reality, which is only a limited reflection of the real dimension of our life.

I asked him whether he wanted to try to access a different space, the Third Space, where it is possible to dialogue with the Inner Physician and contact the Higher Self to find some answers. I invited him to immerse again in the note that had just urged him to let his non-conscious speak and had guided me into focusing on his discomfort. I suggested that he imagine the A as a path or a bridge connecting his microcosm to the macrocosm, where all answers lie, and where he could probably find what he needed if he asked with his heart and not with his mind.

Was it a hazard? Yes, but I was there for him to facilitate his path and help him enter that space. And he did it.

Sometimes we need to reach the point of desperation in order to find the courage to try the unthinkable and have the chance to really listen to what the universe (our Inner Physician, our Higher Self) wants to tell us. We only need to stop covering our ears (metaphorically) and stop trying to hide the voice of our Higher Self with other sounds or buzzes.

Little by little, by talking and by reproducing the A again, the patient started telling me that maybe what he needed was to stop panicking when things were not going as he had expected. In fact, he would need to assess one problem at a time and calmly and humbly try to propose simple actions to face problems with more serenity, giving himself the chance to consider a wide range of answers before establishing the best way to deal with the difficulties.

His tinnitus improved, but it did not disappear completely. However, he was not complaining about it anymore and actually told me that the ringing in his ears was now helping him to always find the space and the moment to tune in and meet himself.

He was more peaceful. It showed on his face and in the way he started smiling after the decisive session. He still had that smile when he came to my office for the last treatment. Before going, he thanked me and told me he now knew how to really feel good.

I had not solved his tinnitus, but I was extremely satisfied.

❧ A CST-CENTERED VISION ❧

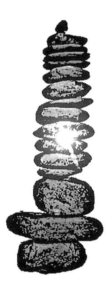

Fig. 24.1. Reproduction of balancing rock art by Michael Grab

Michael Grab, land artist, knows everything about balancing stones. He believes the process of creating these structures made of stones has spiritual and healing properties. He says many cultures from all around the world have practiced the art of balancing stones for centuries. When in balance, their purposes range from marking human presence to showing gratitude to the art of meditative nature.

This artist balances stones until all of their gravity centers are balanced perfectly. Facilitators carry on the same process when they follow the correct disposition of all the systems of the organism until they have restored the natural balance of mind/body/spirit.

CHAPTER 25

A Seven-Step Treatment for the Dying Process

Don't expect anything. All you need to do is trust the patient's consciousness. It knows what they need.

DR. JOHN E. UPLEDGER

This section concerns the first part of the working protocol Facilitators should apply when they need to support an individual in the phase of transition that takes place in the dying process and might also occur during the assistance to a coma patient.

The objective of this treatment is to help all physiological structures to be as functional as possible in facilitating the organism as it goes through the current phase in order to reach the following one (whatever it may be, depending on the patient's will).

The treatment is structured to apply simple and noninvasive techniques that are adaptable to the patient's position. If the patient's situation does not allow us to carry out the techniques in the usual way, we could implement a technique by simply acting on the distal points of the meridians. We could also treat the patient energetically through intention, without placing our hands on their body and palpating the organ involved directly. We might have to work exclusively in the Third Space in connection with all the structures that the patient's Higher Self brings to our attention. This will guide us as we proceed, even in the treatment of one single part of the organism, and enable us to connect with the patient's entire physiological, emotional, and spiritual system.

As we will later see in this chapter, in order to implement the seven-step treatment on patients in this transition/transmutation phase of their Life Cycle, we will apply the following in all cases:

• Start by realigning the vector/axis system (acknowledging its polarity).
• Use the visualization of the Third Space when necessary.

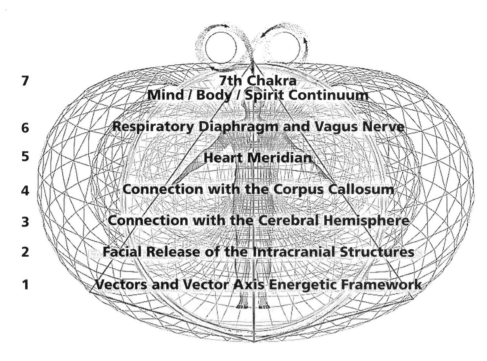

Fig. 25.1. The seven steps

- Perceive the active lesions caused by Energy Cysts and identify their connections with the peculiar characteristics of chakras, including their vibrational quality.
- Connect the two cerebral hemispheres through the corpus callosum, thus connecting with the central nervous system and the RAS.
- Release the entropic energy through the meridians and facilitate the flow of syntropic energy coming in, stabilizing the entire energy flow of the organism.
- Expand the toroidal energetic field of the heart chakra (fourth chakra) in the unity of the Third Space (the healing space connected with the universal energy), fostering the mind-body-spirit connection.
- Reaching the seventh chakra (bregma), enhance access through the energy flow to the information that is useful to the patient and to the functionality of their organs, systems, and entire organism depending on the instructions given by the Higher Self.

We must always connect with and rely on our Higher Self if we want to perceive, deduce, and translate any possible form of dialogue that takes place between our non-conscious and the patient's non-conscious.

Up until this point, we have gathered a huge amount of information as preparatory knowledge that the Facilitator will use in the seven-step treatment through the therapeutic gesture. Before introducing the actual treatment protocol, we will proceed to examine in a concise way (with a brief numerological digression) three crucial elements: synchronicity, synergy, and empathy.

SYNCHRONICITY: BEYOND THE LIMITS OF SPACE-TIME

We often chance upon what we may call "meaningful coincidences." Facilitators know it well. For example, it sometimes happens that immediately after a certain professional specialization course on CST and SER, the next patients coming to you for treatment actually suffer from symptoms that are attributable to the subject of the course you have just attended. Or you get interested in a specific topic related to your own professional growth and—what a coincidence!—a new article has just been published on that topic. A simpler case: you think about someone you have not seen in a long time, and you meet them shortly after. It has probably happened to most of us. Is it by chance? No, it is a phenomenon called synchronicity.

Though the phenomenon was defined coherently only relatively recently, by psychoanalyst Carl Jung, synchronicity was a field of study and research long before. Consider what Arthur Schopenhauer (1788–1860) wrote when he was examining the studies of another philosopher, Immanuel Kant (1724–1804); he actually described what Kant had called "magical effects" as "direct influences of the will that go beyond spatiotemporal limits."

Let us see, then, how this phenomenon is interpreted from a scientific point of view, more than two centuries after Schopenhauer and almost half a century after Jung, through the historical-scientific analysis of Paolo Silvestrini, physicist, researcher, and artist:

> The quantum state does not have a univocal reality unless it is being measured. . . . Through the phenomenon of "quantum entanglement," the "EPR pairs" of photons (or electrons) exist in one single quantum state, which is not determined unless it is being measured. When a measurement is done on the state of one of the particles, this causes the collapse of the collective state so that the other immediately aligns with the corresponding state. . . . We could call this mysterious a-causal link the "principle of synchronicity," a term coined by the great psychologist Carl Gustav Jung, who in 1952 dedicated an entire book to the a-causal links he had observed in the context of subjective perception in psychology. . . . In order to explain the psychology of unconscious processes, Jung introduced a new principle alongside causality. There are parallel phenomena that cannot be connected with each other from a causal [cause-and-effect] point of view; this connection between events seems essentially produced by their relative simultaneity with unconscious

psychological processes—hence the term "synchronicity." . . . The separation of objects and events that we normally use to describe our everyday experience is not reflected in the quantum world, and Jung describes a similar modality of perception of reality in the unconscious phenomena that emerge to conscious awareness.

In an even more explicit way, in his foreword to the English translation of the I Ching—Book of Changes, Jung comments on the efficiency of the Eastern divination methods from a merely psychological standpoint; to him, the I Ching is based on the principle of synchronicity, which in Eastern traditions connects all cosmic events that take place in one specific instant—including the subjective perception of human beings—in a universal phenomenon in which the only connecting element is "temporal synchronicity." It is "time" that permeates and determines the explicit form of the universe, and this form changes because time changes. Jung wrote . . . "The ancient Chinese mind contemplates the cosmos in a way comparable to that of the modern physicist. . . . The microphysical event [in quantum physics] includes the observer just as much as the reality underlying the I Ching comprises subjective, i.e., psychic conditions in the totality of the momentary situation. Just as causality describes the sequence of events, so synchronicity to the Chinese mind deals with the coincidence of events." . . .

This vision is very close to the perspective of the world quantum physics forces us to accept with the evidence of the violation of the principle of local realism in the phenomenon of quantum entanglement. . . . Once again, quantum physics leads to consequences that go far beyond the methodological principles at the foundation of its historical development.[1]

SYNERGY: MIRROR NEURONS

The Facilitator intentionally ascribes to synergy the intention that enables them to pursue the correct attitude in the therapeutic gesture and restores the optimal constructive relations between the particles, organs, and systems of the organism during the treatment. That is how the Facilitator invites all the elements they have assessed to cooperate in order to restore the person's well-being.

Similarly, this entire book is meant as a synergic expression in which all elements add together and complete and strengthen each other, creating a conceptual cognitive substratum that implements the Facilitator's action.

What is far more important is what happens beyond our cognitive speculation and manifests itself in the neural and cellular synergy (entanglement) resulting from the connections that at first are established on an intuitive/perceptive level and then emerge on a conscious level in the people who pursue the search for coherent information coming from the "substance" of the Higher Self.

We believe Dr. Upledger was one of those people.

In order to better define synergy, we rely again on the words of theologian Vito Mancuso:

> The constructive dimension of thought is represented by the logos, which desires logic and produces wisdom and knowledge. Thought as logos-logic is exercised through verbs such as observe, ponder, consider, reconsider, analyze, reflect, and meditate. Thought as logos sometimes becomes a source of inspiration, and in those rare moments it reproduces the logic of creation and generates creativity; the verbs that identify it in this case are realize, devise, discover, and create. . . .
>
> Is it possible to orient the desires of the I without identifying it with the voracity of the ego? . . . Trying to walk on the thin edge, . . . I get a glimpse of the life of the mind, and consequently of existence, which tradition regards in terms of idea and I intend to present through the symbolic image of heavenly love. . . .
>
> First of all, I want to clarify that with this strange expression I refer to ideas (or ideals) and their ability to apply force. With heavenly love I mean the ideas as nonmaterial forces that produce in us an intense attraction. . . . Do you call it psyche? Mind? I? Ego? Self? Selfhood? Consciousness? Soul? Spirit? Call it as you wish, or how your personal education makes you call it; through the symbol of heavenly love I personally want to refer to a real non-material force that has a great attraction and exists outside the ordinary mind . . . constructing thought properly since it arranges the concepts that come from the processing of sensible data in a specific architectural order. The guiding idea is comparable to an orchestra conductor who knows how to manage all the musicians in order to make them create a harmony. . . .
>
> I talk about love because love is the most powerful force there is. I imagine that many people might disagree with this statement, and I have no trouble understanding why. . . . Nonetheless, I believe that only good and love are able to build, give positive energy, infuse life, and last. . . .
>
> According to physics, matter is nothing but solidified energy, therefore everything we see and touch can be reduced to energy. The word "energy" comes from the Greek *energeia,* composed of the preposition *en*—meaning "in"—and the noun *ergon*—meaning "act, action, work"; therefore, energy etymologically means "in action," "working." And if everything is energy, then everything works, or takes action.
>
> Let us now examine a famous sentence by Marcus Aurelius: Gegonamen pros synergian. This expression is usually translated as "we are born to cooperate," but in this context it is more incisive in its literal sense, "we are born for synergy." The sense of human life in itself is not simply to work and produce energy, but its peculiarity consists of eliciting a more refined energy, able to create mutual connections until it reaches the apex of love, and for this reason it is called synergy.[2]

The term *synergy* conceptually means cooperation, or a combined action of principles whose effects add up. However, this concept assumes different connotations depending on the context in which it is examined. For example, sociologist Lester Frank Ward (1841–1913) regarded it as a cosmic principle that produces the structure generated from the cooperation of opposite forces; in the scientific psychology of Théodule-Armand Ribot (1839–1916), it represents the first physiological and unconscious stage of sympathy, one of the foundations of social life; for Maurice Blondel (1861–1949), it is, instead, the unity of the functions of universalization and concretization that belong to thought.

In addition, we need to be reminded that the concept of synergy is derived from that of synergism, which has the same etymological root but takes on different meanings. In theological language, starting from Filippo Melantone (1497–1560), synergism is the doctrine that assigns a specific value to the function of free will and good deeds, as the sign of collaboration of humans in the logic of individual salvation. In biological and medical sciences, synergism can refer to either the functional cooperation of one or more anatomical units in a specific physiological process (movement, chemical reaction, etc.) or a pharmacological process used as therapy and produced by two or more medications that enhance their effect through their combined actions.

Let us now explore summarily the aspect of synergy that is the most relevant in neuroscience. We are going to rely on the expertise of Luciano Rispoli, psychotherapist and founder of functional psychotherapy (neofunctionalism), in the context of the action of mirror neurons:

> We talk a lot about mirror neurons lately; and it is only right to do so since they are a discovery of great scientific value, in addition to being a success entirely accomplished by Italian researchers—Giacomo Rizzolatti and his team.
>
> However, this discovery is deeper and more complex than what is commonly perceived. . . . Neurology used to regard the motor system as being a mere executor with a secondary role. It was believed that human beings acquire data through perception and process them cognitively, and that from this level of cognition "orders" are sent to the motor system. Nonetheless, the study of the functioning of frontal and parietal areas as well as motor and premotor areas of the brain showed a completely different reality: the motor system does not deal with motions, but with actions in their entirety. . . .
>
> In fact, one of the first discoveries that paved the way to this vision was that frontal and parietal areas are strictly connected with visual, auditory, and tactile areas, which entails that cortical areas of perception and cognition are not completely distinct and separate from those of motion. . . .

Another point that helps us understand how the motor system relates to actions with a complex configuration and not just single movements comes from the study of these neurons. . . . As we have already said, these neurons are not connected with movement but with an action that can even be composed of very different motions. . . .

The premotor area can therefore be seen as an actual reservoir of possible actions the individual can make, or, in other terms, a "vocabulary" of actions, each of them is connected with specific neurons. . . .

To clarify the matter, these neurons are defined as bimodal because they are activated both during the actions made by the individual on an object and during the simple observation of that object. What is astonishing is that they are located in the motor area. The object is immediately coded as a series of hypothetical actions. The neurons react not to the form of the object but to the meaning it has for the person.

However, reacting to a meaning means UNDERSTANDING. . . .

Mirror neurons are specific bimodal neurons . . . that are activated when the individual performs an action, but also when they are observing another person performing the action. The individual therefore experiences the same sensations as the person who is carrying out the action, as if they were performing it as well. Anyway, we need to remember that this happens only if the same action is contained in that individual's "vocabulary" of actions. . . .

In order for it to be in the vocabulary, the individual must have experienced it personally before. . . .

The insula is also involved in the resonance of emotions. It is through the insula that sensory inputs are transformed into "visceral" reactions, meaning psychophysiological modes of functioning that "color" emotional responses (either observed or one's own). . . .

The key point is that we are dealing with actual knowledge, an implicit, pragmatic, and nonreflective understanding. . . .

Relying on its motor competence, the brain immediately recognizes the actions of others without reasoning, understanding them with no need to resort to cortical mechanisms. . . .

These discoveries of neuroscience tell us very clearly that treatments need to include motor and sensory elements, not only cognitive ones, since these dimensions are strictly interconnected. . . .

In fact, it is not enough to recognize that these systems are integrated; we also need to better understand how they are integrated. We need to understand how human beings function when they are good and healthy, what happens when they get ill, and especially what happens in the therapeutic process and how the various systems are involved when the patient gets better or recovers completely.

The first point we need to clarify is that illnesses and disorders are alterations of the functioning of all the systems, none excluded. It is also clear by now that the systems lose their complete integration because of the alterations of the various functions, which cause interruptions in their interrelations. . . .

What guides the synergy of the interventions on the various planes of the Self and in various systems is the objective that the individual needs to pursue at every step: the restoration of specific functions that were altered, became lacking, or are blocked. This can be done because each functioning is made of an organized series of functions (specific cognitive and emotional systems but also sensory-motor, neurovegetative, and endocrine apparatuses) all connected in a precise configuration in which it becomes clear what to do and what direction to take.[3]

EMPATHY

We have repeatedly talked about empathizing with the patient, specifying that the empathic attitude of the Facilitator must never become sympathy. It is therefore only right to finally go through the definitions of empathy as opposed to sympathy, the neural implications of empathy, and the clarification about what line must not be crossed if we do not want to nullify the therapeutic act by sympathizing with the patient. Moreover, let us be reminded that the empathic—and not sympathetic—relationship between patient and Facilitator is a protection for the patient to guarantee the impartiality of the therapeutic gesture in the path toward the restoration of their well-being, and it is also useful to prevent the Facilitator (as well as all therapists and caregivers) from accessing the suffering that gives way to the phenomenon called burnout, which can occur when participating too much in other people's feelings.

On the part of neuroscience, we can already anticipate that a part of the cerebral reactions involved in the empathic relationship implies the intervention of mirror neurons. However, some of the most recent research studies brought us a better definition of the cerebral areas involved in the process of empathy, allowing us to discover that they further differentiate from those that we already know are involved in the interaction with the processes activated by mirror neurons. In short, it appears that the choice of the action (gesture) that the subject is about to perform on the observed object (or situation) not only takes place through a simulation (in which the mirror neurons are involved) but also involves the decoding (through other specific neurons) of the value attributed to the object or situation the action or gesture is directed to. In practice, I understand what I need to do to carry out the action; I can also anticipate mentally what I am observing because I have internalized it before, but my action will also depend on the subjective value I attribute to the object or situation I am observing and toward which I need to perform the action (or gesture). All of this seems to occur in yet another neural process that is mainly managed by the amygdala.

Why does this concern us? Because it helps us further delineate the physiological processes involved in the behaviors and emotions of a person on a scientific level. In addition, we can use these tools to substantiate the characteristics of anomalies and dysfunctions, leading them back to specific cerebral areas and their peculiar functions.

We are now going to see how all of this is explained in an article from *MIND—Mente & Cervello*, the Italian edition of *Scientific American*:

> Unlike other mental faculties, the cerebral activity associated with empathy is not limited to one specific part of the brain but involves different areas. Not only that, the areas involved in the emotional participation in the suffering of others are differentiated from those that intervene in the occurrence of a feeling of care toward the person we empathize with. A group of neuroscientists from the University of Colorado in Boulder identified these two circuits.... Psychologists make a distinction between cognitive empathy, which is connected with the conceptual understanding of other people's mental states, and affective empathy, which is the ability to share or "simulate" internally other people's emotions. There is also empathic care, the emotion of concern toward those who are in pain, which makes us take action to alleviate their discomfort.
>
> Affective empathy and empathic care are different, because a state of empathy that is particularly strong and/or lasts for a long time might generate the desire for flight or for burnout, a psychological defense mechanism that translates to insensitive or indifferent behavior and that is quite frequent in health professionals such as physicians or nurses. Yoni K. Ashar and his colleagues studied the reactions of over 200 subjects, using functional magnetic resonance, as they were listening to real stories with a strong empathic charge.... From the results, it emerged that the empathic care system involves the cerebral areas responsible for value estimation and reward, such as the ventromedial prefrontal cortex and medial orbitofrontal cortex.
>
> In contrast, empathic suffering involves the systems that help us imagine what another person feels or thinks, especially the premotor cortex and the primary and secondary somatosensory cortexes.[4]

We are now going to examine the subject of empathy more in depth, this time from a technical-operative point of view coming from Giulia Mayer, occupational and neuromotor therapist. Let us read her honest and constructive remarks:

> Most people believe that the establishment of a healthy relationship between therapist and patient is the foundation of a successful treatment, whether it is

rehabilitative or not. In fact, the trust in the therapist motivates patients to collaborate in the rehabilitative project and encourages them to give their best and face the multiple obstacles disability inevitably entails. . . . We can lay the groundwork for a reflection on two possible ways of relating to the patients: through empathy or through sympathy. . . . A relationship based on sympathy, on "feeling together," makes the therapist participate in all the present, past, and future tribulations their patient deals with. Although a deep identification might seem the most humane way of relating, it is damaging in the long term. When the patient becomes tired and disheartened, the therapist does too. The opposite occurs as well, meaning that the therapist will bring their personal preoccupations, anxieties, and uncertainties into the therapeutic session, searching for reassurance in the patient, as if they were confidants.

It will not take long before the patient understands that the sympathetic relationship does not bring the results they were searching for. They will maybe grow fond of their therapist, but they will prefer to work with someone else, someone they are not familiar with, in order to work better. . . . Empathy allows us to feel and identify in an emotion that is not our own, but still remaining outside. . . . Empathizing consists in finding the right balance between detachment and closeness, allowing the relationship to be really therapeutic. By remaining in empathy, the therapist does not share with their patients their own anxieties and worries, especially personal ones. They try to always bring a certain level of positivity to the life of a person who is obviously going through an extremely negative period. . . . They are not easily convinced that the patient's mental state is an obstacle to the treatment. They listen to them for the right time, but try to go on. This kind of relationship can be summarized with this sentence: "I listen to you and understand you. It is very hard, but we can do it together, so . . . let's work!" . . . It is therefore the duty of all therapists, rehabilitation professionals, physicians, nurses, etc. to make an effort to remain empathic with the patients for the advantage of both.[5]

Yet another perspective on empathy is given by psychologist Daniel Goleman:

Cognitive empathy . . . means that we can understand how the other person is thinking; we see his point of view. . . . Emotional empathy . . . refers to someone who feels within herself the emotions of the person she's with. . . . This lets us feel with the other person—but not necessarily feel for, the prerequisite for compassion. . . . That requires empathic concern, the third variety of empathy. Empathic concern means we not only understand how the other person sees things and feels in the moment, but also want to help them if we sense the need.[6]

Continuing from Goleman's definition of empathic concern, Daniela Dato writes:

> [Empathic concern] naturally leads to empathic action, which, starting from our understanding of the other person, allows us to understand how to help them—not only to understand the other person and feel with them, but also to concretely help them. It is empathy that guides our forms of understanding of the world, our memory, learning, perception, and interpretation of our own emotions and those of others, allowing us to connect cognitive learning with social and systemic learning. In other words, it is about learning to orient and manage our attention.[7]

THE NUMBER 7: THE ALLEGORIC SYMBOLISM OF THE SEVEN STEPS OF TREATMENT

Everything has a meaning. Even numbers can mean something. For example, the number 7 is associated with the steps of the conclusive treatment protocol that summarizes what we have been explaining so far. It is also associated with the major chakras.

Let us review the meaning of number 7, especially as it relates to two structurally antagonistic contexts: numerology and Christian/Catholic symbolism.

> 7. Action in the world. . . . Our plant is now thriving, its actions do not just follow blind automatism; its vital energy is directed toward the world consciously. This is the moment in which the plant accepts its role in the world and accepts to act by pollinating and letting itself be pollinated.[8]

The excerpt above, from the field of evolutionary numerology, refers to an analogy between the development of numbers—in this case, 7—and that of a plant. It is taken from a wider article by Gestalt counselor Alessandro Latrofa on the numerological vision of Alejandro Jodorowsky, essayist, playwright, tarot expert, composer, poet, and film and theater director.

Jodorowsky himself wrote, "The sequence of numbers can be compared to a seed that germinates to engender a plant, which in turn will create a bud, and then a flower that will transform itself into a fruit, the perfect product of the tree that bears it. After reaching maturity the fruit will fall, thereby freeing the seed, which will enter the ground and start the entire process over again."[9]

About the specific analogy we have just described, if we look to biblical references, the correspondence that emerges spontaneously is the words of Jesus as reported in the gospels of the New Testament (John 12:24–25): "Very truly I tell you, unless a kernel of wheat falls to the ground and dies, it remains only a single seed. But if it dies, it produces many seeds. Anyone who loves their life will lose it, while anyone who hates their life in this world will keep it for eternal life."

Let us turn to the words of Sebastiano Arena, electronic engineer, philosopher, poet, and numerology expert, about number 7:

> Number 7 expresses totality, universality, and perfect balance and represents a complete dynamical cycle . . . and the whole, since it is the number of creation. Since ancient times, it was considered a magical and religious symbol of perfection, because it was connected with the moon cycles. Not being produced by any number between 1 and 10, it was considered uncreated and identified with the identical value of the monad. . . . The Babylonians considered any day of the month that is a multiple of 7 to be a festival. This number was considered a symbol for holiness by Pythagoreans. It was called venerable by the ancient Greeks and "anima mundi" by Plato. It also symbolized life in some ancient cultures. Number 7 represents the achievement of perfection accomplished by human nature in its internal union of divine ternary and earthly quaternary. Since it is made of the union of triad and tetrad, number 7 indicates the wholeness of perfection, participating in the double nature of physicality and spirituality, human and divine. It is the invisible center, spirit, and soul of all things. Seven is the number of the pyramid, for it is formed by a triangle (3) and a square (4). Therefore, it is the privileged expression of mediation between human and divine.[10]

Gianfranco Ravasi, Catholic archbishop, biblicist, theologian, and Hebraist, wrote the following on numerology and number 7:

> Even those who are not familiar with the Scripture know that it is scattered with numbers that often do not have to be considered quantitatively, but qualitatively, which means as symbols. . . . Things get more complicated in the following phase of Judaism, with the appearance of a particular numerology called "gematry," a term that is the deformation of the word "geometry." Its objective was to find the hidden and secret meaning of words based on the numerical correspondences of letters. This exercise will become the foundation of the so-called "Qabbalah" (literally "transmitted reality," "tradition"), a mystical Judaic theory that started thriving in the twelfth century and has left its trace in various modern esoteric movements and popular contemporary forms. . . . Behind all the biblical numerology there is always the conviction that the Lord—as we can read in the Book of Wisdom in what is maybe a mention to a sentence by Plato—has "arranged all things by measure and number and weight." . . . Therefore, the fact that in Genesis

the creation of the universe is distributed in the seven days of the week, with its apex in liturgical Saturday, is connected to the fact that seven and its multiples are a symbol for wholeness and perfection.[11]

To conclude this brief analysis, we offer number 7 as described in the Book of Changes, best known as I Ching or Zhou Yi, one of the first classic texts of Chinese culture, written more than 2,000 years ago. The contents of the I Ching were examined also by Carl Jung, whose studies went beyond the common (and often superficial) interpretations that saw it only as a means of consultation with divinatory purposes. Without denying the divinatory character of the text, Jung found connections with psychological interpretative properties, updating its reading through a psychoanalytic approach focused on modification of behavioral peculiarities in the individual.

The divinatory answers of the I Ching make constant reference to the way the Noble One (the consulter) proceeds on the journey of life, facing its occurrences. The Noble Ones are in fact defined as those who objectively accept what happens outside; they fortify themselves from the inside and then start to move toward their objectives consciously, every day, step by step, in order to give shape to their personality in the direction of a new life.

The I Ching is divided in two sections, with the second one providing commentary on the first. It offers sixty-four hexagrams, each made of six lines that are either unbroken (yang) segments or broken (yin) segments. In the first section of the text, each hexagram represents a unit and corresponds to a situation; the second section provides development of the interpretations. Some segments of the hexagram (the muting lines) have the characteristics of being opposable and therefore able to transform their yang quality into its opposite yin quality, changing the character of the hexagram itself and manifesting the transformative potential (corresponding to the mutation) in relation to each situation or event.

As noted earlier in this chapter, by studying the mechanism of consultation, Jung coined the concept of synchronicity (a causal and a temporal connection of one or more significant events). The correspondence of the extraction of the hexagram with the questioned situation, both deemed to be in psychic communication with the personal and collective unconscious, allows the association of the extracted hexagram to the relative question and the issues it poses. According to Jung, the idea of associating to numbers the basic principle to obtain a hexagram derives from Chinese philosophy, which sees numbers as qualitative factors not quantitative ones.

Just to answer curiosity and without any reference to the consultation of the Book of Changes, you will find below (fig. 25.2) the hexagrams corresponding to number 7 and its transformative possibilities.

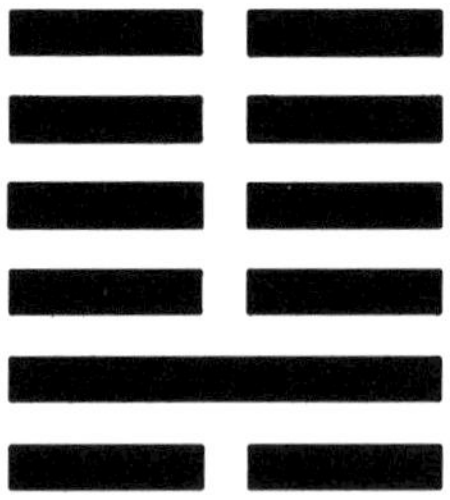

☷
☵

Fig. 25.2. Hexagram of 7 from the Book of Changes

We refer now to the interpretation of this hexagram provided by the blog *Cieloevento*:

> The 7—the Army is another hexagram that explicitly refers to Water. . . . The image represents water flowing underground before emerging from a spring. This is the appearance. However, under the surface there is actually an impetuous river that would crush anything on its way if it came up from underwater. This metaphor represents the military strength implied in farmers even in times of peace; when everything was going fine, they cultivated the field, but in times of war they were called by the emperor and lay down their hoes to become soldiers.[12]

The second line of the hexagram (from the bottom upward) is the muting line that transforms it. It is the line of the Noble One, which stays in the middle of the army. From here, the Noble One incarnates the general that will lead the army to the victory. The transformed hexagram corresponds to number 2. *Cielovento* explains:

> The 2—Receptive is the hexagram that represents the pure Yin principle and the feminine. It is therefore a sign that means we do not have to stay still but rather must understand which way to go, because it is uncertain (all lines are broken). The qualities of the Receptive must be exploited to search inside ourselves for the right way, because only the synchronic action [natural manifestation of the final change] that is spontaneous [meaning it complies to the law of attraction]—is the way of the Tao.[13]

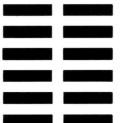

Fig. 25.3. Hexagram of 2 from the Book of Changes

STRUCTURAL PHASES OF THE 7-STEP TREATMENT

Thanks to life, which has given me so much.
It gave me laughter and it gave me tears
So I can distinguish happiness from sadness,
The two materials of my song,
And your song, too, which is the same song,
And everyone's song, which is my very own.
Thanks to life, which has given me so much

VIOLETA PARRA

The techniques we are going to examine now through the sequential development of the treatment protocol synthesize everything that we have analyzed in the previous chapters. They are addressed specifically to Facilitators who need to treat a person in a situation of transition and passage between two different phases of the person's Life Cycle, especially when the passage occurs as a consequence to traumatic factors that are connected with loss, abandonment, separation, bereavement, or even the final transition itself.

As it is proposed, the complete treatment is preparatory to the facilitation of the transformative experience of each person. Even this experience—which might be connected with the situations mentioned above—is often necessary and inevitable for many of us in some crucial phases of our life.

To begin, the protocol requires understanding of all the elements that originated the process. It also requires awareness that the therapeutic and facilitative gesture fulfills its objectives for each element involved through the peculiarities of the CST and SER Facilitator's aptonomic touch.

As noted earlier:

Main objective: to facilitate the homeostasis of the organism in order to induce a greater relaxation in each physical structure involved in the passage from one phase of the Life Cycle to the next.

Technique: Over the course of the seven steps, we will use all the techniques outlined in this book.

Hand placement: If palpation is not possible, rely on the Direction of Energy through the intention at a close distance from the patient's body.

Step 1: Alignment of the Vector/Axis System

When starting the treatment protocol, the first step is to evaluate the patient's energetic framework through the vector/axis system.

The treatment starts from the feet station, placing the hands on each of the patient's insteps or soles. From this position, you are able to start to map the vector/axis system through the landmarks of the major and secondary chakras.

Then proceed to realign the entire vector/axis system, visualizing and assessing it in the Third Space (thought-form) and using all the movements that are necessary to bring the vectors back to their correct position in relation to their axis.

At this stage, you are connected with the following:

- central nervous system
- limbic system
- the three brains (reptilian, mammalian, and neocortex)

MAIN REFERENCES TO THE TOPICS IN THE BOOK

Topic	Chapter(s)
Energetic framework, vector/axis system, vectors	15, 16
Polarity, directional pole	10, 12
Chakras	15, 16
Corpus callosum, cerebral hemispheres	11, 21
Central nervous system	11, 17
Three brains, limbic system	6, 9, 17
Third Space	23

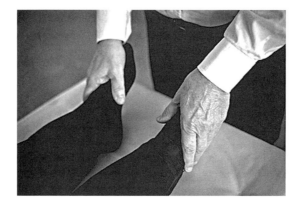

Fig. 25.4. Alignment of the vector/axis system

A Seven-Step Treatment for the Dying Process

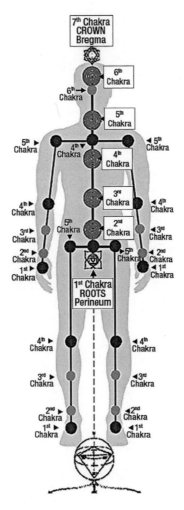

Fig. 25.5. Vector/axis system with polarity and chakras

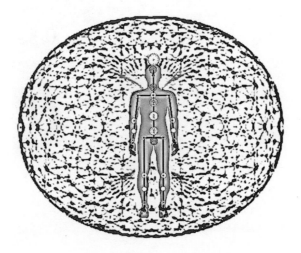

Fig. 25.6. Third Space thought-form

Step 2: Fascial Release of Intracranial Structures

As described in the first level of CranioSacral Therapy practice, you can use one of the three cranial vault holds to perceive the anomalous tensions in the intracranial membranes.

MAIN REFERENCES TO THE TOPICS IN THE BOOK

Topic	Chapter(s)
Cranial vault holds, release of intracranial structures	11, 21
Intracranial membranes, fascia (fascial release)	4, 10
Central nervous system	11, 17

To begin, place your hands on the cranial vault and focus with the intention on the three intracranial membranes:

- dura mater
- arachnoid mater
- pia mater

Following the direction of the barrier, maintain your hand placement until you perceive the release of the membranes. In this way, you remove reciprocal tension and improve the functionality of the entire central nervous system.

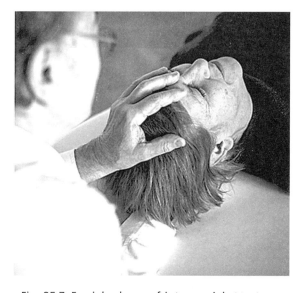

Fig. 25.7. Fascial release of intracranial structures

A Seven-Step Treatment for the Dying Process

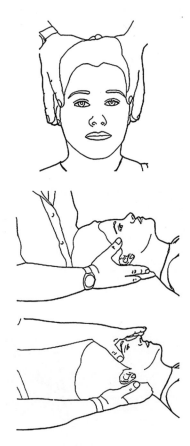

Fig. 25.8. The three cranial vault holds

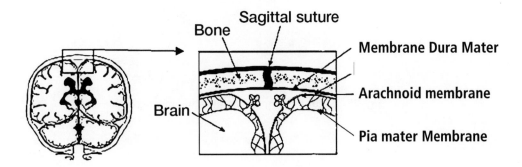

Fig. 25.9. Meninges: dura mater, arachnoid mater, pia mater

Step 3: Connection with the Cerebral Hemispheres

Maintaining the cranial vault hold that you implemented in step 2, or using one of the two other holds (whichever is the most adequate), you will now connect with the two cerebral hemispheres and the central nervous system.

Remaining connected with the Higher Self, use the technique of the Direction of Energy to support the path chosen by the entire system, thus facilitating its passage from one phase to the next.

MAIN REFERENCES TO THE TOPICS IN THE BOOK

Topic	Chapter(s)
Cranial vault holds	11, 21
Cerebral hemispheres	11, 21
Central nervous system	11, 17
Direction of Energy	11, 17

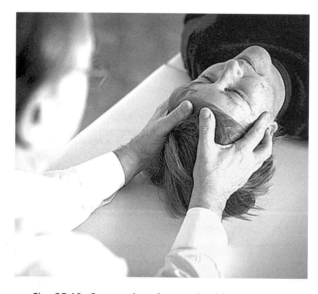

Fig. 25.10. Connecting the cerebral hemispheres

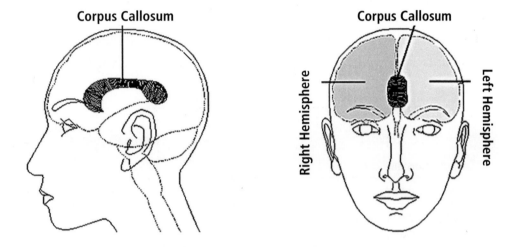
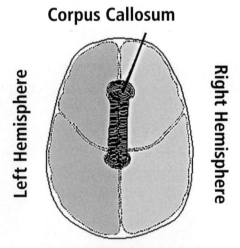

Fig. 25.11. Corpus callosum and cerebral hemispheres

Step 4: Connection with the Corpus Callosum and the RAS

Maintaining your cranial vault hold (or whichever vault hold is most adequate), connect the two cerebral hemispheres through the corpus callosum, transmitting information between the two hemispheres and, at the same time, between the anterior and posterior parts of each hemisphere. In the meantime, maintain the directionality of the vector/axis system.

The corpus callosum allows us to control fear and calm the RAS when it is overexcited, thus facilitating the passage from one phase to the next of the Life Cycle.

MAIN REFERENCES TO THE TOPICS IN THE BOOK

Topic	Chapter(s)
Corpus callosum	11, 21
Vector/axis system	15, 16
Reticular activating/alarm system, reticular formation	6, 11, 17
Life Cycle	2

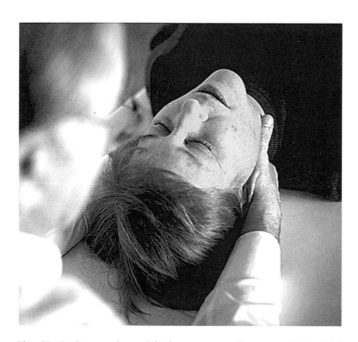

Fig. 25.12. Connection with the corpus callosum and the RAS

A Seven-Step Treatment for the Dying Process 443

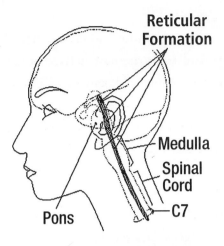

Fig. 25.13. Reticular formation

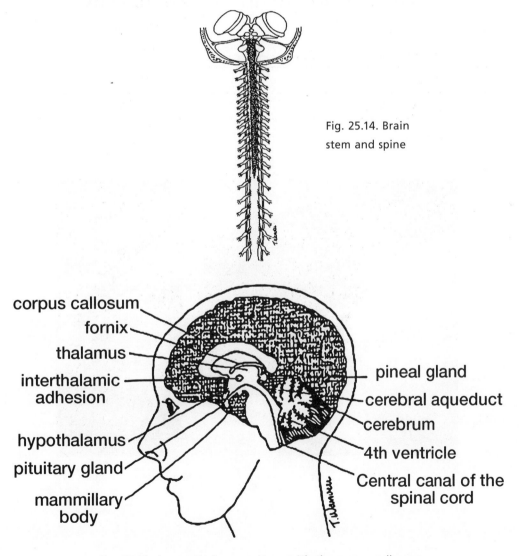

Fig. 25.14. Brain stem and spine

Fig. 25.15. Anatomical connections with the corpus callosum

Step 5: Heart and Pericardium Meridians

To remove energy blockages of the heart and pericardium meridians, use the emptying/filling technique to empty the organism from the destructive energy it withholds (which is probably caused by an Energy Cyst) and fill the meridians with constructive (syntropic) energy.

When treating the heart meridian, try to infuse a sense of love and soothe the fear of losing loved ones. After treating the heart meridian, you may similarly treat the pericardium meridian to soothe the fatigue of the heart.

Afterward, if the position of the patient allows it, you may employ the thoracic inlet technique to improve the entire heart-to-heart venous and arterial blood circulation (as described in the ten-step protocol of Upledger's CS1 techniques).

MAIN REFERENCES TO THE TOPICS IN THE BOOK

Topic	Chapter(s)
Meridians, heart, pericardium	10, 13
Thoracic inlet	21
Energy Cysts	1, 4, 18

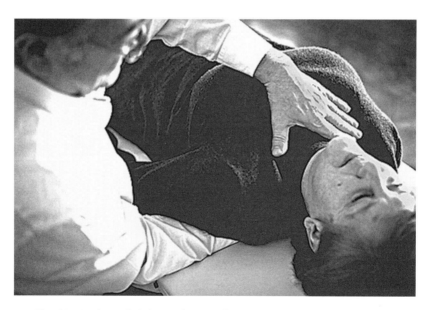

Fig. 25.16. Thoracic inlet technique for pericardium/heart meridians

A Seven-Step Treatment for the Dying Process 445

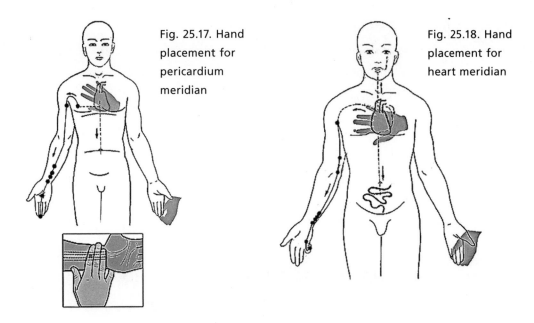

Fig. 25.17. Hand placement for pericardium meridian

Fig. 25.18. Hand placement for heart meridian

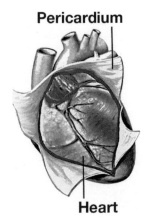

Fig. 25.19. Pericardium and heart (cross-sectional view)

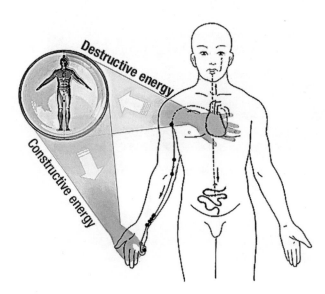

Fig. 25.20. Emptying and filling: transforming destructive energy into constructive energy

Step 6: Respiratory Diaphragm and Vagus Nerve

Release the respiratory diaphragm through the respiratory diaphragm technique. This soothes the fascial tension that inhibits the functionality of the pericardium and the vagus nerve. The vagus nerve allows all the viscera (including lungs, heart, pericardium, etc.) to be sufficiently functional.

If the patient's position or the circumstances do not allow it (e.g., if the patient is hypersensitive due to physical pain or if medical monitoring constitutes an obstacle), use the third chakra technique with Direction of Energy, keeping one hand at a close distance from the solar plexus. In addition, you can work on the liver meridian (one hand on the organ, the other on the distal point).

MAIN REFERENCES TO THE TOPICS IN THE BOOK

Topic	Chapter(s)
Respiratory diaphragm	21
Pericardium, lungs, heart	13
Vagus nerve, vagus system	17, 20
Chakras	15, 16

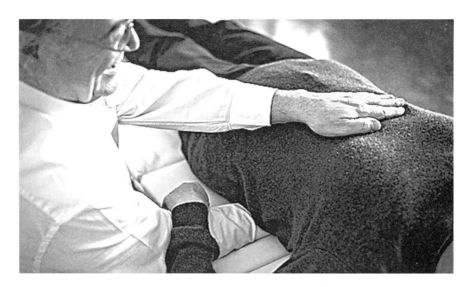

Fig. 25.21. Vagus nerve and respiratory diaphragm release

A Seven-Step Treatment for the Dying Process 447

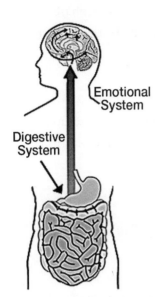

Fig. 25.22. Connection of the emotional system to the digestive system

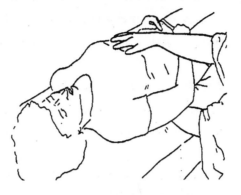

Fig. 25.23. Hand placement for the respiratory diaphragm release

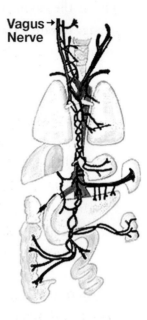

Fig. 25.24. Vagus nerve

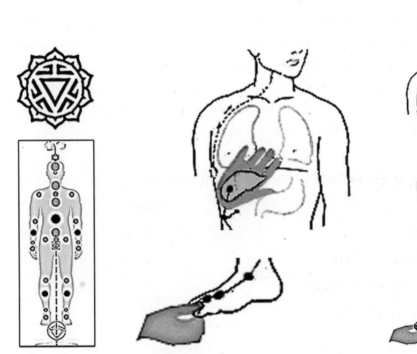

Fig. 25.25. Third chakra and liver meridian (map and technique)

Step 7: The Seventh Chakra and the Mind-Body-Spirit Continuum

This is the culmination of the treatment, when you work to facilitate the phase of passage toward a transformative or final experience of the Life Cycle. In the request you make to the universe for the patient's sake, focus on the following:

- opening every cell to the cosmic energy received by the center
- letting the center convey all information and induce the structure to relaxation
- connecting this cosmic energy from the center through the heart and to sacrum
- stabilizing the RAS
- harmonizing the direction of the vectors between Earth and sky
- letting the pons be free from any obstacle
- allowing the spirit to accept the answer of the universe (Higher Self) or allowing it to leave the body, if it wishes to do so

All this must be done with respect for the individual's free will and through connection with the Higher Self.

Place one hand on the bregma or about four inches from it. Energetically connect the body with the channel for cosmic energy, and let the latter come in. Then connect with the pineal gland and the center, thus enhancing the energy flow that enters (syntropic energy) and leaves (entropic energy) the organism.

Connecting with the seventh chakra (crown chakra), use the technique of energetic reharmonization and make use of the systemic model of energetic-therapeutic vibrations to reassess the organism and perceive whether there still are dissonances. Then, by sending the correct vibration, proceed to release, facilitate, and support the energy flow to enhance the mind-body-spirit continuum in relation to the universal energy, depending on the instructions of the Higher Self.

MAIN REFERENCES TO THE TOPICS IN THE BOOK

Topic	Chapter(s)
Chakras	15, 16
Anatomical structures	16, 17, 20
Mind-body-spirit continuum	24
Therapeutic vibrations	22

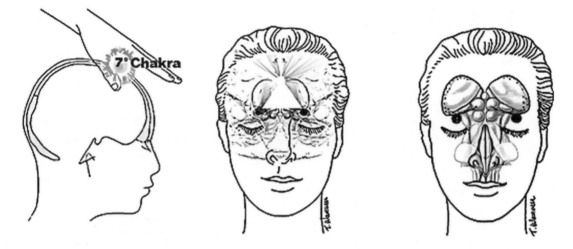

Fig. 25.26. Seventh chakra, center, and pons

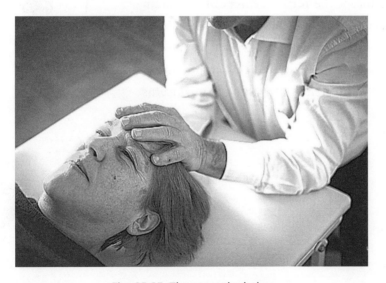

Fig. 25.27. The seventh chakra

The main structures involved in this phase are the following:

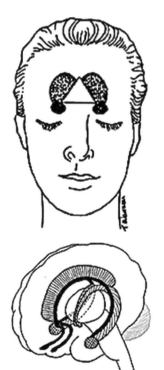

Center: Receives the spiritual energy of the universe through the crown (seventh) chakra and sends it into the areas of the organism that need it.

Pons: Connects the higher centers of the brain with the entire body. When our physical body ceases to exist, our spirit is free to float upward through the pons. It also perceives cosmic information and is involved in everything that concerns vital choices.

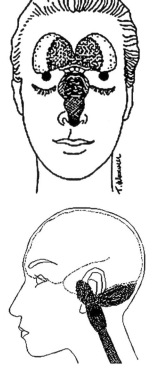

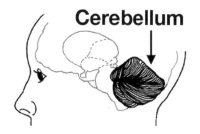

Cerebellum: Can stop the heart and breathing through the vagus system when it perceives that it is the proper time to die.

Reticular formation: All inputs to and outputs from the brain pass through here.

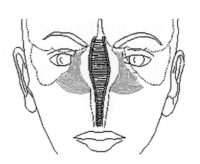

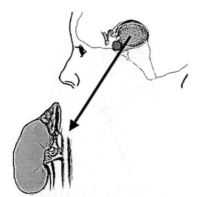

Reticular activating/alarm system (RAS): Responds to stimuli connected with fear; influences all the other anatomical and emotional systems of the human body.

Amygdala: Holds the memory and fear of what occurs in situations of survival.

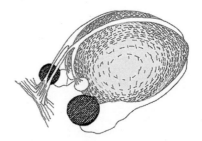

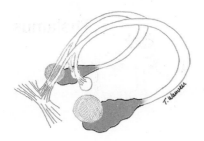

Hippocampus: Plays a fundamental role in recent memory and the emotion of fear; holds the emotional memory of olfactory events, especially those connected with fear. A dysfunction here can be a main cause for anxiety in the overall system.

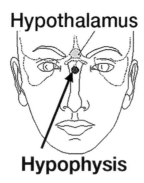

Hypophysis (pituitary gland): Interprets the cosmic symbols received from the universe through the pineal gland and translates them into concrete action.

Pineal gland: Orchestrates the integration of the body with the mind and the spirit. Serves as a mediator between individual consciousness and the universe.

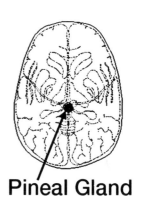

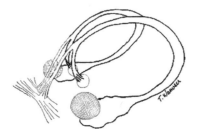

Fornix: Connects the cerebral hemispheres and constitutes the main seat of trust.

Thalamus: Selects the sensory impulses that are transmitted to the brain, especially emotional ones. Functions in long-term memory and stimulates us to reflect on the first memory of our existence.

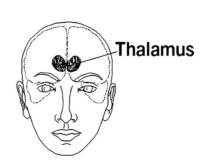

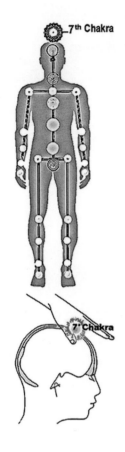

Seventh (crown) chakra: The seat of enlightenment in which the individual "I" unites with the cosmic universal "I," the channel of the Higher Self. Determines the mystical experiences of peace and blessing. It is the main conductor of divine energy from the cosmos to the human spiritual universe.

✷ ✷ ✷

The seven-step treatment for the passage from a known phase of the Life Cycle—which is ending—to a new unknown phase in the universal energy continuum is a further tool that can enrich your knowledge, abilities, and therapeutic skills. You can use it consciously anytime life allows you to do so.

> *It would be possible to describe everything scientifically, but it would make no sense; it would be without meaning, as if you described a Beethoven symphony as a variation of wave pressure.*
> ALBERT EINSTEIN

> *This coverage of the finished product is far from inclusive of all we know or don't know about brains and how they work. But it should give you a background and a feel for things so that you have a better chance of keeping abreast of some of the advances in neuroscience and how they can affect you and your loved ones and/or your patients and clients.*
> DR. JOHN E. UPLEDGER

> **Personal Growth Exercise:
> Understanding the Mind-Body-Spirit Continuum**

In light of the information you have received and based on your own experience up until now, we invite you to answer a few brief questions.

How do you imagine your intervention through CST in support of someone who is dying?

_____
_____
_____
_____
_____

If you have already had this experience, what do you remember about it?

_____
_____
_____
_____
_____

What were your difficulties?

_____
_____
_____
_____
_____

What do you feel has changed in your perception after reading this book?

_____

_____

_____

_____

What do you think now of the cyclus vitae (life in its cycle of birth and death)?

_____

_____

_____

_____

Clinical Observations

More than thirty years ago, a friend of mine, who at the time lived with me in Liverpool and was a member of the cycling club I frequented, asked me to make an assessment of his mother, who had been manifesting the signs of unusual chronic fatigue and eyestrain for a long time.

When I went to visit her, his mother immediately reassured me that there was nothing to worry about and that her "discomforts" were just connected to her old age. I asked her whether she wanted to tell me something about the traumatic events of her life or any other thing she deemed to be useful as a clue to her current state. She started talking but did not say anything particular, or at least anything that could be connected with her symptoms.

She accepted treatment anyway, though I believe that she did so only to please her son and not because she really thought she needed it.

At this first session, I treated her with just some relaxation techniques to reestablish an optimal craniosacral rhythm and to enhance her blood circulation and oxygenation. After the session, she was grateful and told me she already felt reinvigorated. I treated her two more times in the following weeks.

Her well-being, however, was sadly not destined to last for long. Two days after the last session, her son called to tell me that just a few hours after each treatment, even though she said she was satisfied with the treatments and complimented my skills, the fatigue came back.

Something was not clear. And yet every time I treated her, she smiled and said she was feeling better.

I decided to tell her son to consult with a physician who could give her a diagnosis for her symptoms and/or carry out some clinical tests. We soon found out that the woman had a brain cancer.

When I saw her again, she told me she had been expecting that news, but she did not want to cause her to son worry. She decided not to undergo any conventional therapy and convinced her son to accept her wish. He was desperate but came to terms with her decision and asked me to go on with the treatments once a week.

It was my first time witnessing a person's final phase of life.

She soon developed ptosis, the drooping of the upper eyelids. I tried to take care of her as much as my knowledge and abilities allowed me to, but I was wondering more and more often what my role actually was in this scenario, which could lead to nothing but death.

Both the patient and her son were always so grateful for what I was doing that I wanted to continue. Now I know that I was not yet aware of what life was offering to me through that experience.

One day, when I went to her house for the usual treatment, the woman told me she wanted to leave her earthly life because she felt she could not deal with the agony she was going through anymore and could not stand her son's suffering. I started treating the seventh chakra, though at this point that decision was based simply on intuition, since at that time I was not conscious of why I was doing it. Furthermore, I did not have a great knowledge of the various parts of the brain and their functions. I only knew that the seventh chakra was connected with the Divine. In retrospect, I realize I needed that connection as well in that moment.

I remember I thought that if the spirit had to get out of the body, it would certainly do it through that chakra. At the end of the treatment, before I left, the woman gave me a hint of a grateful smile.

The next day, her son called me to tell me that his mother had died quietly in her sleep, apparently without suffering, and that her expression was the most relaxed he had seen on her face over those last days. He thanked me again for taking care of her.

In fact, his voice sounded serene. When I asked him how he was feeling, he answered that he was extremely relieved because his mother had finally stopped suffering, and especially because she had not been in pain when she died.

During the first years after I came back to Italy, I was on the best of terms with a colleague of mine and all of her family. When this Facilitator's mother was diagnosed with cancer, their choice was between allopathic medicine (considered invasive by all the family members and my colleague's mother in particular) and all the possible alternative treatments, including CranioSacral Therapy. Because of the mutual affection and trust I shared with the entire family, I was asked to give my opinion as well.

My colleague's mother came to her own decision about how to deal with her disease, and her decision was not to be treated with allopathic medicine but to resort to alternative care through various methods of treatment, including CranioSacral Therapy. She said her trust in allopathic medicine had always been inversely proportional to the trust she had in its alternatives.

Therefore, her daughter and I started treating her with CST, homeopathy, and naturopathy, and she also started a macrobiotic diet.

We initially took care of her together through multi-hands treatments. Later, because of my work schedule—which caused me to go out of town very often—she was treated mainly by my colleague, while I took part in the treatments when I could. Nonetheless, we kept in contact every day to discuss all the results.

We had not established an actual protocol, but since my colleague was an expert therapist—and especially since I knew her mother well—there was no need to do that. It was more important to communicate and give each other mutual support in the therapy.

We focused partly on the daily assessments and partly on the sensations my colleague's mother reported having (she was a very sensitive woman, good at listening to her body), but we worked almost always on the intracranial fascial system and the diaphragms of the body, the relevant chakras and meridians to reinforce the organs, and the central nervous system. I almost exclusively took care of the emotional side of the work because my colleague was too directly involved to carry out that part of the treatment.

At the time, I could not know that the treatments on my colleague's mother were the beginning of what would later become—through my other experiences with terminal patients—the seven-step treatment protocol.

As time went by, my colleague and I realized that her mother was slowly fading away. There was no healing to be done.

Nonetheless, I must say that thanks to CST, her daughter's unconditional love, and the support of all her family members, my colleague's mother lived that period of her life without suffering physical pain, without having to resort to morphine, and without losing her hair, throwing up, or having blue skin and lips because of chemotherapy.

She passed away gradually and with great dignity, like she deserved. In the very last period of her life she started communicating verbally less and less. I remember that after some months, during which she barely spoke at all, I received a phone call from her. She wanted to ask me how I was doing. On that occasion, I was the one who was speechless because of the surprise and the joy. After that call, she went back to her silence.

But there was still something we could do.

It might sound like nonsense, but in connecting with her mother's Higher Self during the last treatment, I clearly perceived that there was something holding her back, making her live beyond her physical strength. When I asked her Higher Self for an explanation, since I could not communicate verbally with her anymore, it was clear that she could not die serenely in the presence of her loving daughter who was taking care of her. Out of love, she was not able to leave the image in her mind of her daughter's eyes in the instant in which the last transition would occur.

> Therefore, my colleague had to leave the house where she was living with her dying mother. Despite my colleague's resistance, we decided to bring her to my next seminar as an assistant. She joined me in Milan, and it was there that she received the phone call announcing the death of her mother, who had peacefully left her earthly life.

⚜ A CST-CENTERED VISION ⚜

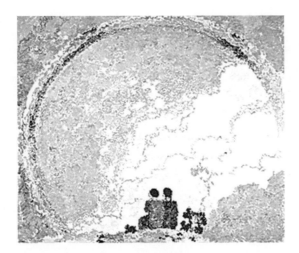

Fig. 25.28. *Rainbow,* by Augusto Giacometti

Swiss painter Augusto Giacometti, who lived in the nineteenth and twentieth centuries, was initially inspired by art nouveau and later strongly influenced by the paintings of Fra Angelico before being drawn to abstract art and taking part in the Dada movement.

In his painting *Rainbow* (fig. 25.28), in the circle that seems to accept and support the pictorial space, the seven colors of the rainbow are delineated like the seven steps of the treatment protocol for the vital energy continuum of the Life Cycle. The two figures sit in a golden space, between Earth and sky, as they contemplate the colors and the shape of the rainbow, which suggests a perfect circle. It looks as if they are contemplating the "becoming."

CHAPTER 26

Ode to Life

Open-System Human Being

Love life, and love it even if it does not give you what it might, love it even if it is not the way you want it to be,
love it when you are born and every time you are about to die.
Never love without love, never live without life.

ANJEZË GONXHE BOJAXHIU
(MOTHER TERESA OF CALCUTTA)

Be the change you want to see in the world.

MOHANDAS KARAMCHAND GANDHI
(MAHATMA GANDHI)

All the techniques described in this book have been structured to reflect the specific sensitivities and attitudes of CST and SER Facilitators in order to encourage and enhance the training of the correct attitude implemented by all Facilitators and to present it to nonpracticing readers.

The constant training of a systemic perspective on existential subjects connected with experiences of separation, abandonment, loss, and bereavement must always be carried out with the awareness of all the structures and functions involved in the treatment, which are all useful to support the patient in:

- activation of all the self-balancing mechanisms of the organism
- facilitation of the transformation
- achievement of mind-body/psyche-soma (conscious/non-conscious) unity

All the elements we share in this text bring us back to the fundamental existential attitude a Facilitator must aim for: *a sincere, authentic gratitude to life.*

TELEONOMY IN CRANIOSACRAL THERAPY AND SOMATOEMOTIONAL RELEASE

We feel good because we believe that we are all born with the natural gift to help each other heal. . . . We would like you to use this innate ability.

DR. JOHN E. UPLEDGER

For a CST and SER Facilitator, it is not hard to perceive, experience, and prove gratitude. And gratitude is nothing but the perceived, experienced, and felt expression of joy. To support, help, and assist the various phases of the Open-System Human Being—which takes back its own innate self-healing ability day by day, upholding regularly the process of finalistic organization of the structures of its own organism (teleonomy)—cannot but produce joy.

The aim of the Facilitator is for such perception to be similarly experienced by people who receive the treatment.

Why teleonomy and not teleology? The purpose is the same: the process of development of a structure tending (either consciously or unconsciously) toward an action that (in a more or less immediately obvious fashion) supports the innate predisposition toward prosperity and vitality or that orients an organism toward an adequate position to protect life and well-being.

However, the ideological and conceptual premises of the two paths are different. Teleonomy is more focused on the strictly biological aspect of development finalized for the conservation of the species, whereas teleology puts first the aspect of biological development that in nature pursues a transcendent project.

This conceptual difference has been investigated and reported on in a great volume of literature, and there is still a very intense debate on the matter between philosophers, scientists, pedagogues, biologists, et cetera. In order to understand it better, let us review the definitions of both terms and the analysis of a Nobel Prize winner, also known as the father of scientific ethology, Konrad Zacharias Lorenz.

Teleonomy

Teleonomy: Finalistic organization of the structures of living organisms (from the Greek word τέλος, *télos*, "aim, purpose," and the suffix *-nomia*, "government, orderly administration").

In biology, teleonomy was first mentioned in 1970 by biologist Jacques Monod in his theory that considered the existence of a finalistic action inside the structure of living beings caused by natural selection and directed to the enhancement of vital functions and elimination of any other function that could be an obstacle—a natural selection privileging structures and functions meant to preserve the species by removing those that are not adequate.

Teleology

Teleology: Philosophic doctrine of finalism (from the Greek word τέλος, *télos*, "aim, purpose," and λόγος, *logos*, "discourse, thought") that conceives the existence of the finality of life not only in the common voluntary human activity meant to achieve an objective but also in the actions that are involuntary and unconscious and nonetheless accomplish an objective.

Teleology is any philosophical conception that sees the entire universe as organized according to a purpose, whether it depends on a divine or providential will or is immanent in nature as an active principle moving the entirety of becoming.

Gratitude to Life

Let us now rely on the words of Konrad Lorenz and the joy that transpires from being able to observe the action of nature (including, of course, human nature) and to participate in it. Though Lorenz, always a scientist, was completely aware of the destructive phenomena of nature, including those caused by human actions, he never stopped expressing his gratitude to life and giving his contribution to improve the collective future with his knowledge.

After all, is not unconditional love a conscious act of love made in the full awareness of both the qualities and flaws of the other person?

The following paragraphs come from Lorenz's book *The Waning of Humaneness*, the title of which is coherent with some of the topics it treats but might be deceiving in respect to the multiple constructive propositions that can be found in it. In the book, Lorenz dedicates much space to teleonomy but does not overlook the spiritual approach to life. He writes:

> Many people believe that the course of universal history follows a pre-established path directed toward a precise destination. In fact, the evolution of organic creation takes place in unpredictable ways. Both our faith in the possibility of a creative evolution and our faith in freedom and human "responsibility" are based on the awareness of this fact. . . . It is necessary to prove convincingly that the subjective processes of our internal experience hold the same degree of reality as anything that can be expressed with the terminology of natural sciences. . . . Today the "eternal active force that beneficially creates" mentioned by Goethe can act only in one way, through human sensitivity to certain values. . . . Human history has been undoubtedly influenced by human knowledge, . . . even the history of other living species in general is influenced in a decisive way by the acquisition of information.

. . . Even the smallest modification that is useful for the adaptation of a species to the environment it lives in changes the following phylogenetics irreversibly. . . . The distinction between teleonomy and teleology is explained through the distinction of the teleonomic question, "What type of adequateness to the purposes guarantees the conservation of the species?" as opposed to the teleological question, which investigates the meaning of existence itself. . . . Perception is an "activity" since any form of cognition is also an action, like every other explorative behavior, . . . and scientific behaviors in the human being develop both phylogenetically and ontogenetically from explorative or curious behaviors. Therefore, science in its essence is strictly connected with art, just as much as curious behaviors are strictly connected with playing. These activities are a condition that is essential for their functioning; they both need . . . a great "extension of scope." . . . In fact, a scientist does not need a strictly defined objective, just like life forms in phylogenetics. . . . Borrowing the meaning Pietschmann gave to these terms, those who are convinced that the theory of natural evolution is both "exact" and "true" will never be able to share the epistemological point of view of scientists or that of their critics, and will probably remain convinced that our ability to perceive forms is indispensable for the scientific study of nature. Nonetheless, they realize that with the perception of forms, the scientific work is only at its start since it is necessary to prove the "exactness" of this "true" perception. . . . This means that scientism and its opposite are inverse mistakes. . . . The analytical scholars criticized by Pietschmann and Chargaff are often evidently lacking the ability to "see" the connections inside complex and integrated systems. Goethe, on the contrary, was the exact opposite, and it was not by chance that he criticized analytical reasoning and its outcomes. . . . An almost infinite number of things are absolutely natural and yet escape the understanding of our brain. . . . Anyway, on an emotional level, and especially in evaluative sensations, there are common elements, emotions that all normal individuals feel in response to a certain external situation. . . . The qualities of our experiences cannot be defined, but we are able to express what is not describable. At least artists can. Musicians do not even need to pronounce any word since they create sounds that speak directly to their audience's hearts. However, the indescribable can be expressed even with words, as proved by poetry. . . . No one could deny that between these processes that take place inside the body and our external form there is a tight connection, and . . . this issue corresponds to that of the relationship between soul and body. . . .

More importantly, the love for everything that is alive can awaken the sense of solidarity of human beings. . . . The love for all living things is an indispensable feeling . . . and there are implicit values in the universe that require respect and can almost endlessly produce higher values. . . . It seems almost impossible to make esoteric symbolists understand that the effort to understand the world in the most complete way possible, in all its earthliness, does not imply a renunciation to all forms of transcendent reality.... From a geological point of view, we have "just come out" from the stage of anthropomorphous apes, therefore I know what dangers there were for the human spirit in such a quick development and that many of these dangers are the univocal consequence of diseases that are theoretically curable.... A closed system with predictable processes would be terrible, but it is by definition a non-living system, therefore it does not exist. It was not biology that set us free from the terrible idea of a closed system, but it was modern physics. To grasp what is the relationship between human freedom and the unpredictability of universal occurrences is a task that exceeds the faculties of human reasoning.... If the claim that man was created in the image and likeness of God holds any truth, this makes reference to the creative activity of man.[1]

SYSTEMIC PERSPECTIVE

Science tells us what we can know, but what we can know is little, and if we forget how much we cannot know we become insensitive to many things of very great importance.

BERTRAND RUSSELL

A premise: systemic perspective = holistic vision of the human being = prevention = well-being.

A holistic vision implies the understanding of things, being aware and conscious of them, being able to insert them in a context, and establishing the nature of the relationships that exist between them.

The holistic vision of the individual is the natural expression of the authenticity that characterizes any personal experience.

For the Facilitator, this perspective cannot and must not remain a meaningless theory to apply only during treatments. The authenticity of this view is the real intention that comes from the Facilitator's hands; it is life energy offering itself as a sincere support to the well-being of another person during the dialogue between Higher Selves.

Dr. Upledger, describing "the whole," had this to say:

By the whole, I mean our consciousness, our behaviors and our responses. When I say consciousness, I mean all levels of consciousness. There are several levels of consciousness of which we are aware, and there are many, many levels of consciousness of which we are unaware. At the present time, we are just beginning to scratch the surface of a true understanding of consciousness at any of its levels. There have been many theories of consciousness which have turned out to be invalid. The problem is so difficult to research, partially because we have to use our own consciousness to research consciousness . . .[2]

Dr. Upledger also noted:

Whether the image and the cellular consciousness that it implies are valid or not matters very little to me. What does matter is that, for whatever reason, the patient is much better and happier now.[3]

CST AND SER ARE ALWAYS AN ODE TO LIFE

People who say it cannot be done should not interrupt those who are doing it.

ADAPTED FROM
PUCK MAGAZINE, 1902

The sense of the vital energy continuum in our existence and experience merges with sensations of strength, stability, awareness, empowerment, well-being, and joy.

Gratitude to life is the feeling constituted by our perception and awareness of the vital energy continuum. It is our joy in being alive.

From their first moment of life, from the encounter of ovum and sperm, human beings go through passages from one phase to the next, transforming their limits and following their self-organization and self-transcendence, two innate abilities of the Open-System Human Being.

The body is a unit. In the relationship between Facilitator and patient, in the dialogue between Higher Selves, all Facilitators following Dr. Upledger's simple and clear instructions are able to:

- facilitate the activation of the natural self-correcting mechanism in another person's organism
- support the organism in the way and to the extent it feels appropriate
- listen to the inner wisdom of the patient's Higher Self and comply with it
- communicate with every structure, function, system, and cell
- support other human beings in any situation, condition, or phase (even in the very last phase of passage) of their Life Cycle

Let us quickly review the subjects of this text:

- We have gone through some of the phases of our Life Cycle together.
- We have revisited our own scenarios of separation/loss/abandonment/bereavement.
- We have been in contact with the destructive energy connected with these scenarios.
- We have learned to identify our potential and transform it into constructive energy that can be useful in our lives, assessing any possibility and opportunity that loss might offer.
- We have refined our attitude in the listening/perception of therapeutic energy to be able to help people who are living through situations/scenarios of loss.
- We have reviewed the techniques that we already know in order to reevaluate their efficiency and potential support to the human life continuum.
- We have assimilated new methods of approach and a deeper knowledge about the self-organization and self-transcendence of the Open-System Human Being.
- We have reiterated the correct approach the Facilitator should use in order to support passages to new phases of the human Life Cycle (including the final passage in the last phase of life) thanks to the dialogue with the Higher Self.
- We have developed the awareness of the gift we were given, which is the ability to do all of this and to pass it on.

Based on these premises, in brief, we can now undeniably deem to have the tools that are needed to propose our Ode to Life.

Ode to Life means being reminded, even as we are living through scenarios of loss and bereavement, or even in the face of death, that we owe gratitude to life for the resources and beauty it gave us, which we are observing now and in every "here" and "this day."

> *You don't get to choose how you're going to die. Or when. You can only decide how you're going to live. Now.*
>
> JOAN BAEZ

Genealogical-Emotional Tree

Over the following pages, you are asked to fill in a peculiar genealogical tree, the "genealogical-emotional tree" of your Life Cycle. Unlike a common genealogical tree, you will not consider only family connections. This specific genealogical tree starts at the roots and proceeds upward to the branches, where the fruits are.

The **roots** represent the most meaningful people, situations, objects, scenarios, and/or experiences that have caused you strong emotions over the course of your life, so much so that they actually took root in you.

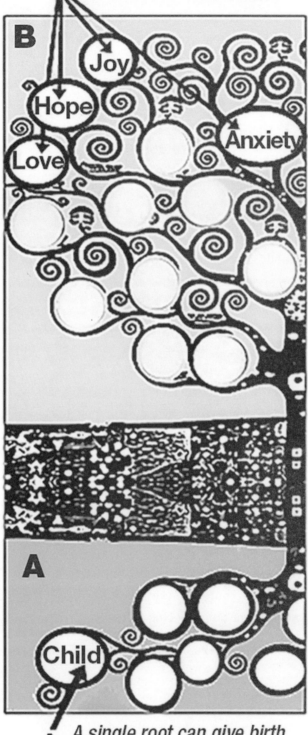

Fig. 26.1. The genealogical-emotional tree

The **fruits** on your tree represent the emotions that have developed in you and remained there, to be recalled when you want or need them. They come from your roots, they blossom, and they become the fruitful and integrated part of your Life Cycle.

The idea is that anything that took root in us and is retraceable to an emotion that remains vivid in time, thanks to a person or a formative experience in our growth, has been and therefore will always be an integral part of our Life Cycle (vital energy continuum).

Roots

Your roots might include:

- people you shared part of your life with (parents, relatives, spouses, partners, friends, acquaintances, employers, colleagues, etc.)
- public figures you were inspired by—those you have considered as your guides and/or who have enriched your life (writers, artists, politicians, activists, teachers, athletes, actors, singers, etc.)
- situations, experiences, places, changes, and/or meaningful actions you encountered (travel experiences, landscapes, a city connected with your cultural background, a specific gesture, a transformation, etc.)
- any other objective or subjective source, such as animals, natural elements, or objects (a pet, a wild animal, a fascinating natural element, a piece of music, etc.)

Fruits

The fruits of the tree are all the emotions that come from events or encounters with elements that followed you for a period of your life, appeared only briefly, or became an integral part of you and transformed your perception of life.

They might be emotions that are either stronger or weaker, constructive or destructive, or even a series of opposite and contrasting emotions. They are always attributable to one of your roots and are therefore meaningful (note that one or more of your emotions might be connected to the same root; see fig. 26.1).

- Fill in the genealogical-emotional tree of your Life Cycle, using fig. 26.2 on the following page.

Good work and . . . good emotions!

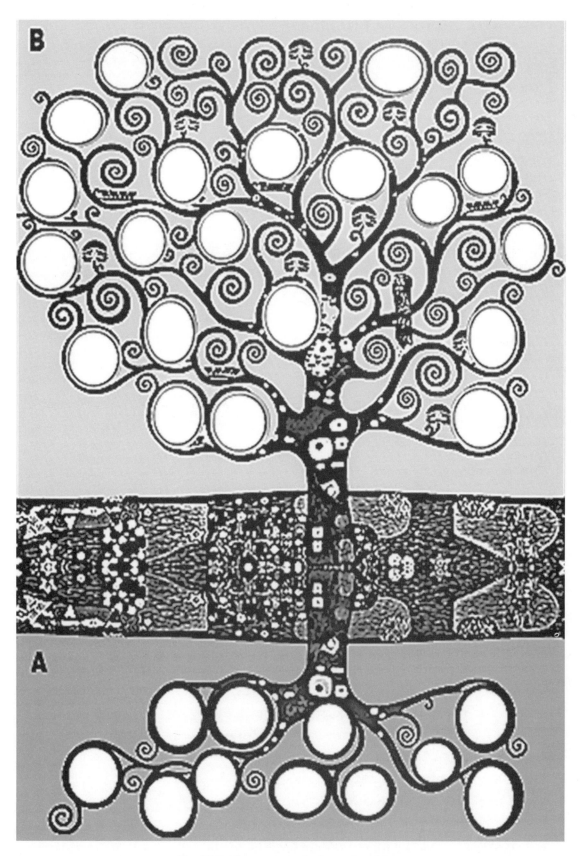

Fig. 26.2. The genealogical-emotional tree

Curriculum Vitae of the Vital Energy Continuum

When I went to school, they asked me what I wanted to be when I grew up. I wrote down "happy."

They told me I didn't understand the assignment, and I told them they didn't understand life.

SOURCE UNKNOWN

The peculiar CV of this exercise is meant to be filled with both objective and subjective, both rational and emotional, data in order to acquire a better awareness about your path in your Life Cycle (cyclus vitae) from your birth until this very day. The exercise is meant to help you realize whether you have fulfilled your ambitions, what scenarios or people allowed you to do it, and how your experiences might have influenced your Biological Process.

On both analytical and emotional levels, it will be a chance to highlight relevant passages between the phases of your Life Cycle in order to understand the importance they bore in maintaining or modifying your vital energy continuum.

In this process, you will be able to evaluate how each event or passage might have led you to be who you are now by:

- influencing your choices
- implementing your knowledge, abilities, and skills
- presenting you with stimuli and models (either to follow or to avoid)
- eventually making you the person you are now

Through this peculiar CV, you can see how separation and/or loss in the various phases of your life might have been favorable physiological events that were necessary in order to drive you to change. You also can see how they allowed you to orient toward your future until this very moment.

From this particular perspective, you can discover the premise needed to transform the negative/destructive elements of various situations/events, implementing your will to transform through a constructive thought-form that can support you and project you into the next intriguingly unknown phase of your life.

Remember, every situation or person that appears as a negative/destructive form/energy/substance could be useful for helping you understand that you do not want to indulge that destructive energy, and you can make use of the awareness of your potential—your self-confidence—to choose a positive/constructive personal environment for your future well-being.

In order to do all of that, follow the structure of the CV, which asks you to reflect on information that is personal, information connected with your profession, and elements that might have influenced your personal growth and vital energy continuum.

Consider this extremely personal curriculum vitae as an outline of the energy continuum of your Life Cycle. While you fill it in, think of it as an actual CV providing the requirements you need to introduce yourself to a new, demanding, and very peculiar employer: your Higher Self.

⸎ The Curriculum Vitae of My Life Cycle ⸎

PERSONAL INFORMATION
Name: Write your first and last name

_____

_____

Spelling: When you say your name, do people understand it immediately and write it correctly, or do you need to spell it for them? If you need to spell it, does that bother you? Briefly explain why.

_____

_____

_____

_____

Aliases: Do you like your name and identify with it, or would you prefer another name? If you prefer another name, what would you like it to be? Why?

_____

_____

_____

_____

Nicknames: Do people call you by a nickname? Who calls or has called you by a nickname? Does that name have a particular meaning? Do you like that people call you by this nickname? Why?

_____

_____

_____

Family: Your last name generally indicates the family you come from, whether it is your mother's or your father's. Do you like your last name, or would you prefer to have a different one? Why?

_____

_____

_____

Address: Write your address—street, house or apartment number, city, state, zip code, country.

_____

Residence: What is the main reason you live there?

_____

_____

_____

Residence Satisfaction: Are you satisfied with the place where you live? Would you like to live anywhere else? Why?

_____

_____

_____

Means of Communication: Write down your phone number(s), email address(es), social media acounts (Facebook, Instagram, LinkedIn, etc.), and any other means of communication you use.

_____

_____

_____

Functional Contact: How often do you have social interaction through the means of communication listed above? (That is, is it at least once an hour, once a day, only every now and then when you need it?)

_____

_____

_____

Communication Use and Satisfaction: Do you think these ways of contacting you are useful? Do you think these means of communication and the time you spend using them are necessary and irreplaceable elements? Do you think any of them might be unnecessary or a counterproductive distraction? Why? Do they distract you from your interests? Are some of them surrogates for other kinds of relationships with people? Why?

_____

_____

_____

_____

Birthday: Write your birth month, day, and year.

_____

Perceived Age: Do you think your biological age corresponds to the age you feel you are? Do you think you have the same level of energy that is commonly associated with your age? Why? Is your feeling about this always the same, or does it change?

_____

_____

_____

_____

Birthplace: Write down the city, state/region, and country in which you were born.

_____

Belonging to Your Birthplace: Do you feel that you belong, on a cultural and emotional level, to the place where you were born and where your origins or roots reside? Why?

_____

_____

_____

Belonging to Another Place: Do you feel that you belong to a place that is not where you were born? Why?

_____

_____

_____

Relationship Status: Write down whether you are single, living with someone, married, separated, divorced, etc.

_____

Quality of Relationship with Self: How is your relationship with yourself? Is it excellent, good, okay, poor, or bad? Why?

_____

_____

_____

Quality of Relationship with Others/Significant Other: How is your relationship with your significant other? If you are single, how are your relationships with other people in general? Is it excellent, good, okay, poor, or bad? Why?

_____

_____

_____

Family: How is the relationship with your family in general? Is it excellent, good, okay, poor, bad, or nonexistent (for objective or subjective reasons?

_____

Family Members: Is your relationship with any of the members of your family problematic? Has it been so in the past? Might it be so in the future? Why?

_____

_____

_____

_____

WORKING EXPERIENCE

Current Job: What is your current job and when did you start it?

_____

Other Working Experiences: List the three most significant and satisfying jobs you have had and why they were so significant and satisfying.

1. _____

_____

_____

_____

2. _____

_____

_____

_____

3. _____

_____

_____

_____

Professional Predispositions: Do you think you have any particular predisposition for a job that would make you feel fulfilled? What are they, and why?

_____

_____

_____

Professional Aspirations: Do you think you can fulfill your professional aspirations and/or improve your professional position? Why?

_____

_____

_____

_____

EDUCATION AND TRAINING

Level of Education: When was the last time you received any kind of officially recognized diploma, what was it, and where did you obtain it?

_____

_____

Desired Education: Do you want or would you have preferred to obtain other diplomas? Why?

_____

_____

_____

Other Qualifications/Certifications: In addition to the diplomas you have, did you receive other qualifications of some kind that you deem to be important for their concrete, personal, or emotional value? What are they and why are they so important? (Write about up to three of them.)

_____

_____

_____

_____

Professional Training Events: Have you attended any course, seminar, or workshop that was useful for your professional training? What were they and why were they useful?

_____

_____

_____

_____

Formative Events: Have you attended any courses, seminars, or workshops that were relevant or useful for your personal growth? What were they and why were they useful?

_____

_____

_____

_____

Knowledge, Competencies, and Skills: What do you think are the greatest knowledge, competencies, and skills you have acquired thanks to your formative path?

_____

_____

_____

Teachers: Who do you think have been your best teachers, on a professional or personal level, from among all of your instructors, colleagues, family members, friends, and acquaintances? Why?

_____

_____

_____

PERSONALITY AND SOCIAL SKILLS

Qualities: What do you think are your best qualities on a personal level? Why do you think they are the best ones? (List up to three of them.)

_____

_____

_____

_____

Flaws: What do you think are your worst flaws or deficiencies on a personal level? Why do you think they are the worst ones? (List up to three of them.)

_____

_____

_____

_____

General Social Skills at Work: What social skills do you think are necessary for an individual within the working environment? Why? (List up to three of them.)

_____

_____

_____

_____

Personal Social Skills at Work: Do you think you have these skills? Why?

_____

_____

_____

General Social Skills in Personal Interactions: What social skills do you think are necessary for an individual within personal interactions and relationships, whether with strangers, acquaintances, relatives, or friends? Why? (List up to 3 of them.)

_____

_____

_____

_____

Personal Social Skills in Personal Interactions: Do you think you have these skills? Why?

_____

_____

_____

_____

Social Situations or Experiences: Name up to three important situations or experiences you have or had in working and/or personal interactions. Are they now in a positive/constructive phase? Have they changed or ended? Why?

_____

_____

_____

_____

PASSIONS AND HOBBIES

Recreational and/or Cultural Interests and Experiences: To live all experiences completely as they are taking place, consciously and with no agenda or specific utilitarian objectives, means allowing yourself to grow. These moments often find their place in play (an essential part of hobbies) and/or in moments of discovery (an essential part of cultural growth). Describe three situations you have experienced in your life that gave you a sense of lightness and/or growth.

_____

_____

_____

_____

Recreational Experiences: Briefly describe what activities most stimulate your imagnation and/or give you a light heart, pleasure, satisfaction, and completeness.

_____

_____

_____

Cultural Experiences: Antonio Gramsci said, "Culture is not a storehouse full of information, but rather the ability of our minds to understand life, our place in it, and our relationships with other people."[4] Briefly describe one or more daily or occasional experiences that enrich you and give you satisfaction, independence, and the will to cultivate relationships and enhance your knowledge, thus building solid foundations for your personal growth.

_____

_____

_____

FREEDOM

Your Life Choices: Freedom is the condition in which you can think, express, and act without constraints, following your will and creativity and choosing freely the means and tools you deem useful. Briefly describe your life choices and how you intend to pursue them.

_____

_____

_____

_____

_____

_____

If something in your CV displeases you, know that we cannot change our past, but we can try to improve our future with the constructive and transformative choices we make.

Personally, I put my efforts into being aware of the choices I want to make and try to keep in mind a statement by historian Carlo M. Cipolla: "Stupid people are those who damage another person or a group of people without accomplishing any personal gain or even causing themselves a loss."[5]

Have a good life!

Clinical Observations

One treatment that will remain impressed in my memory I received in Florida when I traveled there for a convention organized by Upledger Institute International called Beyond the Dura.

Dr. Upledger often invited some of us, Instructors and friends, to his house for a lunch of Thai food, which he loved. Before lunch, we would exchange multi-hands treatments.

Each of those treatments was informal, meaning that it did not comply with a specific protocol designating a conductor among the participating Facilitators. They occurred in a harmonic environment in which we treated each colleague on the bodily part we felt most drawn in that moment. It had always been a pleasant habit that none of us would ever turn down.

However, on that particular occasion something very peculiar happened that opened my eyes to yet another facet of Dr. Upledger's modality of treatment, interpretation of the therapy, and creativity in the implementation.

It was my turn to be treated. Let me start by saying that before this moment, all the treatments I had received during these social gatherings had been carried out in total silence. All the Facilitators took their places to treat me, and Dr. Upledger placed his hands on my head as the others (among them I remember Ken Koles, Tim Hutton, and Hank Meldrum) placed theirs on other parts of my body.

After a few minutes, Dr. Upledger started to hum a song we all knew. It was a tune very similar to one sung by Boy Scouts at their meetings, and all the participants started humming as well.

Since I had raised my son in England, I knew that song, which came from an Anglo-Saxon cultural context. It was very similar to some songs I had learned at the Italian orphanage where I had spent my childhood, and they were connected to pleasant moments, the field trips in particular. Therefore, at first I was pleased to hear my colleagues humming lightheartedly while they were treating me.

After a while, remembering that treatments had always before taken place in complete silence and concentration, I started worrying and even getting a little irritated. In fact, I was wondering why no one seemed to be focused on me, and everyone was acting so frivolously during *my* treatment. It seemed disrespectful.

I wanted to say something, but I realized I would not know what to say without coming across as rude. And it was Dr. Upledger himself who had initiated the humming.

I took courage anyway and expressed my discontent. In response, he helped me understand that I was missing a good opportunity to keep quiet, telling me, "Haven't you understood anything about the therapy? Don't you know we listen and treat with our hands? Don't you remember we are led by the patient's Inner Physician? Try to enjoy *your* treatment."

I realized I could do nothing but shut up and thank Dr. Upledger and my colleagues at the end of the treatment.

It was only later, after several hours of teaching new students, that I fully comprehended the meaning of that event and that specific treatment.

To grow up in an orphanage is not a pleasant experience. It can be very sad. I had found a way to stay strong and fight the sadness by becoming an altar boy so that I could sing during all masses. In addition, I had volunteered to become part of the orphanage band as first trumpeter, and later as second tenor horn. I played in marches during city events, and when we went to holiday camps in the Alps I sang with the other children the songs of the Alpini, the Italian alpine troopers, every time we went trekking in the woods. All that singing and playing had always brought me a type of joy that encouraged me to consider life as something wider, something that certainly was beyond the orphanage.

As I was teaching my students and encouraging them to never forget how much searching for joy and being grateful to life can help us and allow us to help other human beings, stressing the fact that all conscious moments of joy and gratitude give us the strength to do that, I realized what Dr. Upledger and my colleagues had wanted me to understand through the treatment I received in Florida.

I understood that in *our* treatment, my friend and mentor Dr. John was bringing to my awareness what my non-conscious wanted to tell me: *I made it!*

I had been treated by therapists who were completely focused on me, and I was (and am) one of them. I was part of something that in my wildest imagination I never could have thought I would be when I was a child playing simple marches and singing as I walked in the mountains in rare moments of joy, which I held in my heart as I waited to get out of the orphanage.

It is hard to get rid of the sense of insecurity, the inferiority complex, and the constant sense of need we sometimes experience in life. They all stay inside us, but Dr. John and my colleagues had tried to make me understand it was time to let go of that attitude, replace it with my potential and the empowerment it would bring, and start to rely on my self-confidence, offering it to life itself, which would guide me to make good use of it. Happiness is a birthright, but it depends on our correct attitude; it is not just a stroke of luck.

What more can I say? *Thanks to life, which has given me so much!*

❧ A CST-CENTERED VISION ❧

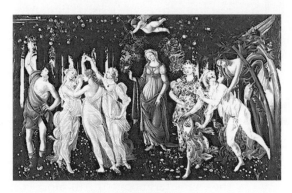

Fig. 26.3. *Primavera*, by Sandro Botticelli

Primavera (fig. 26.3), by Sandro Botticelli, is one of the most famous works of the Italian Renaissance artist. The word *primavera* means spring, the season in which life awakens, the new beginning that allows nature to manifest, with its complexity and beauty, an Ode to Life. Venus, in the center of the painting, represent humanitas, the spiritual activities of the human being. To her right (our left), we see humanitas at work in the form of the three Graces, and reason guiding human actions and chasing away passion and intemperance in the form of Mercury. Spring is nature itself, meaning a cyclical universal force with a regenerative power, as embodied by the group to the left of Venus, in which we see Zephyrus, Chloris, and Flora.

The overall meaning of the work connects with our contemplation of life and reflection on the wonders and power of the natural order of the universe.

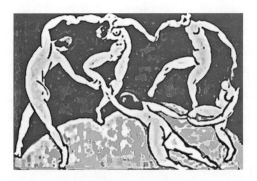

Fig. 26.4. Reproduction of *Dance*, by Henri Émile Benoît Matisse

Dance (fig. 26.4) is one of Matisse's great masterpieces. The painting can be seen as an allegory of human life, made of constant movement in communion with other individuals. All of this happens on the edge of the world, in a space between being and nonbeing. The circular vortex of the dancers has both the joyous aspect of an animated life and the sense of anguish of being forced to dance endlessly.

In this painting, through the synthesis of contents and form, Matisse expresses some profound truths not only about humankind but also about the entire universe. He does not describe a matter of fact but expresses the relentlessness of life, its constant renewal, and its eternal movement through composition and color.

❧

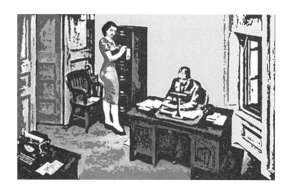

Fig. 26.5. Reproduction of *Office at Night,* by Edward Hopper

Edward Hopper's evocative art is permeated with a strong realism, resulting in a synthesis of figurative vision combined with a poetic view of everyday life. The artist himself declared that he painted not what he saw but what he felt.

In scenarios that represent forced uniformity (just like the model for a CV) but also an emotional space, the characters appearing in Hopper's paintings, like *Office at Night* (fig. 26.5), emerge from the neutrality of the background with their own identity thanks to the light that spreads on their bodies and on their faces. The same might be said of an SER treatment.

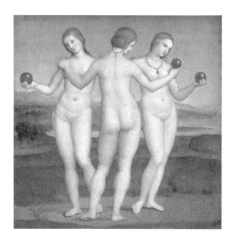

Fig. 26.6. *Three Graces,* by Raffaello Sanzio (Raphael)

The Graces embody beauty, grace, and charity (meaning love that is given, received, and returned) and infuse joy in the hearts of gods and men. In the representation of the Graces by Raphael (fig. 26.6), they are the reward for men who have accomplished their goals after choosing between an ephemeral and easy life (*voluptas*) and the harder path that envisions no material goods but leads to moral salvation (*virtus*). The apples in the hands of the Graces are the gift of the Hesperides to humankind; they are a symbol of immortality as a reward for virtue. The embrace between the three young women represents the gift of grace as a spiritual and emotional quality.

Within the context of the holistic vision, when Facilitators need to deal with existential subjects, which are often very hard to face, they take the patient back to their well-being through their intention and the fundamental existential attitude that they have learned through a work that is virtuous only when it implies a sincere and authentic gratitude to life.

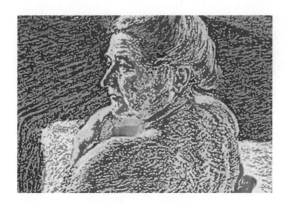

Fig. 26.7. Reproduction of *Nude from Behind,* by Umberto Boccioni

The woman portrayed In Umberto Boccioni's *Nude from Behind* (fig. 26.7) is his mother. The light on her skin looks like it is fragmented into thousands of shards, infinite specks of pure color, one next to the other, as is typical in the painting technique of divisionism. The effect of oblique light softly glowing on the mature woman's body proves that it is possible to transcend pure matter through a vision of profound love, like the love of a son.

The most intimate beauty of a person is manifested in all phases of their life. Authentic beauty can be found even where, to inattentive eyes, the transformation of matter modifies physical forms and takes away its true light. The Facilitator is trained to perceive the authenticity of a person's experience and can therefore contact the dimension of the human being meant to be an open system, bringing the patient to a space in which they can freely express their natural and innate self-healing, self-transcendence, and natural beauty.

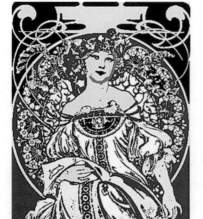

Fig. 26.8. Reproduction of *Daydream,* by Alfons Maria Mucha (Alphonse Mucha)

Alphonse Mucha is considered the greatest exponent of Art Nouveau. His style made him the initiator of a new pictorial language, an innovative visual art accessible to everyone. With its ornamental lines and structures, Art Nouveau represents an actual attempt at reforming life. Its primary source of inspiration is nature, admired for its formal perfection. In his painting *Daydream* (fig. 26.8), sinuous lines incarnate a lively vision of the world as an eternal creative and natural phenomenon within a constant biological regeneration.

Strength, stability, well-being, awareness, and joy in life are all elements that in therapy, just like in art, represent the eternal creative and natural phenomenon of regeneration.

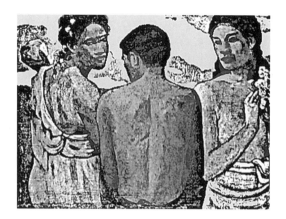

Fig. 26.9. Reproduction of *Three Tahitians,* by Paul Gauguin

French painter Paul Gauguin was initially part of the Impressionism movement, but he detached himself from it later on, accentuating the pictorial abstraction of his art in a style called Synthetism. A controversial and restless man, constantly traveling in search of the origins of human civilization, Gauguin was able to portray in his paintings the harmony of landscapes and the simple rituality of life through bright colors painted in wide blocks.

For Facilitators, the journey toward origins is the constant training of the correct attitude in the relationship with the patient, which brings them to the origin of the language of the Higher Self, allowing them to listen to and comply with every part of the organism of the patient, just like the painter grasps the simplicity of the language of the forms that are able to narrate harmony.

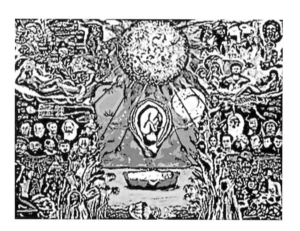

Fig. 26.10. Reproduction of *Moses (Nucleus of Creation),* by Frida Kahlo

Frida Kahlo's paintings were influenced by her physical suffering and politic engagement. Her art expresses her interior state and her way of relating to the world. In *Moses,* which she called *Nucleus of Creation* (fig. 26.10), the subject is Moses as a baby in his cradle with a third eye (wisdom) on his forehead. Above him is the representation of a fetus in a womb and, above that, the sun. The sun and the water at the bottom both symbolize sources of life. On the two sides are emblematic figures of humanity touched by sunlight and embraced by death. The drops of water in the middle symbolize the cycle of love, whereas the new branches on the dead tree trunks stand for the cycle of life.

Kahlo's painting appears as a complete, although dreamlike, representation of the continuum of the universal Life Cycle that humankind belongs to, between life, love, and death.

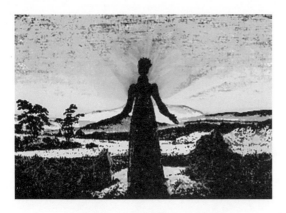

Fig. 26.11. Reproduction of *Woman before the Rising Sun,* by Caspar David Friedrich

As an exponent of Romanticism, Caspar David Friedrich was one of the most important symbolic landscape artists. He considered the landscape a divine work and used it to represent the feeling of sublime, the reunion with the spiritual Self through the contemplation of nature. He wrote, "Close your bodily eye, that you may see your picture first with the eye of the spirit. Then bring to light what you have seen in the darkness, that its effect may work back, from without to within."[6]

In *Woman before the Rising Sun* (fig. 26.11), we sense the wonder felt by the woman standing before the grandness of nature and creation in front of the sun that is emerging from behind the hill. It might be compared to the wonder we feel for the great revelation of life that is inside each human, even in the phase of sunset.

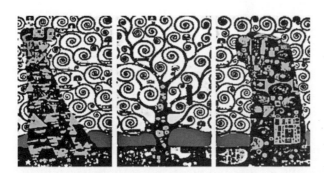

Fig. 26.12. Reproduction of the *Stoclet Frieze,* by Gustav Klimt

Gustav Klimt's *Stoclet Frieze* (fig. 26.12) is constituted by three panels: the central one with the Tree of Life, a panel titled *Expectation* (or the Wait) on the left, and a panel titled the *Embrace* (or Accomplishment) on the right. The floral pattern and the death of vegetation on the ground, leaving the seed that allows rebirth in the cycle of seasons, represent regeneration and life energy. The tree, a reference to the biblical "tree of knowledge," holds on one of the branches a black bird symbolizing the threat of death, contrasted by the thriving branches and fruits. This scene tells the story of a woman waiting for love near the tree of life. She fulfills her dream in the passion of an embrace in which the male part makes the completion of the unity of unconscious, spirit, and matter possible.

In Klimt's artwork, we can see life in its most significant phases: the interruption of the energy continuum in the life cycle, transformation, and fulfillment, including the natural occurrence of death. Each person and each emotion is a seed that can take root in the ground of our life, producing sprouts, branches, flowers, and fruits. It is up to us to reinvigorate our tree by getting rid of the bad roots and the dead branches, giving more strength and vitality to the entire plant so that it can produce flowers (spirit/intellect) and good fruits (physicality/actions).

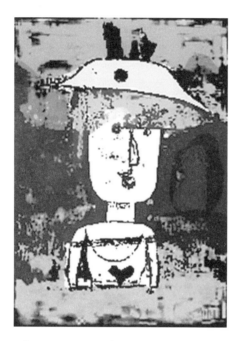

Fig. 26.13. Reproduction of *Portrait of Mrs. P. in the South,* by Ernst Paul Klee

Ernst Paul Klee was an eclectic artist who produced music, poetry, literature, and painting. As an exponent of abstract art, he represented through color and shapes the emotional impression of reality on his spirit, sometimes using only simple lines and blocks of color. For him, art was research into the hidden mechanisms of nature, the ability to see beyond a spiritual practice in which the image is just the final result of a reflection on oneself and one's own thinking. Klee famously said, "Art does not reproduce the visible but makes it visible." He believed that what we see is just a proposition, a possibility, an aid to get to what lies beyond the visible. In his *Portrait of Mrs. P. in the South* (fig. 26.13), we see a heart shape on Mrs. P.'s chest—a symbol that appears frequently in his work. The motif bridges the organic and inorganic worlds by symbolizing life forces while serving as a mediating form between incorporeal nature and physical matter.

How much of SomatoEmotional Release can we find in the description of art given by Klee? Very much. Let us just replace the word *art* with *body* or *symptom* and read the sentence again. The analogy with SER will be clear. Moreover, how much of the meaning of the heart shape in the painting can we associate with the therapeutic Third Space as the mediating space between the organic world and that of the unconscious? Think about it! Now ask yourself, *How can I not be happy or grateful for a therapy that, just like art—one of the highest expressions of humankind—is able to express all of that?*

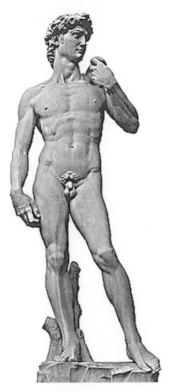

Fig. 26.14.
Reproduction of *David*,
by Michelangelo Buonarroti

Michelangelo's *David* (fig. 26.14) is widely considered a masterpiece of sculpture. It is one of the most recognized symbols of the Italian Renaissance. The artist represented David, the biblical hero, as he is about to fight Goliath, his gigantic Philistine enemy. His frowned expression and penetrating stare show his concentration, expressing the intellectual power that helps the physical one. In his right hand David holds the stone wrapped in the slingshot he is about to use to defeat the enemy. The fierce look in his eyes is that of a hero who is aware of his own strength, a strength that is represented by Michelangelo with connotations that are not limited to religious faith.

In the statue, the head stands for reason (the mind), the means that makes it possible for humans to set themselves apart from beasts, whereas David's hands symbolize the tool that reason uses to take action and create.

We chose this image to represent what the Facilitator and the patient are about to face when they start the process of transformation of destructive energy into constructive energy. The patient is David, whereas the Facilitator is his slingshot. With the weapon, the individual gets ready to address the destructive energy causing their problems. The destructive energy is Goliath, the enemy of the patient's well-being. In David, we can find the patient's determination in facing their own issues and the Facilitator's correct attitude and self-confidence used as a means to facilitate and support the actions of the patient in this fight. We all know the (biblical) epilogue: David defeats Goliath.

David Kracov built *Book of Life* (fig. 26.15, next page) with metal, a material in which the artist sees a surprising lightness. Colorful butterflies soar out from the pages of a book, like words that come to life. Kracov created the work as a tribute to Rabbi Yossi Raichik, who was the director of Chabad's Children of Chernobyl nonprofit organization. His tireless activities contributed to save and give new hope to 2,500 children affected by the nuclear catastrophe of Chernobyl in 1986.

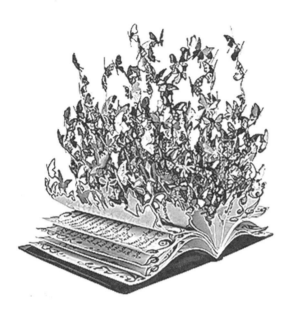

Fig. 26.15. *Book of Life,* by David Kracov

The words of all the scientists, physicians, therapists, researchers, scholars, philosophers, and knowledgeable people quoted and mentioned in this text similarly come to life through the Facilitator and are transformed into actions and gestures that are able to help patients "come out from their cocoon" and open up to the new phases of their Life Cycle.

PARTING

Panta Rhei
Everything Flows

Nothing is created, nothing is destroyed, everything transforms.
ANTOINE LAVOISIER

Everything flows. This principle regulates the phenomena of reality. Greek philosopher Heraclitus defined this principle as *panta rhei* 2,500 years ago; French chemist Antoine Lavoisier reestablished it in 1700 with the physical law of conservation of mass. Dr. John Upledger and his son John Matthew Upledger taught it to all Facilitators through their lives.

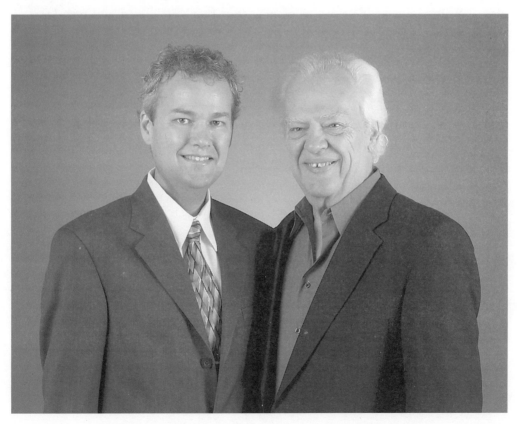

John Matthew Upledger and his father, Dr. John Edwin Upledger

Dr. John Edwin Upledger was one of the major developers of alternative medicine and the founder of CranioSacral Therapy and SomatoEmotional Release. Without him, the world would not have received these methods, and none of the phases of my work (in my Life Cycle) as a Facilitator, osteopath, and CST and SER Instructor and communicator would have occurred.

John Matthew Upledger was the administrator of Upledger Institute International and made Dr. John's projects possible. Thanks to his eternal enthusiasm, dedication, and tireless work of supervision and management, CST and SER are implemented today in over 170 countries. It was he who facilitated the work of all of those who use Dr. Upledger's techniques today.

We all have the task and honor of being at the same time witnesses and protagonists of evolution. In even the smallest and apparently insignificant actions, we determine changes and transformations within our own Life Cycle and in the universal energy continuum we belong to. As Edward Norton Lorenz famously asked, "Does the flap of a butterfly's wings in Brazil set off a tornado in Texas?" If we pursue the correct attitude and awareness, I am certain that we can bring our renewed constructive energy to life.

The aim of this book is to offer the opportunity to develop further knowledge about CranioSacral Therapy and SomatoEmotional Release not only to insiders (the Facilitators) but also to those who wish to approach the information Dr. Upledger left us. With this text, I intend to plant a seed that will sprout and give fruit as actions following your reading.

Although some of the information and concepts given in this text might seem hard to process, know that CST and SER transform them into simple reality. Dr. Upledger knew how to make any kind of complexity understandable and accessible to everyone, on both a didactic and a practical level. This was one of his greatest gifts.

As was the case for me in writing this book, thanks to the information I researched and transcribed, I hope that reading and learning about the authors I have mentioned may be a stimulus for further research and personal growth and awareness.

The most important thing I can offer to you, which I hope has emerged from this book, is what Dr. Upledger left as a legacy to his students when during the lessons I attended he said, "Remember first and foremost that you are Facilitators. Your role is to facilitate the self-healing mechanism of patients and offer empathy, through the touch of their hands, with the guidance of the Higher Self."

If even just one little part of this work helps someone to any extent, I will feel like I have honored both you who have read this book and the work of Dr. Upledger, without whom I could never have written anything.

In conclusion, any information you might need is already available to your hands. Therefore, I cannot help but quote once again Dr. Upledger's words:

"Trust your hands. They know what they are doing."

Acknowledgments

A big thank you to all the experts I have quoted and/or mentioned; their knowledge was one of the foundations that enabled me to write this book. If you ask me why I chose the selections I did, know that I wish I could mention many other writings, articles, and essays by people I wanted the reader to meet, but the space of a book can be limiting.

Thanks to Dawn Langnes Shear, Kathy Woll, and Alex Jozefyk, who with their hard work represent wholeheartedly Upledger Institute International and who believed in the idea of this book, promoting its international diffusion.

I am also grateful for the sincere and productive participation of Pierpaolo Bon, the Italian publisher who took care of all the aspects that were necessary to print the book in Italian, as well as Giada Pianigiani, who accepted to translate it from Italian to English, and Rossella Bagnardi, who accurately revised the translation.

Another thank you goes to all my current and past fellow Facilitators and Instructors from Upledger Institute International. Through their experiences, I have learned, shared, and studied the aspects of CST and SER both as a therapist and as a student—and now an Instructor.

Thank you to all the patients and students who have been my life coaches in my work and to all the colleagues and friends that I mentioned in the book for sharing with me their working experiences and their time.

Special thanks go to Thea Keber, Euro Piuca, and Patricia Quirini. Thea, my co-president at Upledger Italy, patiently transcribed all the chapters of this book. Euro gave an entire chapter to it. Patricia used her precision and dedication to correct my mistakes and suggest any possible improvement. Thanks also to Monica, who, with her preparation and knowledge, was the first person to inspire the writing of this book.

Once again I would like to mention Dawn Langnes Shear for the enormous help she has given me. Without her help I certainly would not have been able to publish the English edition of this book. Dawn was the "guardian angel" who worked together with the editorial team of Healing Arts Press—together with my editor, Meghan MacLean, in particular—to guide and support me along the way toward the realization of my intent.

Thanks again to life for allowing me to meet each of these people and share with them the important phases of my Life Cycle.

Ode to Life! For all the experiences it made me go through and how they formed me for what I am now (for better or worse)—thank you.

A CST-CENTERED VISION

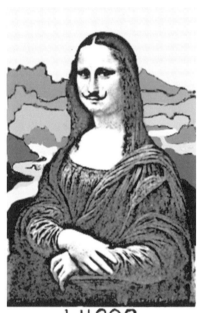

Reproduction of *L.H.O.O.Q.*, by Marcel Duchamp

This artwork is a ready-made by one of the French artists who founded the Dadaist movement. The acronym L.H.O.O.Q., used by Duchamp to title this piece, when read in French, purposely creates a vulgar and provocative expression echoed by the moustache and goatee drawn on the painting *Mona Lisa*. These elements are the reason why this artwork has always been considered a manifesto against conformism. Note that with this piece, Duchamp did not intend to reject or desecrate Leonardo's art but rather to honor it in a very personal way, with the intention of ridiculing superficial and ignorant admirers, who define Mona Lisa as beautiful only to conform.

Dare to think out of the box, allow yourself to be visionary, and follow your Higher Selves. Visions give birth to intuition, which produces ideas, which in turn transform projects into action and are able to change constructively your energy and your life.

A personal thank you to all of those who already believe that.

Notes

1. A BRIEF HISTORY OF CRANIOSACRAL THERAPY (CST) AND SOMATOEMOTIONAL RELEASE (SER)

1. Covey 1989.
2. Robbins 1991.

3. THE PATIENT-FACILITATOR RELATIONSHIP IN CST

1. Ostaseki, 2006, p. 42 (trans. from Italian).

4. FOUNDATIONAL TECHNIQUES

1. Figari 2016 (trans. from Italian).

5. EGO

1. Edelstein 2006 (trans. from Italian).
2. Jung, as quoted by Psicologi Junghiani 2011 (trans. from Italian).
3. Istituto di Gestalt HCC Italia 2012 (trans. from Italian).
4. Bonacchi 2015 (trans. from Italian).
5. Assagioli, Taylor, Crampton 1966, p. 4 (trans. from Italian).

6. BIOLOGICAL PROCESSES IN THE LIFE CYCLE

1. Bencivenga et al. 2015 (trans. from Italian).
2. Riggs, Martienssen, and Russo 1996
3. Aiello 2013.
4. Lansberger and Kilstrup-Nielsen 2008 (trans. from Italian).
5. Sgarrella, n.d. (trans. from Italian).
6. Rispoli 1987 (trans. from Italian).
7. Bioenergetica Italia 2004 (trans. from Italian).
8. Becherucci et al. 2018 (trans. from Italian).
9. Treccani, n.d., "Entelechia" (trans. from Italian).

10. Grassi Zucconi 2000 (trans. from Italian); Leotta 2019 (trans. from Italian).
11. Onelli 2013, p. 65 (trans. from Italian).
12. Forestiero 2007 (trans. from Italian).
13. di Giorgi 2016 (trans. from Italian).

7. SEPARATION AND LOSS

1. HumanTrainer, n.d. (trans. from Italian).
2. Gardini 2018 (trans. from Italian).
3. Le Scienze 2012 (trans. from Italian).
4. Gardini 2018 (trans. from Italian).
5. Munch 2002 (trans. from Italian).

8. MEASURING STRESSORS

1. Upledger 2010b, pp. 377–78.
2. Simone 2014 (trans. from Italian).
3. Fatica 2017, p. 39 (trans. from Italian).

9. PROCESSING EMOTIONS

1. Upledger 1990, p. 136.
2. Aquino 2013b (trans. from Italian).
3. Trevisani 2013.
4. Associazione Nazionale Orientatori 2019 (trans. from Italian).
5. Solms and Turnbull 2002.
6. Mauri 2018 (trans. from Italian).
7. Aquino 2013b (trans. from Italian).
8. Aquino 2013b (trans. from Italian).
9. eLEAS 2016.
10. Ascolese 2014 (trans. from Italian).
11. Il Diogene, n.d. (trans. from Italian).
12. Aquino 2013b (trans. from Italian).
13. Aquino 2013b (trans. from Italian).
14. Frattini 2019 (trans. from Italian).

10. CONSTRUCTIVE AND DESTRUCTIVE ENERGY

1. Treacy 2016 (trans. from Italian).
2. Guardini 1997, p. 10 (trans. from Italian).
3. Vadalà 2004.
4. Di Muro 2018 (trans. from Italian).
5. Tradizione Sacra, n.d. (trans. from Italian).

6. Filosoficamente 2016 (trans. from Italian).
7. Sapere.it, n.d., "I principi primi e l'intelligenza suprema" (trans. from Italian).
8. Blasi 2017 (trans. from Italian); Three Initiates [pseud.] 1908, chapter 2.
9. Bertoldi, n.d. (trans. from Italian).
10. Miranda 2014 (trans. from Italian).
11. Cavaleri 2003, pp. 117–18 (trans. from Italian).
12. Istituto Psicoterapia Gestalt Espressiva, n.d. (trans. from Italian).
13. Viglienghi, n.d. pp. 6–7 (trans. from Italian).
14. Treccani, n.d., "Polarità" (trans. from Italian).
15. Oliveri 2006 (trans. from Italian).
16. Treccani, n.d., "Polarità" (trans. from Italian).
17. Ergymax, n.d. (trans. from Italian).
18. Oliveri 2006 (trans. from Italian).
19. Sapere.it, n.d., "Polarità" (trans. from Italian).
20. Sapere.it, n.d., "Polarità" (trans. from Italian).

11. THE CEREBRAL HEMISPHERES

1. Riza.it, n.d., "Emisfero destro e sinistro del cervello" (trans. from Italian).
2. Cavalcanti 2018 (trans. from Italian).
3. Manzelli 2017, p. 1 (trans. from Italian).
4. Manzelli 2018a (trans. from Italian).
5. Sacchetti 2018 (trans. from Italian).
6. AIPRO 2017, pp. 1–2 (trans. from Italian); HealthQE 2017.
7. AIPRO 2017, pp. 2–4 (trans. from Italian); HealthQE 2017.
8. Pomodoro 2014 (trans. from Italian).
9. Upledger 2010b, p. 17.

12. TRANSFORMATION

1. Montalto 2010 (trans. from Italian).
2. Ferrucci 2014 (trans. from Italian).
3. Assagioli 1993.
4. Ferrucci 2009 (trans. from Italian).
5. Paternoster 2016 (trans. from Italian).
6. Batfroi 2007, p. 158 (trans. from Italian).

13. SEATS OF EMOTIONS

1. AIPRO 2017, p. 8 (trans. from Italian).
2. Tradizione Sacra, n.d. (trans. from Italian).
3. AIPRO 2017, pp. 9–10 (trans. from Italian).
4. Di Stefano 2013 (trans. from Italian).

5. Centro Studi Eva Reich, n.d. (trans. from Italian).
6. Goleman and Dalai Lama 2003.
7. Goleman and Dalai Lama 2003.

14. SMALL DEATHS

1. Valcarenghi 2014 (trans. from Italian).
2. Jendrzej 2009, pp. 1–5 (trans. from Italian).
3. Rasini 2018 (trans. from Italian).
4. D'Alisa 2016 (trans. from Italian).

15. ENERGETIC FRAMEWORK OF THE HUMAN BODY

1. Lucarelli 2015 (trans. from Italian).
2. Cremaschini 2018 (trans. from Italian).
3. La Mente è Meravigliosa 2019 (trans. from Italian).
4. Skuola.net, n.d. (trans. from Italian).
5. Mastrobisi 2017, pp. 35–61 (trans. from Italian).
6. Cilento 2018 (trans. from Italian).
7. Valesini 2016 (trans. from Italian).
8. La Mente è Meravigliosa 2019 (trans. from Italian).
9. Tradizione Sacra, n.d. (trans. from Italian).
10. Treccani 2010c (trans. from Italian).
11. Upledger 1990, 67.

16. CHAKRAS

1. Bihar, as quoted in Bihar and Daniel 2014 (trans. from Italian).
2. Bergamaschi 2011 (trans. from Italian).
3. Eliade 1999, p. 223 (trans. from Italian).
4. Fayenz 2012 (trans. from Italian).
5. Burrini 2016 (trans. from Italian).
6. White 2003, p. 222.
7. Magicamente Colibrì 2018; Pert 1988, p. 131.
8. Stranieri and Tulli, n.d., "Il sistema energetico e I corpi sottili" (trans. from Italian).
9. Annica 2011 (trans. from Italian).
10. Bettoschi, n.d. (trans. from Italian).
11. Pascale, n.d. (trans. from Italian).
12. Ascoltare la vita 2013 (trans. from Italian).
13. Tradizione Sacra, n.d. (trans. from Italian).
14. Fairymoon [pseud.] 2013 (trans. from Italian).
15. Wallis 2016.

17. CST AND SER IN GRIEF

1. Levi-Montalcini 2017.
2. Valentino 2017 (trans. from Italian).
3. Galimberti 2005 (trans. from Italian).
4. Garaventa 2017 (trans. from Italian).
5. Mapelli 2014 (trans. from Italian).
6. Mattalucci and Pinkus 2000 (trans. from Italian).
7. Pastel 2016.

18. ENTROPY AND SYNTROPY

1. Vecchia 2017 (trans. from Italian).
2. Vecchia 2017 (trans. from Italian).
3. Riflessioni.it, n.d. (trans. from Italian).
4. Vecchia 2017 (trans. from Italian).
5. Bersani Greggio 2017 (trans. from Italian).
6. Di Renzo Editore, n.d. (trans. from Italian).
7. Minotti 2018 (trans. from Italian).
8. Minotti 2018 (trans. from Italian).
9. Rita 2019 (trans. from Italian).
10. Caligiuri 2022 (trans. from Italian).
11. Ascheri, n.d. (trans. from Italian).
12. Vannini 2006 (trans. from Italian).
13. Vannini 2006 (trans. from Italian).
14. Licata 2013 (trans. from Italian).
15. More 1998.
16. Kelly 2009.
17. Pagliaro 2016 (trans. from Italian).

19. MAJOR STRESSORS

1. Treccani 2010a (trans. from Italian).
2. Istituto A. T. Beck, n.d. (trans. from Italian).
3. Lunghi, Baroni, and Alò 2017, pp. 18–21 (trans. from Italian).
4. Guazzelli and Gemignani 2012, pp. 97–98 (trans. from Italian).
5. Chetta 2008, pp. 2–4, 10–11, 21 (trans. from Italian).
6. Folino, Onorati, and Sepe 2018 (trans. from Italian).
7. Brunetti 2018 (trans. from Italian).
8. Bratina 2009 (trans. from Italian).

20. CST AND SER IN DEATH

1. Pacilli 2017 (trans. from Italian).
2. Epicurus, n.d.
3. Pascal 1932, p. 97.
4. Mazzocchi 2011 (trans. from Italian).
5. Liucci 2018 (trans. from Italian).
6. Fey 2010 (trans. from Italian).
7. ANAPACA, n.d. (trans. from Italian).
8. Gelati 2013 (trans. from Italian).
9. Pasin 2016 (trans. from Italian).
10. Carmignani 2018 (trans. from Italian).
11. Salgado 2016 (trans. from Italian).

21. THE FINAL TREATMENT

1. Upledger, 2010b.
2. Gazzola 2003 (trans. from Italian).
3. Zilio 2016, pp. 117–150 (trans. from Italian).
4. Brunetti 2018 (trans. from Italian).
5. De Fanis 2017 (trans. from Italian).
6. Mancuso 2007 (trans. from Italian).
7. Paparoni 1982 (trans. from Italian).

22. THERAPEUTIC VIBRATIONS

1. Upledger 2010b.
2. Upledger 2010b, p. 381.
3. Cenacolo di Andrea 2015 (trans. from Italian).
4. Musto, n.d. (trans. from Italian).
5. Manzelli 2018b (trans. from Italian).
6. Treccani, n.d. "Fonone" (trans. from Italian).
7. University of Turin Department of Geology, n.d. (trans. from Italian).
8. Treccani, n.d., "Fonone" (trans. from Italian).
9. University of Turin Department of Geology, n.d. (trans. from Italian).
10. Giardi 2017 (trans. from Italian).
11. Crepaldi 2013 (trans. from Italian).
12. Geymonat 1970 (trans. from Italian).
13. Head and Librale, n.d. (trans. from Italian).
14. Crotti 2010 (trans. from Italian).
15. Crotti 2014 (trans. from Italian).
16. Fiscaletti 2016 (trans. from Italian).
17. Fiscaletti 2016 (trans. from Italian).

18. Manzelli 2018c (trans. from Italian).
19. Abbà 2018 (trans. from Italian).
20. Uberti, n.d. (trans. from Italian).
21. Stefanelli, n.d. (trans. from Italian).

23. FORM OF THE THIRD SPACE

1. Fanpage.it 2018 (trans. from Italian).
2. Mistretta, n.d. (trans. from Italian).
3. Losa 2017 (trans. from Italian).
4. Venuti 2012 (trans. from Italian).
5. Bianciardi, n.d. (trans. from Italian).
6. Di Corpo and Vannini 2010 (trans. from Italian).
7. Manzelli 2018a (trans. from Italian).
8. Consapevoli.net 2014 (trans. from Italian).
9. Essere il Cambiamento 2012 (trans. from Italian).
10. Losa 2019 (trans. from Italian).
11. Silva 2016 (trans. from Italian).
12. Jung 2014, p. 423.

24. MIND-BODY-SPIRIT CONTINUUM

1. Upledger 2010b, p. 17.
2. Biason 2018 (trans. from Italian).
3. Mancuso 2007 (trans. from Italian).
4. McMahon 1993.

25. A SEVEN-STEP TREATMENT FOR THE DYING PROCESS

1. Silvestrini 2017 (trans. from Italian).
2. Mancuso 2017 (trans. from Italian).
3. Rispoli 2017 (trans. from Italian).
4. Le Scienze 2017 (trans. from Italian).
5. Mayer 2019 (trans. from Italian).
6. Goleman 2009.
7. Dato 2016 (trans. from Italian).
8. Latrofa 2019 (trans. from Italian).
9. Latrofa 2019 (trans. from Italian).
10. Arena 2017, p. 11 (trans. from Italian).
11. Ravasi 2012 (trans. from Italian).
12. *Cieloevento* editorial staff 2015 (trans. from Italian).
13. *Cieloevento* editorial staff 2015 (trans. from Italian).

26. ODE TO LIFE

1. Lorenz 2017 (trans. from Italian).
2. Upledger 2010a, p. 313.
3. Upledger 2010a, p. 30.
4. Gramsci 2014 (trans. from Italian).
5. Cipolla 2002 (trans. from Italian).
6. Friedrich 2001 (trans. from Italian).

References

Abbà, M. 2018. "Psicoacustica musicale." https://www.ideegreen.it/psicoacustica-musicale-109698.html.

Aiello, F. 2013. "Is the epigenetics another dimension in evolution?" http://www.scienceonthenet.eu/content/article/francesco-aiello/epigenetics-another-dimension-evolution/febbraio-2013.

AIPRO. 2017. *Le basi dell'elettrodinamica quantistica in medicina (QED)*. Aprilia, Italy: Associazione Italiana Prevenzione Respirazione Orale. https://www.aipro.info/wp/wp-content/uploads/2017/08/elettrodinamica_quantistica_medicina.pdf.

ANAPACA. n.d. "Comprendere la morte, accompagnare la vita." https://www.anapaca.it/comprendere-la-morte-accompagnare-la-vita/.

Anderson, Susan and Scott. 2008. "Vibrational Frequency List." *Just a List* (blog), March 13, 2008. http://justalist.blogspot.com/ 2008/03/vibrational-frequency-list.html.

Annica. 2011. "I 12 meridiani cinesi e la loro relazione coi 7 chakra." *Sezione Aurea* (blog). http://www.sezioneaureastudio.it/2011/04/i-12-meridiani-cinesi-e-la-loro.html.

Aquino, P. 2013a. "La neuropsicologia delle emozioni." https://www.neuroscienze.net/la-neuropsicologia-delle-emozioni/.

Aquino, P. 2013b. "Le emozioni e le neuroscienze affettive." https://www.neuroscienze.net/le-emozioni-e-le-neuroscienze-affettive/.

Arena, S. 2017. "Il significato e la simbologia esoterica dei Numeri." https://www.accademiaopera.it/wp-content/uploads/2017/12/txt-186.pdf.

Ascheri, V. n.d. "Luigi Fantappiè." http://disf.org/autori/luigi-fantappie.

Ascolese, A. 2014. "L'importanza delle emozioni positive–Psicologia Positiva." *State of Mind* (online), February 27, 2014. https://www.stateofmind.it/2014/02/emozioni-positive/.

Ascoltare la vita. 2013. "Descrizione dei Chakra." http://ascoltarelavita.blogspot.com/2013/04/descrizione-dei-chakra.html.

Assagioli, R. 1974. *The Act of Will*. Baltimore: Penguin Books.

———. 1993. *Psicosintesi: Per l'armonia della vita*. Redacted by Marialuisa Macchia Girelli. Rome: Astrolabio Ubaldini.

Assagioli, R., G. C. Taylor, and M. Crampton. 1966. "Dialogo con Roberto Assagioli." www.psicoenergetica.it/scritti%20Assagioli/14%20IL%20SE'%20E%20IL%2 0SUPERCOSCIENTE/Dialogo%20con%20Roberto%20Assagioli.doc.

Associazione Nazionale Orientatori. 2019. "Intelligenza emotiva: sviluppare consapevolez-za di sé per avere conoscenza degli altri." https://www.asnor.it/intelligenza-emotiva-sviluppare-consapevolezza-di-se-per-avere-conoscenza-degli-altri/.

Avico, R. 2019a. "Giovanni Liotti, trauma da attaccamento, dissociazione: da un recente articolo di Benedetto Farina." http://www.psychiatryonline.it/node/8008.

Avico, R. 2019b. "La ricerca di sicurezza: teoria polivagale e PTSD." http://www.psychiatryonline.it/node/7871.

Batfroi, S. 2007. *La via dell'alchimia cristiana.* Translated by P. Faccia. Rome: Edizioni Arkeios.

BBC News. 2019. "First image of Einstein's 'spooky' particle entanglement." https://www.bbc.com/news/uk-scotland-glasgow-west-48971538.

Becherucci, P., S. Bernasconi, E. Bozzola, F. Cerutti, S. Cianfarani, et al. 2018. "La valutazione auxologica in età evolutiva." https://www.area-pediatrica.it/archivio/2881/articoli/29051/.

Bencivenga, S., D. Borgese, M. Gandini, F. Rubettino, S. Sardiello, and S. Venturi. 2015. "Nuove Arti Terapie, n. 26." https://www.nuoveartiterapie.net/la-rivista/numero-26/.

Bergamaschi, G. 2011. "Disciplina logica ed elementi di psicologia junghiana: un'analisi critica." http://www.gianfrancobertagni.it/materiali/meditazione/bergama schi.pdf.

Bersani Greggio, F. 2017. "L'entropia nella fisiologia umana." Blog on the *Scienza Conoscenza* website, July 26, 2017. https://www.scienzaeconoscenza.it/blog/scienza_e_fisica_quantistica/l-impronta-dell-entropia-nella-fisiologia-umana-prima-parte.

Bertoldi, F. n.d. "Hegel." http://www.filosofico.net/hegel542.htm.

Bettoschi, G. n.d. "Capire il corpo attraverso i Chakra." https://www.lifegate.it/persone/stile-di-vita/capire_il_corpo_attraverso_i_chakra.

Bianciardi, G. n.d. "Geometria frattale: un'introduzione." http://www.larchivio.com/xoom/bianciardi-frattali.htm.

Biason, A. 2018. "Anima e coscienza: intervista a Massimo Teodorani." *Altro Giornale,* January 15, 2018. https://www.altrogiornale.org/anima-e-coscienza-intervista-a-massimo-teodorani/.

Bihar, A., and S. Daniel. 2014. *Corpo, mente e spirito: la trilogia.* REI (Rifreddo).

Bioenergetica Italia. 2004. "Bioenergetica." https://www.bioenergetica.eu/bioenerg.asp.

Blasi, I. 2017. "Il gioco delle polarità, un'altalena tra essere e non essere." https://www.psicologa.lecce.it/polarita/.

Bolelli, R. 2018. "Siamo musica." http://www.ilgiornaledellefondazioni.com/content/siamo-musica.

Bonacchi A. 2015. "Rappresentazioni del senso di identità in psicosintesi." http://www.centrosynthesis.it/2015/05/rappresentazioni-del-senso-di-identita-in-psicosintesi/.

Bratina, E. 2009. "Corso di teosofia. Quattordicesima parte." https://www.teosofica.org/all/Corso_di_Teosofia_14.pdf.

Brown, H. J., Jr. 1991–1995. *The Complete Life's Little Instruction Book.* Nashville, Tenn.: Rutledge Hill Press.

Brunetti, G. 2018. "L'anima: dalla metafisica alle neuroscienze. Concezione trinitaria della persona." https://www.riflessioni.it/finestre-anima/anima-dalla-metafisica-alle-neuroscienze.htm.

Burigana, F., C. Cuomo, amd P. Véret. 2016. "Una voce a cinque sensi–Sonorità e Benessere." Blog on the *Scienza Conoscenza* website, January 1, 2016. https://www.scienzaeconoscenza.it/blog/consapevolezza/una-voce-a-cinque-sensi-sonorita-e-benessere548.

Burrini, G. 2016. "Chakra astrali e centri eterici secondo l'antroposofia." https://docplayer.it/11102837-Chakra-astrali-e-centri-eterici-secondo-l-antroposofia.html.

Caligiuri, L. M. 2022. "Che cos'è l'Entanglement." Blog on the *Scienza Conoscenza* website,

August 29, 2022. https://www.scienzaeconoscenza.it/blog/scienza_e_fisica_quantistica/cos-e-entanglement-meccanica-quantistica.

Capocci, M., and R. Costa. 2015. "Ricci, geni ed epigenetica." *Le Scienze,* August 3, 2015. http://www.lescienze.it/archivio/articoli/2015/08/03/news/ricci_geni_ed_epigenetica-2713108/.

Carmignani, U. 2018. "La sindrome del gemello scomparso." https://www.lacittadellaluce.org/it/notizia/2018/04/13/la-sindrome-del-gemello-scomparso.

Cavalcanti, G. 2018. "Nel cervello si 'viaggia' con la fibra ottica. Parlano I ricercatori italiani pubblicati su Nature." https://www.sanitainformazione.it/salute/cervello-fibra-ottica-ricercatori-nature/7.

Cavaleri, P. A. 2003. *La profondità della superficie. Percorsi introduttivi alla psicoterapia della Gestalt.* Milan: Franco Angeli.

Cenacolo di Andrea. 2015. "Tutto è vibrazione–come il suono e frequenze influenzano il nostro corpo." http://infocenacolo.altervista.org/linfluenza-del-suono-e-delle-vibrazioni-sul-nostro-corpo/.

Centro Studi Eva Reich. n.d. "Il perché delle emozioni che proviamo." http://www.enzasansone.it/download/emozioni_perche.pdf.

Chetta, G. 2008. "Stress e benessere–educazione mentale nell'ambito della psico-neuro-endocrino-connettivo immunologia." https://www.giovannichetta.it/documentaz/stress_benessere_giovanni_chetta.pdf.

Cieloevento editorial staff. 2015. "I Ching for Daphne—hexagram 7.2." *Cielovento* (blog), December 1, 2015. http://cieloevento.blogspot.com/2015/12/i-ching-per-dafne-esagramma-72-2.html.

Cilento, F. 2018. "L'intelligenza intuitiva e il ruolo delle emozioni per la crescita dell'io." http://www.crescita-personale.it/intelligenza/950/intelligenza-intuitiva.html/.

Cipolla, C. M. 2002. "Le leggi fondamentali della stupidità umana." http://www.giovis.com/cipolla.htm.

Ciranna-Raab, C., and A. Manzotti. 2019. *La medicina osteopatica in pediatria.* Milan: Edra.

Consapevoli.net. 2014. "La teoria del tutto di NassimHaramein." http://www.consapevoli.net/la-teoria-del-tutto-di-nassim-haramein.php.

Cotov, M. n.d. "Le emozioni distruttive." https://www.criticamentepsi.it/unipi/articolo/le-emozioni-distruttive.

Covey, Stephen R. 1989. *The 7 Habits of Highly Effective People: Powerful Lessons in Personal Change.* New York: Free Press.

Cremaschini, M. 2018. "Il thin-slicing o giudizio intuitivo." http://www.marilenacremaschini.it/il-thin-slicing-o-giudizio-intuitivo/.

Crepaldi, F. 2013. "Alle origini della sonoterapia." https://www.cicap.org/n/articolo.php?id=275550.

Crotti, E. 2010. "Cimatica: interazione tra corpo e suono." https://www.musica-spirito.it/musica-scienza/cimatica-corpo-suono/.

Crotti, E. 2014. "Cimatica: lo studio delle onde sonore." https://www.musica-spirito.it/guarigione-2/cimatica-studio-delle-onde-sonore/.

D'Alisa, P. 2016. "Morire costantemente a se stessi." https://giardinaggiointeriore.net/morire-costantemente-a-se-stessi/.

Dato, D. 2016. "Emozioni e preoccupazione empatica. Una via pedagogica per imparare a prestare attenzione al mondo." https://hdl.handle.net/11369/341406.

De Fanis, F. 2017. "L'horror vacui nell'epoca dei social network tra arte, filosofia e psicologia." http://www.artspecialday.com/9art/2017/11/15/horror-vacui-social-network/.

Di Corpo, U., and A. Vannini. 2010. "Sintropia: una terza via nel dibattito sull'evoluzione.: https://www.ariannaeditrice.it/articolo.php?id_articolo=30406.

Di Giorgi, P. 2016. "Fisica quantistica e processi mentali." http://www.istitutoeuroarabo.it/DM/fisica-quantistica-e-processi-mentali/.

Di Giovanni, A. 2009. *Il mondo dell'acustica e della Psicoacustica. Scenari applicativi.* Lulu Editore.

Di Muro, C. 2018. "Il fenomeno della polarità: dall'universo alle nostre emozioni." Blog on the *Scienza Conoscenza* website, January 2, 2018. https://www.scienzaeconoscenza.it/blog/psicologia-quantistica/fenomeno-della-polarita.

Di Renzo Editore. n.d. "Entropia e Informazione." https://www.direnzo.it/it/energia-entropia.

Di Stefano, M. 2013. "Candace Pert: la golden girl delle neuroscienze." https://www.medicinaintegratanews.it/candace-pert-la-golden-girl-delle-neuroscienze/.

Edelstein, A. 2006. "Cos'è l'ego? Intervista a James Hollis su Jung." https://www.ariannaeditrice.it/articolo.php?id_articolo=1641.

Educazione & Scuola. 2013. "Neuroscienze: 'il peso emotivo.'" http://www.edscuola.it/archivio/interlinea/neuroscienze.htm.

eLEAS. 2016. "Levels of Emotional Awareness Scale." https://eleastest.net/the-levels-of-emotional-awareness-scale.

Eliade, M. 1999. *Lo yoga: immortalità e libertà.* Milan: Biblioteca Universitaria Rizzoli.

Epicurus. n.d. "Epicurus: Letter to Menoeceus." https://newepicurean.com/suggested-reading/letter-to-menoeceus/.

Ergymax. n.d. "Approfondimento: vibrazione e polarità cellulare." http://www.medika.it/ergymax/prodotti/lega-ergymax-bozza/approfondimento-vibrazione-e-polarita-cellulare/.

Essere Il Cambiamento. 2012. "Il toroide." https://www.essereilcambiamento.it/il-toroide.

Fairymoon [pseud.]. 2013. "Chakra secondari." *Moonboulevard* (blog). https://moonboulevard.wordpress.com/2013/07/01/chakra-secondari/.

Fanpage.it. 2018. "Che cosa significa frattale, il termine che ha messo in crisi gli studenti al Test di medicina 2018."

Fatica, A. 2017. *Epigenetica: il complesso mondo della regolazione genica.* Rome: Carocci Editore.

Fattiroso, M. 2014. "La memoria cellulare: le cellule, gli organismi, il corpo e l'acqua." https://www.crescita-personale.it/articoli/competenze/intelligenza/memoria-cellulare.html.

Fayenz, D. 2012. "Chakras mantra e mandala." https://www.riflessioni.it/teosofia/chakras-mantra-mandala.htm.

Ferrucci, Piero. 2009. *Crescere: teoria e pratica della psicosintesi.* Rome: Astrolabio Ubaldini.

Ferrucci, Piero. 2014. *La nuova volontà: un'indagine teorica e pratica.* Rome: Astrolabio Ubaldini.

Fey, A. 2010. "Comprendere la morte, accompagnare la vita." https://www.angefey.it/attivita/formazione/comprendere-la-morte-accompagnare-la-vita.

Figari, R. 2016. "Appunti sui vettori." Edited by Alberto Clarizia. University of Naples Federico Department of Physics. http://people.na.infn.it/~clarizia/appunti_sui_vettori.pdf.

Filosoficamente. 2016. "Eraclito: il divenire e l'unità degli opposti." https://filosoficamente.altervista.org/123-2/.

Fiscaletti, D. 2016. "Che cos'è il suono?" Blog on the *Scienza Conoscenza* website, January 1, 2016. https://www.scienzaeconoscenza.it/blog/scienza_e_fisica_quantistica/che-cos-e-il-suono-in-fisica.

FisicaQuantistica.it. 2013. "Memorie cellulari." https://www.fisicaquantistica.it/fisica-quantistica/memorie-cellulari.

Folino, F., A. Onorati, and D. Sepe. 2018. "Pensare positivo." https://www.neuroscienze.net/pensare-positivo/.

Forestiero, S. 2007. "Evoluzione biologica: quadro generale." https://www.treccani.it/enciclopedia/evoluzione-biologica-quadro-generale_%28Enciclopedia-della-Scienza-e-della-Tecnica%29/.

Fotia, F. 2018. "Ricerca, memoria cellulare: così il nostro corpo si ricorda come combattere le malattie." http://www.meteoweb.eu/2018/01/ricerca-memoria-cellulare-cosi-il-nostro-corpo-si-ricorda-come-combattere-le-malattie/1029639/.

Frattini, I. 2019. "Le neuroscienze e la regolazione affettiva." http://www.esserecon.it/2019/10/05/le-neuroscienze-e-la-regolazione-affettiva/.

Friedrich, C. 2001. *Scritti sull'arte.* Translated by L. Rubini. Milan: Abscondita.

Galimberti, U. 1999. *Psicologia.* Turin: Garzanti.

Galimberti, U. 2005. "Se il dolore si mostra in televisione." https://www.feltrinellieditore.it/news/2002/07/17/umberto-galimberti-se-il-dolore-si-mostra-in-televisione-255/.

Garaventa, R. 2017. "Equivocità del nulla in Karl Jaspers." http://www.consecutio.org/2017/04/equivocita-del-nulla-in-karl-jaspers/.

Gardini, S. 2018. "Epigenetica: come l'ambiente e il menoma si influenzano a vicenda." https://www.genomeup.com/2018/07/30/epigenetica-come-lambiente-e-il-genoma-si-influenzano-vicenda/.

Gazzola, F. 2003. "Antiriduzionismo." http://www.naturalismedicina.it/articolo.asp?i=373.

Gelati, M. A. 2013. "Vita e morte, meglio prenderle con filosofia." https://www.ilfattoquotidiano.it/2013/12/20/vita-e-morte-meglio-prenderle-con-filosofia/820932/.

Geymonat, L. 1970. *Storia del pensiero filosofico e scientifico.* Milan: Garzanti Editore.

Giardi, D. 2017. "Il Big Bang della musica: la nascita del suono nella storia dell'uomo." https://auralcrave.com/2017/03/06/il-big-bang-della-musica/.

Giardinaggio Interiore. 2016. "Morire costantemente a se stessi." https://giardinaggiointeriore.net/morire-costantemente-a-se-stessi/.

Goethe, Johann Wolfgang von. 1908. *The Maxims and Reflections of Goethe.* Translated by T. B. Saunders. 2nd rev. ed. London: Macmillan and Co.

Goleman, Daniel. 2009. "'Empathy'—Who's Got It, Who Does Not." *HuffPost,* June 2, 2009. https://www.huffpost.com/entry/empathy-whos-got-it-who_b_195178.

Goleman, D., and Dalai Lama. 2003. *Emozioni distruttive* [*Destructive Emotions*]. Translated by R. Cagliero. Milan: Mondadori

Gramsci, A. 2014. *Quaderni del carcere.* Milan: Einaudi.

Grassi Zucconi, G. 2000. "Ritmo biologico." http://www.treccani.it/enciclopedia/ritmo-biologico_%28Universo-del-Corpo%29/.

Guardini, R. 1997. "Opposizione polare (estratti)." https://ilcristo.it/images/stories/Opposizione_polare.doc.

Guazzelli, M., and A. Gemignani. 2012. *Stress e disturbi da somatizzazione.* Milan: Sprinter.

Head, S., and A. Librale. n.d. "Armonic Overtones. Brevi accenni di storia del suono." http://www.eurekacentro.com/files/armonicovertones.pdf.

HealthQE. 2017. "Quantum Electodynamic Coherence." http://www.healthqe.cloud/2017/02/19/hello-world/.

Hegel, G. W. F. 1977. *Phenomenology of Spirit*. Oxford, U.K.: Oxford University Press.

Holmes, T., and R. Rahe. 1967. "The Social Readjustment Rating Scale." *Journal of Psychosomatic Research* 11 (2): 213–18.

HumanTrainer. n.d. "John Bowlby." http://www.humantrainer.com/wiki/John-Bowlby.html.

Huxley, Aldous. 1933. *Texts and Pretexts: An Anthology with Commentary*. New York and London: Harper & Brothers.

Il Diogene. n.d. "Antonio Damasio." http://www.filosofico.net/damasioantonio.htm.

In Arte Salus. 2019. "Emiliano Toso, il biologo molecolare che scopre il potere della sua musica." http://www.inartesalus.it/2019/07/31/emiliano-toso-il-biologo-molecolare-che-scopre-il-potere-della-sua-musica/.

Istituto A. T. Beck. n.d. "La via neuroendronica: il ruolo dell'asse ipotalamo-ipofisi-surrene nel trauma." https://www.istitutobeck.com/via-neuroendocrina-trauma.

Istituto di Gestalt HCC Italia. 2012. "Il now-for-next in psicoterapia–La società della Gestalt raccontata nella società post-moderna." http://www.gestalt.it/it/libri-psicologia-psicoterapia-teoria-gestalt-clinica-psichiatria/presentazione_libro/100.pdf.

Istituto Psicoterapia Gestalt Espressiva. n.d. "La Gestalt espressiva." https://www.psicoterapiadellagestalt.it/psicoterapia-della-gestalt.

Jendrzej, E. 2009. "Fare esperienza di se stessi: fra soggettività e oggettività." *3D* 6(2): 120–30. http://www.isfo.it/files/File/2009/Jendrzej09.pdf.

Jung, C. G. 1949. "Foreword." (Foreword to the I Ching.) https://www.iging.com/intro/foreword.htm.

Jung, Carl. 1970. "Psychological Aspects of the Mother Archetype." Lecture, 1938, reproduced in *Four Archetypes: Mother, Rebirth, Spirit, Trickster,* translated by R. F. C. Hull. Princeton, N.J.: Princeton University Press.

Jung, C. G. 2014. *Civilization in Transition*. Vol. 10 of *C. G. Jung: The Collected Works*. Translated by R. F. C. Hull. New York: Routledge.

Kelly, K. 2009. "Extropy." http://kk.org/thetechnium/extropy/.

Kübler-Ross, E. 2009. *On Death and Dying: What the Dying Have to Teach Doctors, Nurses, Clergy and Their Own Families*. Abingdon, U.K.: Routledge.

Kundera, Milan. 1984. *The Unbearable Lightness of Being*. Translated by M. H. Heim. New York: Harper & Row.

La Mente è Meravigliosa. 2019. "L'intuito è l'anima che ci parla." *La Mente è Meravigliosa* (blog), October 15, 2019. https://lamenteemeravigliosa.it/intuito-anima-ci-parla/.

Lansberger, N., and C. Kilstrup-Nielsen. 2008. "Epigenetica." *Enciclopedia della Scienza e della Tecnica* (online). http://www.treccani.it/enciclopedia/epigenetica_%28Enciclopedia-della-Scienza-e-della-Tecnica%29/.

Latrofa, A. 2019. "Numerologia evolutiva dei Tarocchi Jodorowsky." https://www.cristobaljodorowsky.it/numerologia-evolutiva-dei-tarocchi-jodorowsky/.

Leotta, V. 2019. "Ritmo circadiano, il nostro orologio biologico." https://violettaleottalim.com/2019/01/09/ritmo-circadiano-orologio-biologico/.

Le Scienze. 2012. "Dai neonati ai centenari, cosa cambia nelle cellule." *Le Scienze,* June 13, 2012. http://www.lescienze.it/news/2012/06/13/news/epigenoma_epigenetica_neonato_centenario_invecchiamento_metilazione_cambiamento_espressione_geni-1085236/.

Le Scienze. 2017. "I circuiti cerebrali dell'empatia e della cura." *Le Scienze,* June 8, 2017. http://www.lescienze.it/news/2017/06/08/news/circuiti_cerebrali_empatia_sofferenza_cura_-_embargo_h_18-3558423/.

Levi-Montalcini, R. 2017. *Elogio dell'imperfezione.* Milan: Baldini Castoldi.

Licata, I. 2013. "Teoria degli Universi e Sintropia. Luigi Fantappié, ricordo di un matematico." *Altro Giornale,* August 10, 2013. https://www.altrogiornale.org/teoria-degli-universi-e-sintropia-luigi-fantappia-ricordo-di-un-matematico/.

Liucci, R. 2018. "Sulla morte e i suoi luoghi comuni." http://www.accademiametafisica.com/sulla-morte-e-i-suoi-luoghi-comuni/.

Lorenz, K. 2017. *Il decline dell'uomo.* Milan: Piano B.

Losa, G. A. 2017. "La geometria frattale in biologia." http://www.ticinolive.ch/2017/01/29/la-geometria-frattale-biologia-medicina-gabriele-losa/.

Losa, G. A. 2019. "Leonardo da Vinci: se la pittura è scienza o no." http://www.ticinolive.ch/2019/05/01/leonardo-da-vinci-se-la-pittura-e-scienza-o-no/.

Lucarelli, G. 2015. "La verità, vi prego, su emisfero destro, emisfero sinistro e creatività." https://www.wired.it/scienza/2015/04/30/emisfero-destro-sinistro-creativita/.

Lunghi, C., F. Baroni, and M. Alò. 2017. *Il ragionamento clinico osteopatico. Trattamento salutogenico e approcci progressivi individuali.* Milan: Edra.

Magicamente Colibrì. 2018. "Candace Pert e le molecole di emozioni: la biologia degli stati della mente." http://www.magicamentecolibri.it/wordpress/candace-pert-e-le-molecole-di-emozioni-la-biologia-degli-stati-della-mente/.

Mancuso, V. 2007. "Il silenzio interiore e l'esperienza dello spirito." https://lapoesiaelospirito.wordpress.com/2007/06/26/il-silenzio-secondo-vito-mancuso/.

Mancuso, V. 2017. *Il bisogno di pensare.* Milan: Garzanti.

Manzelli, P. 2017. "Biofotoni e la vita." http://www.edscuola.eu/wordpress/wp-content/uploads/2017/06/BIOVITA.pdf.

Manzelli, P. 2018a. "Biologia quantica: biofotoni e biofononi." http://www.edscuola.eu/wordpress/?p=100607.

Manzelli, P. 2018b. "Energia elettromagnetica nella medicina energetica e per la biologia quantica." http://www.edscuola.eu/wordpress/?p=99980.

Manzelli, P. 2018c. "Epigenetica delle relazioni quantiche mente-cervello." http://www.bioquantica.org/epigenetica-delle-relazioni-quantiche-tra-mente-cervello/.

Manzelli, P. 2018d. "Il suono e i suoi effetti." https://www.neuroscienze.net/il-suono-e-i-suoi-effetti/.

Manzelli, P. 2018e. "Le tracce mnesiche." https://www.edscuola.eu/wordpress/?p=100410.

Manzelli, P. 2018f. "Suono, voce, fononi." https://www.edscuola.eu/wordpress/?p=99019.

Mapelli, M. 2014. "Riassunto il dolore che trasforma. Attraversare l'esperienza della perdita e del lutto." https://www.studocu.com/it/document/universita-degli-studi-di-milano-bicocca/educazione-permanente-e-degli-adulti/riassunti/riassunto-il-dolore-che-trasforma-attraversare-lesperienza-della-perdita-e-del-lutto/470988/view.

Mastrobisi, G. J. 2017. "Il virtuale della fenomenologia nella fisica: temporalità e cinestesi alla prova della teoria della relatività. Dai manoscritti di Einstein e Husserl." http://www.scienzaefilosofia.com/wp-content/uploads/2018/03/res710647_03-MASTROBISI-1.pdf.

Mastronardi, Luigi. 2016. *La mente che guarisce. Tecniche psicologiche per favorire la salute.* Turin: Edizioni L'Etàdell'Acquario.

Mattalucci, C., and L. Pinkus. 2000. "Lutto–universo del corpo." http://www.treccani.it/enciclopedia/lutto_%28Universo-del-Corpo%29/.

Mauri, M. 2018. "La 'doppia via' di LeDoux: i due diversi modi di reagire agli stimoli del cervello." https://www.tsw.it/journal/ricerca/doppia-via-ledoux-come-reagisce-cervello-a-stimoli/.

Mayer, G. 2019. "Empatia e simpatia." http://www.giuliamayer.it/empatia-e-simpatia/.

Mazzocchi, A. 2011. "Morire di paura. Perché non dobbiamo temere la morte." http://www.informasalus.it/it/articoli/morire-di-paura.php.

McMahon, P. 1993. *The Grand Design: Reflections of a Soul/Oversoul.* New York: Regency Press.

Minotti, R. 2018. "L'entropia della mente." https://www.neuroscienze.net/gestalt-e-fisica-quantistica/.

Miranda, C. 2014. "Oltre la polarità, l'equilibrio nell'integrazione." http://tuttosottoilcielo.com/oltre-le-polarita/.

Mistretta, R. n.d. "La spirale cosmica: sezione aurea dell'universo." No longer available, originally published on the Bocconi website.

Montalto, P. 2010. "Discutere oggi sull'essere e il divenire a partire da Parmenide e Eraclito." http://www.literary.it/dati/literary/m/montalto_pasquale/discutere_oggi_sullessere.html.

Morandi, A. 2018. "Good Vibrations o God Vibrations?" https://www.ayurvedicpoint.it/storia-dell-ayurveda/618-good-vibrations-o-god-vibrations.

More, M. 1998. "The Extropian Principles. Version 3.0: A Transhumanist Declaration." https://mrob.com/pub/religion/extro_prin.html.

Moreau, P., E. Toninelli, T. Gregory, R. R. Aspden, P. A. Morris, and M. J. Padgett. 2019. "Imaging Bell-type nonlocal behavior." *Science Advances* 5(7): eaaw2563.

Munch, E. 2002. *Il grido: scritti sull/arte e sull/amore.* Pistoia: Via del Vento Edizioni.

Musto, R. n.d. "Elementi di riflessione sulla psicoacustica." https://www.esonet.it/News-file-categories-op-newindex-catid-91.html.

Oliveri, D. 2006. "Cos'è la polarità cellulare?" https://www.vialattea.net/content/2433/.

Onelli, A. 2013. [The evolutionary path of our mind: Multidisciplinarity and Multiculturality in the helping relationship]. Rome: Armando Editore.

Ostaseki, F. 2006. *Saper accompagnare.* Translated by Letizia Baglioni. Milan: Mondadori.

Pacilli, A. M. 2017. "La paura della morte è paura della vita? Riflessioni in filosofia." https://www.nelfuturo.com/paura-della-morte-paura-della-vita.

Pagliaro, G. 2016. "Buddismo, fisica quantistica e guarigione." Blog on the *Scienza Conoscenza* website, January 1, 2016. https://www.scienzaeconoscenza.it/blog/consapevolezza-spiritualita/buddhismo-fisica-quantistica-e-guarigione.

Palumbo, M. 2016. "Il lutto: fasi, reazioni e trattamento." *State of Mind* (online), November 4, 2016. https://www.stateofmind.it/2016/11/lutto-reazioni-trattamento/.

Pannocchia, A., F. Pavone, et al. 2013. *Analisi delle migliori pratiche e tecnologie disponibili nei settori della misurazione e registrazione del rumore e in quello della psicoacustica. Introduzione alla psicoacustica e ai possibili campi di impiego nell'acustica ambientale.* Turin: Provincia di Torino Area Risorse Idriche e Qualità dell'Aria and ARPA Piemonte Dipartimento Provinciale di Torino.

Paparoni, D. 1982. *Mimmo Paladino e il pane.* Vicenza: Neri Pozza.

Pascal, B. 1932. *Pascal's Pensées.* Translated by W. F. Trotter. London: Dent & Sons.

Pascale, F. n.d. "La riarmonizzazione energetica e i chakra." http://www.dhyana.it/benessere/riarmonizzazione-energetica/445.

Pasin, C. 2016. "La sindrome del gemello superstite: quando i concepimenti non si conoscono." https://www.eticamente.net/49913/la-sindrome-del-gemello-superstite-quando-i-concepimenti-non-si-conoscono.html.

Pastel, R. H. 2016. "Upledger CranioSacral Immersion Report for Dr. John E. Upledger Program for Military Post-Traumatic Stress." https://www.upledger.com/docs/2016-CranioSacral-Immersion-Program-Results.pdf.

Paternoster, R. 2016. "Dall'uovo del mondo all'uovo pasquale." http://www.storiain.net/storia/dalluovo-del-mondo-alluovo-pasquale/.

Pert, C. B. 1988. "The Wisdom of the Receptors: Neuropeptides, the Emotions, and Bodymind." *Advances* 8, no. 8 (Summer): 8-16. https://candacepert.com/wp-content/uploads/2017/07/Advances-v8-198-Wisdom-of-the-Receptors1.pdf.

Pomodoro, A. 2014. *Forma, segno, spazio.* Edited by Stefano Esengrini. Falciano: Maretti.

Pompas, M. 2017. "La magia del suono." https://www.karmanews.it/16406/la-magia-del-suono/.

Pompas, R. 2013. "Rudolf Steiner: il pensiero, il colore, l'arte." https://www.karmanews.it/71/rudolf-steiner-il-pensiero-il-colore-larte/.

Psicologi Junghiani. 2011. "La teoria della personalità secondo Jung." https://psicologijunghiani.wordpress.com/2011/07/19/la-teoria-della-personalita-secondo-jung/.

Psychiatry on line Italia. 2013. "Scale di valutazione: Eventi psicosociali stressanti." http://www.psychiatryonline.it/node/3677.

Pulvirenti, E. 2016. "Tutta l'arte attorno all'uovo." https://www.didatticarte.it/Blog/?p=5575.

Rasini, V. 2018. "Antropologia della soggettività. Il destino dell'ente "patico" e l'uomo." http://www.scienzaefilosofia.com/2018/03/25/antropologia-della-soggettivita-il-destino-dellente-patico-e-luomo/.

Ravasi, G. 2012. "La salvezza in una cifra." https://www.avvenire.it/agora/pagine/bibbiaenumeri.

Riflessioni.it. n.d. "Entropia." *Dizionario Filosofico.* https://www.riflessioni.it/dizionario_filosofico/entropia.htm.

Riggs, A. D., R. A. Martienssen, and V. E. A. Russo. 1996. "Introduction." In *Epigenetic Mechanisms of Gene Regulation,* edited by V. E. A. Russo, et al., 1–4. Cold Spring Harbor, N.Y.: Cold Spring Harbor Laboratory Press.

Rispoli, L. 1987. "La vegetoterapia carattero-analitica e il caso di Emma." *Psicoterapia e Scienze Umane* 4. http://www.lucianorispoli.it/745-2/.

Rispoli, L. 2017. "Neuroni specchio in psicoterapia." http://www.lucianorispoli.it/luciano-rispoli-neuroni-a-specchio-in-psicoterapia.

Rita, V. 2019. "Ecco la prima immagine dell'entanglement quantistico." *Wired.* https://www.wired.it/scienza/lab/2019/07/15/prima-immagine-entanglement-quantistico/.

Riza.it. n.d. "Cos'è l'ego? Ego significato psicologico." https://www.riza.it/psicologia/tu/6766/ego-cos-e-il-vero-significato-in-psicologia.html.

Riza.it. n.d. "Emisfero destro e sinistro del cervello." https://www.riza.it/psicologia/tu/2368/cervello-emisfero-destro-e-sinistro.html.

Robbins, Tony. 1991. *Awaken the Giant Within: How to Take Immediate Control of Your Mental, Emotional, Physical & Financial Difficulties.* New York: Summit Books.

Romanò, N. 2017. "Tieni il tempo: una breve introduzione ai ritmi biologici." https://www.fondazioneveronesi.it/magazine/i-blog-della-fondazione/il-blog-di-airicerca/tieni-il-tempo-una-breve-introduzione-ai-ritmi-biologici.

Sabater, Valeria. 2021. "Neurobiologia dell'intuito: I presentimenti." *La Mente è Meravigliosa* (blog), November 15, 2021. https://lamenteemeravigliosa.it/neurobiologia-dellintuito-i-presentimenti/.

Sacchetti, A. 2018. "La coerente unità e diversità della vita." http://www.associazione-eco.it/362-2/.

Salgado, Sebastião. 2016. *Kuwait: un deserto in fiamme*. Edited by Lélia Wanick Salgado. Taschen.

Sapere.it. n.d. "I principi primi e l'intelligenza suprema: Uno, Diade e Demiurgo." http://www.sapere.it/sapere/strumenti/studiafacile/filosofia/La-filosofia-antica/Platone/I-principi-primi-e-l-intelligenza-suprema-Uno-Diade-e-Demiurgo.html7.

Sapere.it. n.d. "Polarità." http://www.sapere.it/enciclopedia/polarit%C3%A0.html.

Sapere.it. 2004. "Energia: consumo e produzione." http://www.sapere.it/sapere/medicina-e-salute/il-medico-risponde/guida-alla-Biologia-cellulare/la-cellula/Fisiologia-cellulare/energia-consumo-e-produzione.html.

Savardi, M. 2015. "Dare un senso al lutto: perché il lutto non diventi una perdita di senso." http://maurosavardi.altervista.org/joomla/78-home/lutto/165-dare-un-senso-al-lutto-perche-il-lutto-non-diventi-una-perdita-del-senso.

Sgarrella, M. C. n.d. "PNEI: psico-neuro-endocrino-immunologia." https://www.amadeux.net/sublimen/dossier/psiconeuroendocrinoimmunologia___pnei.html.

Signorini, G. F. 2005. "L'entropia è disordine?" http://www.chim.unifi.it/~signo/did/etc/entropia/entropia.pdf.

Silva, A. 2016. "I pensieri sono energia, intervista a Bruce Lipton." Blog on the *Scienza Conoscenza* website, January 1, 2016. https://www.scienzaeconoscenza.it/blog/medicina-non_convenzionale/bruce-lipton-pensieri-cellule-energia-ambiente.

Silvestrini, P. 2017. "Sincronicità ed entanglement quantistico." https://www.paolosilvestrini.com/sincronicita-ed-entanglement-quantistico/.

Simone, M. 2014. "Disturbo post-traumatico da stress." https://www.nienteansia.it/articoli-di-psicologia/atri-argomenti/disturbo-post-traumatico-da-stress/8628/.

Skuola.net. n.d. "Husserl, Edmund - Fenomenologia (3)." https://www.skuola.net/filosofia-contemporanea/edmund-husserl-fenomenologia.html.

Solms, M., and O. Turnbull. 2002. *The Brain and the Inner World: An Introduction to the Neuroscience of Subjective Experience*. New York: Other Press.

Stefanelli, M. n.d. "Cakra, chakra e chakras: i vortici di energia vitale." https://www.amadeux.net/sublimen/dossier/chakras_onde_e_risonanza.html.

Stranieri, D., and R. Tulli. n.d. "Il sistema energetico e i corpi sottili." http://digilander.libero.it/isolachenonce/terapie/bioenergetica/chakra/sistema_energ.html.

Stranieri, D., and R. Tulli. n.d. "I corpi sottili." https://digilander.libero.it/isolachenonce/terapie/bioenergetica/chakra/corpi_sottili.html.

Terzani, T. 2018a. *Un altro giro di giostra*. TEA.

———. 2018b. *Un indovino mi disse*. TEA.

———. 2019a. *Un idea di destino*. TEA.

———. 2019b. *Lettere contro la guerra*. TEA.

———. 2021. *La fine è il mio inizio*. Longanesi.

Three Initiates [pseud.]. 1908. *The Kybalion*. As reproduced in "The Kybalion Chapter II: The Seven Hermetic Principles." http://www.kybalion.org/kybalion.php?chapter=II.

Toffler, Alvin. 1970. *Future Shock*. New York: Random House.

Tradizione Sacra. n.d. "L'anatomia energetica umana." http://www.tradizionesacra.it/anatomia_energetica_umana.htm.

Treacy, I. 2016. "La polarità come strutura del reale." Loescher.

Treccani. n.d. "Entelechia." http://www.treccani.it/enciclopedia/entelechia/.

Treccani. n.d. "Fonone." http://www.treccani.it/enciclopedia/fonone/.

Treccani. n.d. "Polarità." http://www.treccani.it/enciclopedia/polarita/.

Treccani. 2010a. "HPA (sigla dell'ingl. Hypothalamic-Pituitary-Adrenal axis, asse ipotalamo-ipofisi-surrene)." *Dizionario di Medicina*. http://www.treccani.it/enciclopedia/hpa-sigla-dell-ingl-hypothalamic-pituitary-adrenal-axis-asse-ipotalamo-ipofisi-surrene_%28Dizionario-di-Medicina%29/.

Treccani. 2010b. "Ovocito (o ovocita)." *Dizionario di Medicina*. http://www.treccani.it/enciclopedia/ovocito_%28Dizionario-di-Medicina%29/.

Treccani. 2010c. "Propriocezione." *Dizionario di Medicina*. http://www.treccani.it/enciclopedia/propriocezione_(Dizionario-di-Medicina)/.

Treccani. 2013. "Yoga." *Lessico del XXI Secolo*. http://www.treccani.it/enciclopedia/yoga_%28Lessico-del-XXI-Secolo%29/.

Trevisani, D. 2013. "Aristotele–ethos, logos, pathos–le tre categorie di analisi della comunicazione persuasiva, del primo vero scienziato della comunicazione." https://studiotrevisani.it/2013/10/08/aristotele-ethos-logos-pathos-le-tre-categorie-di-analisi-della-comunicazione-persuasiva-del-primo-vero-scienziato-della-comunicazione/.

Troiano, R. 2002. "La teoria analitica di Carl Gustav Jung." https://www.viaggio-in-germania.de/jung.html.

Uberti, M. n.d. "Psicoacustica." http://www.maurouberti.it/psicoacustica/psico acustica.html.

Unilibro. 2018. "Suono quantico." Special issue, *Scienza e conoscenza* 66. https://www.unilibro.it/libro/scienza-e-conoscenza-vol-66-suono-quantico/9788878694699.

University of Turin Department of Geology. n.d. *Le vibrazione nei cristalli*. https://geologia.campusnet.unito.it/didattica/att/7a8e.0278.file.pdf.

Upledger, J. E. 1987. *CranioSacral Therapy II: Beyond the Dura*. Seattle: Eastland Press.

Upledger, J. E. 1990. *SomatoEmotional Release and Beyond*. Palm Beach Gardens: UI Publishers.

Upledger, J. E. 1997. *Your Inner Physician and You*. Berkeley, Calif.: North Atlantic Books.

Upledger, J. E. 2010a. *A Brain Is Born: Exploring the Birth and Development of the Central Nervous System*. Berkeley, Calif.: North Atlantic Books.

Upledger, J. E. 2010b. *Cell Talk: Transmitting Mind into DNA*. Berkeley, Calif.: North Atlantic Books.

Upledger, J. E., and J. D. Vredevoogd. 1983. *CranioSacral Therapy*. Seattle: Eastland Press.

Vadalà, G. 2004. "Il benessere come equilibrio tra le polarità psicocorporee." http://www.drvadala.it/articoli/11-psicologia/26-il-benessere-come-equilibrio-tra-le-polarita-psicocorporee.html.

Vadi, M. 2016. "I ricordi traumatici vengono registrati nella memoria cellulare." https://www.generazionebio.com/notizie/7014-ricordi-traumatici-memoria-cellulare.html.

Valcarenghi, M. 2014. "Il cambiamento e l'arte di saper andare via." https://www.ilfattoquotidiano.it/2014/11/08/il-cambiamento-e-larte-di-saper-andare-via/1200509/.

Valentino, V. 2017. "Neurobiologia delle emozioni: le strutture neurali implicate nella regolazione emotiva." *State of Mind* (online), December 20, 2017. https://www.stateofmind.it/2017/12/neurobiologia-emozioni/.

Valesini, S. 2016. "L'intuizione 'batte' il ragionamento analitico." *La Repubblica,* April 4, 2016.

Vannini, A. 2006. "Capitolo 4: energia negativa, sintropia e sistemi viventi." *Syntropy* 3: 70–78. http://www.sintropia.it/journal/italiano/2006-it-3-05.pdf.

Vecchia, A. 2017. "L'entropia." https://www.cosediscienza.it/entropia.

Venuti, P. 2012. "Frattali e caos in medicina." http://www.studiodentisticovenuti.it/2012/12/30/frattali-caos/.

Viglienghi, V. n.d. "Il mistero dell'ovoide di Assagioli." https://www.psicoenergetica.it/scritti/Il%20mistero%20dell'Ovoide%20di%20Assagioli.doc.

Vinci, M. 2012. "Le Uova." http://eurekariflessioni.blogspot.com/2012/02/biologia-dello-sviluppo-parte-i-le-uova.html.

Wallis, H. 2016. "The Real Story on the Chakras." Christopher Wallis personal blog, February 5, 2016. https://hareesh.org/blog/2016/2/5/the-real-story-on-the-chakras.

White, D. G. 2003. *Kiss of the Yogini: "Tantric Sex" in Its South Asian Contexts.* Chicago: University of Chicago Press.

Wikiwand. n.d. "Omeostasi." https://www.wikiwand.com/it/Omeostasi.

Wilde, Oscar. 1909. *De Profundis.* New York: G. P. Putnam's Sons.

Wolfe, A. 2017. "An Expert Take on Performing under Pressure." *Wall Street Journal,* February 3, 2017.

Zilio, F. 2016. "Tra riduzionismo e antiriduzionismo. Lo statuto della neurofilosofia e il contributo di Georg Northoff." http://tesi.cab.unipd.it/56251/1/Tra_riduzionismo_e_antiriduzionismo_-_Federico_Zilio.pdf.

Figure Credits

Dedication. Dr. John E. Upledger and Dr. Diego Maggio, courtesy of Upledger Institute International

Contents. Dr. Diego Maggio courtesy of Upledger Institute International

Preface. Dr. Diego Maggio in Liverpool; *artist*: T. Keber

Preface. Dr. John E. Upledger, courtesy of Upledger Institute International

Fig. I.1. Dr. John E. Upledger with photo of Diego Maggio's graduation *artist*: Angelica D'onofrio, courtesy of Diego Maggio

Fig. 1.1. The craniosacral system, courtesy of Upledger Institute International

Fig. 1.2. *Vitruvian Man,* by Leonardo da Vinci; *source*: Wikiwand

Fig. 2.1. From atom to human being; *artist*: T. Keber, courtesy of Upledger Italia, partially a reproduction of the Pixabay image 254133

Fig. 3.1. The Third Space in the patient/Facilitator relationship; *artist*: T. Keber, courtesy of Upledger Italia

Fig. 3.2. Reproduction of *Eye with a View*; *artist*: T. Keber, adapted from the original by Salvador Dalí

Fig. 4.1. The three cranial vault holds; *artist*: Frank Lowen, courtesy of Upledger Institute International

Fig. 4.2. Evaluation with the Arcing technique, courtesy of Upledger Italia

Fig. 4.3. Energy Cyst and the vibrational field; *artist*: T. Keber, adapted from a Microone–Freepik image

Fig. 4.4. Evaluation with the Significance Detector, courtesy of Upledger Italia

Fig. 4.5. Therapeutic Imagery and Dialogue, courtesy of Upledger Italia

Fig. 4.6. Diagram of the vector/axis system; *artist*: T. Keber, adapted from Freepik image 766045

Fig. 4.7. Reproduction of *The Song of Love*; *artist*: T. Keber, adapted from the original by Giorgio de Chirico

Fig. 4.8. *Over the Town,* by Marc Chagall; *source*: Wikiart

Fig. 5.1. *Seers,* by Egon Schiele; *source*: Wikimedia

Fig. 5.2. Reproduction of *Transfer*; *artist*: T. Keber, adapted from the original by René Magritte

Fig. 6.1. Reticular formation in the brain stem; *artist*: T. Keber, adapted from an image by Frank Lowen, courtesy of Upledger Institute International

Fig. 6.2. The brain stem and spine; *artist*: Tad Wanveer, courtesy of Upledger Institute International

Fig. 6.3. Biological Process in the Life Cycle; *artist*: T. Keber

Fig. 6.4. Circadian rhythm; *artist*: T. Keber, adapted from a biological clock image from Wikimedia

Fig. 6.5. Circadian rhythm—our biological clock; *artist*: T. Keber

Fig. 6.6. Diagram of MacLean's triune brain; *artist*: T. Keber

Fig. 7.1. *The Three Ages of Woman,* by Gustav Klimt; *source*: Google Arts and Culture

Fig. 7.2. *Separation*, by Edvard Munch; *source*: Wikimedia

Fig. 9.1. Amygdala; *artist*: T. Keber, adapted from Frank Lowen's image, courtesy of Upledger Institute International

Fig. 9.2. Thalamus; *artist*: T. Keber, adapted from Frank Lowen's image, courtesy of Upledger Institute International

Fig. 9.3. Cerebral cortex; *artist*: T. Keber, adapted from on Frank Lowen's image, courtesy of Upledger Institute International

Fig. 9.4. *Day and Night,* by Maurits Cornelis Escher; *source*: photo by D. Maggio at Salone degli Incanti in Trieste, July 2020

Fig. 10.1. The symbols for Tao and for yin and yang; *artist*: T. Keber

Fig. 10.2. The major and minor chakras and their energy field; *artist*: T. Keber

Fig. 10.3. Energy meridians; *artist*: T. Keber

Fig. 10.4. Assagioli's ovoid (Egg Diagram); *artist*: T. Keber

Fig. 10.5. Gastrulation; *artist*: T. Keber

Fig. 10.6. The oocyte; *artist*: T. Keber

Fig. 10.7. The (polar) structure of an atom; *artist*: T. Keber

Fig. 10.8. The (polar) structure of a water molecules; *artist*: T. Keber

Fig. 10.9. Magnetic field lines created by the poles of a solenoid; *artist:* T. Keber, adapted from a Wikimedia image

Fig. 10.10. Magnetic field lines; *artist*: T. Keber

Fig. 10.11. Toroidal magnetic field of the human body; *artist*: T. Keber

Fig. 10.12. Direction of the fascia in the human body, courtesy of Upledger Institute International

Fig. 10.13. Earth's meridians and parallels; *artist*: T. Keber

Fig. 10.14. Restrictions in the fascia caused by an Energy Cyst; *source*: Freepik

Fig. 10.15. Color is produced by the meeting of light and darkness; *artist*: T. Keber

Fig. 10.16. *Composition No. IV with Red, Blue, and Yellow,* by Piet Mondrian; *source*: Wikiart

Fig. 11.1. Right and left hemispheres and corpus callosum; *artist*: T. Keber, adapted from Frank Lowen's images, courtesy of Upledger Institute International

Fig. 11.2. Nervous system; *artist*: T. Keber, adapted from a Wikiwand image

Fig. 11.3. EEG; *artist*: T. Keber, adapted from a Wikimedia image

Fig. 11.4. The three cranial vault holds; *artist*: Frank Lowen, courtesy of Upledger Institute International

Fig. 11.5. Self-listening exercise, courtesy of Upledger Italia

Fig. 11.6. *Big Sphere,* by Arnaldo Pomodoro; *source*: Flickr, image 12109204215

Fig. 11.7. Reproduction of a piece from the Feeling Material series; *artist*: T. Keber, adapted from the original by Antony Gormley

Fig. 12.1. Assagioli's Egg Diagram; *artist*: T. Keber

Fig. 12.2. The cosmic egg shaped by the god Ptah; *artist*: T. Keber, adapted from an image featured in an ancient Egyptian tomb

Fig. 12.3. Details of *Brera Madonna,* by Piero della Francesca; *source*: Wikiart

Fig. 12.4. *Concert in the Egg,* by Hieronymus Bosch (or a follower); *source*: Wikipedia

Fig. 13.1. Arc of movement of Energy Cysts and craniosacral movement; *artist*: T. Keber, adapted from Frank Lowen's image, courtesy of Upledger Institute International

Fig. 13.2. Pericardium and heart; *artist*: T. Keber, adapted from a Freepik image

Fig. 13.3. Lungs; *artist*: T. Keber, adapted from a Freepik image

Fig. 13.4. Kidneys; *artist*: Bruce Blaus *source*: WikiJournal of Medicine

Fig. 13.5. Spleen; *artist*: T. Keber

Fig. 13.6. Liver; *artist*: T. Keber

Fig. 13.7. Hand placement for the pericardium meridian; *artist*: T. Keber

Fig. 13.8. Hand placement for the heart meridian; *artist*: T. Keber

Fig. 13.9. Hand placement for the lungs meridian; *artist*: T. Keber

Fig. 13.10. Hand placement for the kidneys meridian; *artist*: T. Keber

Fig. 13.11. Hand placement for the spleen meridian; *artist*: T. Keber

Fig. 13.12. Hand placement for the liver meridian; *artist*: T. Keber

Fig. 13.13. Meridian emptying and filling technique; *artist*: T. Keber

Fig. 13.14. Reproduction of cosmogram on the Cyprus stele of the Hologram of Europe installation; *artist*: T. Keber, adapted from a photograph of Diego Maggio's of Marko Pogačnik's sculpture

Fig. 14.1. Reproduction of *Yesterday, Today, Tomorrow*; *artist*: T. Keber, adapted from the original by Lucille Clerc

Fig. 15.1. The energetic framework of the human body; *artist*: T. Keber, courtesy of Upledger Italia

Fig. 15.2. Vector/axis system and polarity; *artist*: T. Keber

Fig. 15.3. Polarity and map of the vector/axis system, with chakras; *artist*: T. Keber

Fig. 15.4. Map of the vector/axis system through the chakras; *artist*: T. Keber

Fig. 15.5. Wave expansion generated by Energy Cysts; *artist*: T. Keber

Fig. 15.6. Vectors along their axis before and after being realigned; *artist*: T. Keber

Fig. 16.1. Mapping the vector/axis system with the chakras; *artist*: T. Keber, courtesy of Upledger Italia Chakra symbols in chapter 16; *artist*: T. Keber

Fig. 16.2. Spinal Cord; *artist*: T. Keber, adapted from Frank Lowen's image, courtesy of Upledger Institute International

Fig. 16.3. Hypophysis; *artist*: T. Keber. adapted from Frank Lowen's image, courtesy of Upledger Institute International

Fig. 16.4. Hypothalamus; *artist*: T. Keber, adapted from Frank Lowen's image, courtesy of Upledger Institute International

Fig. 16.5. Pineal gland; *artist*: T. Keber, adapted from Frank Lowen's image, courtesy of Upledger Institute International

Fig. 16.6. The seven major chakras; *artist*: T. Keber

Fig. 16.7. Mapping the vector/axis system through the chakras; *artist*: T. Keber

Fig. 16.8. Misalignment of vectors caused by an Energy Cyst at the level of the fifth chakra; *artist*: T. Keber

Fig. 16.9. Using chakras to realign the vectors; *artist*: T. Keber

Fig. 16.10. The vector/axis system after realignment; *artist*: T. Keber

Fig. 16.11. Vector/axis system realignment through the chakras; *artist*: T. Keber, courtesy of Upledger Italia

Fig. 17.1. Occiput and atlas; *artist*: T. Keber, adapted from Frank Lowen's image, courtesy of Upledger Institute International

Fig. 17.2. Compression triad; *artist*: T. Keber, adapted from Frank Lowen's image, courtesy of Upledger Institute International

Fig. 17.3. Vagus system; *artist*: T. Keber, adapted from Frank Lowen's image, courtesy of Upledger Institute International

Fig. 17.4. Third ventricle; *artist*: T. Keber

Fig. 17.5. Amygdala; *artist*: T. Keber, adapted from Frank Lowen's image, courtesy of Upledger Institute International

Fig. 17.6. Fornix; *artist*: T. Keber, adapted from Tad Wanveer image, courtesy of Upledger Institute International

Fig. 17.7. Hippocampus; *artist*: T. Keber, adapted from Älice Quaid image, courtesy of Upledger Institute International

Fig. 17.8. Medulla oblongata; *artist*: T. Keber, adapted from Frank Lowen's image, courtesy of Upledger Institute International

Fig. 17.9. Cerebral cortex; *artist*: T. Keber, adapted from Frank Lowen's image, courtesy of Upledger Institute International

Fig. 17.10. Locus coeruleus; *artist*: T. Keber

Fig. 17.11. Thalamus; *artist*: T. Keber, adapted from Frank Lowen's image, courtesy of Upledger Institute International

Fig. 17.12. Cerebellum; *artist*: T. Keber, adapted from Tad Wanveer's image, courtesy of Upledger Institute International

Fig. 17.13. Vagus nerve; *artist*: T. Keber

Fig. 17.14. Limbic system; *artist*: T. Keber, adapted from Älice Quaid image, courtesy of Upledger Institute International

Fig. 17.15. CranioSacral Therapy to support the family unit, courtesy of Upledger Italia

Fig. 17.16. CST and SER support to bereavement; *artist*: T. Keber, courtesy of Upledger Italia

Fig. 17.17. *There Is Always Hope,* by Banksy; *source*: photo from The Walkman Magazine Blog

Fig. 17.18. Reproduction of *Guernica,* by Pablo Picasso; *source*: murals & street art—*fair use* for a work of public and free exhibition. The photographical reproduction of this work is covered under the article 35.2 of the Royal Legislative Decree 1/1996 of April 12, 1996, and amended by Law 5/1998 of March 6, 1998—CC BY-SA 3.0

Fig. 17.19. Reproduction of *Our Present Image,* by David Alfaro Siqueiros; *source*: murals & street art—*fair use* for a work of public and free exhibition. The photographical reproduction of this work is covered under the article 35.2 of the Royal Legislative Decree 1/1996 of April 12, 1996, and amended by Law 5/1998 of March 6, 1998—CC BY-SA 3.0.

Fig. 17.20. Mural, Montreal, Canada, 2014, by Julien Malland (aka Seth Globepainter); *source*: murals & street art—*fair use* for a work of public and free exhibition. The photographical reproduction of this work is covered under the article 35.2 of the Royal Legislative Decree 1/1996 of April 12, 1996, and amended by Law 5/1998 of March 6, 1998—CC BY-SA 3.0

Fig. 17.21. *Dream of a Sunday Afternoon,* by Diego Rivera; *source*: murals & street art—*fair use* for a work of public and free exhibition. The photographical reproduction of this work is covered under the article 35.2 of the Royal Legislative Decree 1/1996 of April 12, 1996, and amended by Law 5/1998 of March 6, 1998—CC BY-SA 3.0

Fig. 17.22. *Enjoy Your Life,* by Banksy; *source*: murals & street art—*fair use* for a work of public and free exhibition. The photographical reproduction of this work is covered under the article 35.2 of the Royal Legislative Decree 1/1996 of April 12, 1996, and amended by Law 5/1998 of March 6, 1998—CC BY-SA 3.0

Fig. 17.23. Untitled work by Keith Haring; *source*: murals & street art—*fair use* for a work of public and free exhibition. The photographical reproduction of this work is covered under the article 35.2 of the Royal Legislative Decree 1/1996 of April 12, 1996, and amended by Law 5/1998 of March 6, 1998—CC BY-SA 3.0

Fig. 17.24. *Kiss Me,* by Mr. Savethewall; *source*: murals & street art—*fair use* for a work of public and free exhibition. The photographical reproduction of this work is covered under the article 35.2 of the Royal Legislative Decree 1/1996 of April 12, 1996, and amended by Law 5/1998 of March 6, 1998—CC BY-SA 3.0

Fig. 17.25. Untitled work by Jean Michel Basquiat; *source*: murals & street art—*fair use* for a work of public and free exhibition. The photographical reproduction of this work is covered under the article 35.2 of the Royal Legislative Decree 1/1996 of April 12, 1996, and amended by Law 5/1998 of March 6, 1998—CC BY-SA 3.0

Fig. 17.26. *Dancer,* by Martin Whatson; *source*: murals & street art—*fair use* for a work of public and free exhibition. The photographical reproduction of this work is covered under the article 35.2 of the Royal Legislative Decree 1/1996 of April 12, 1996, and amended by Law 5/1998 of March 6, 1998—CC BY-SA 3.0

Fig. 17.27. *For All Liverpool's Liver Birds,* by Paul Curtis. *artist*: photo by Diego Maggio

Fig. 17.28. *Dragonfly and Chrysanthemums,* by Utagawa Hiroshige; *source*: Honolulu Museum of Art

Fig. 18.1. The release of the entropic energy held in an Energy Cyst; *artist*: T. Keber

Fig. 18.2. Entropy and syntropy/negentropy; *artist*: T. Keber

Fig. 18.3. Release of entropic energy retained by an Energy Cyst through the aptonomic touch; *artist*: T. Keber

Fig. 18.4. The structure of an atom; *artist*: T. Keber

Fig. 18.5. From atom to energy; *artist*: T. Keber

Fig. 18.6. Reproduction of *Starry Night*; *artist*: T. Keber, adapted from the original by Vincent van Gogh

Fig. 18.7. Reproduction of *Water Lilies*; *artist*: T. Keber, adapted from the original by Claude Monet

Fig. 18.8. Reproduction of *Portrait of Félix Fénéon*; *artist*: T. Keber, adapted from the original by Paul Signac

Fig. 19.1. HPA axis; *source*: Wikimedia

Fig. 19.2. HPA organs; *artist*: T. Keber, adapted from Frank Lowen's image, courtesy of Upledger Institute International and National Cancer Institute of the U.S. National Institutes of Health

Fig. 19.3. The HPA axis response to stress; *artist*: T. Keber

Fig. 20.1. DNA holds genetic information on the end of life; *source*: Freepik

Fig. 20.2. Pons; *artist*: Tad Wanveer, courtesy of Upledger Institute International and *artist*: T. Keber, adapted from Frank Lowen's image, courtesy of Upledger Institute International

Fig. 20.3. Vagus nerve; *artist*: T. Keber

Fig. 20.4. Cerebellum; *artist*: T. Keber, adapted from Tad Wanveer's image, courtesy of Upledger Institute International

Fig. 20.5. The pons, crown chakra, and center; *artist*: T. Keber, adapted from Tad Wanveer's image, courtesy of Upledger Institute International

Fig. 20.6. Reproduction of *Kuwait: A Desert on Fire*; *artist*: T. Keber, adapted from the original by Sebastião Salgado

Fig. 20.7. Reproduction of *Black and White*; *artist*: T. Keber, adapted from the original by Man Ray (aka Emmanuel Radnitzky)

Fig. 20.8. Reproduction of *The Tetons and the Snake River*; *artist*: T. Keber, adapted from the original by Ansel Adams

Fig. 20.9. Reproduction of *Nude, Baie des Anges*; *artist*: T. Keber, adapted from the original by Bill Brandt

Fig. 20.10. Reproduction of *Shell*; *artist*: T. Keber, adapted from the original by Edward Weston

Fig. 20.11. Reproduction of *A Certain Oppression*; *artist*: T. Keber, adapted from the original by Rodney Smith

Fig. 20.12. Reproduction of *Tranquility*; *artist*: T. Keber, adapted from the original by Hengki Koentjoro

Fig. 20.13. Reproduction of *Self-Portrait*; *artist*: T. Keber, adapted from the original by Andy Warhol

Fig. 21.1. Diego Maggio treating the respiratory diaphragms, courtesy of Upledger Italia

Fig. 21.2. The three cranial vault holds; *artist*: Frank Lowen, courtesy of Upledger Institute International

Fig. 21.3. Shem Ha Meforash; *artist*: Devid Caressa

Fig. 21.4. Hei Vav Hei Yud; *artist*: Devid Caressa

Fig. 21.5. The energetic framework of the human body; *artist*: T. Keber

Fig. 21.6. Hand placement for the respiratory diaphragm release; *artist*: T. Keber, adapted from Frank Lowen's image, courtesy of Upledger Institute International

Fig. 21.7. Hand placement for the thoracic inlet release; *artist*: T. Keber, adapted from Frank Lowen's image, courtesy of Upledger Institute International

Fig. 21.8. First vault hold; *artist*: Frank Lowen, courtesy of Upledger Institute International

Fig. 21.9. Second vault hold; *artist*: Frank Lowen, courtesy of Upledger Institute International

Fig. 21.10. Third vault hold; *artist*: Frank Lowen, courtesy of Upledger Institute International

Fig. 21.11. Reproduction of *Zenith* (the original features a horse; here, we substitute the human figure); *artist*: T. Keber, adapted from the original by Mimmo Paladino

Fig. 22.1. Assessment of energy vortex frequencies and reharmonization, courtesy of Upledger Italia

Fig. 22.2. Chakra landmarks and musical notes based on the 432 hertz grid; *artist*: T. Keber

Fig. 22.3. Experiments on water crystals with the vibrations of sounds; *artist*: T. Keber, adapted from images from Masaru Emoto's experiments

Fig. 22.4. Chladni figures, formed by the vibrations of sound; *source*: Wikipedia

Fig. 22.5. Hans Jenny's experiments of cymatics; *artist*: T. Keber

Fig. 22.6. Vortex of movement of Energy Cyst; *artist*: T. Keber, adapted from Frank Lowen's image, courtesy of Upledger Institute International

Fig. 22.7. Sketches of sculptures; *artist*: T. Keber, adapted from the originals by Fausto Melotti

Fig. 23.1. Thought-form as Third Space; *artist*: T. Keber

Fig. 23.2. Fractal forms in the nautilus; *artist*: T. Keber

Fig. 23.3. Fractal structures in neuronal ramifications; *artist*: T. Keber

Fig. 23.4. Butterfly-shaped fractal structures; *artist*: T. Keber

Figure Credits 523

Fig. 23.5. Mandelbrot set; *source*: Wikipedia

Fig. 23.6. Fractals in the organic structure of a plant; *artist*: T. Keber

Fig. 23.7. Toroidal magnetic field; *artist*: T. Keber

Fig. 23.8. Toroidal magnetic field of the da Vinci's *Vitruvian Man*; *artist*: T. Keber

Fig. 23.9. Emptying and filling; *artist*: T. Keber

Fig. 23.10. Reproduction of *Demeter*; *artist*: T. Keber, adapted from the original by Hans Jean Arp

Fig. 23.11. Reproduction of a mandala; *artist*: T. Keber, adapted from the original by James Brunt

Fig. 24.1. Reproduction of *Ascending Movement*; *artist*: T. Keber, adapted from the original by Michael Grab

Fig. 25.1. The seven steps; *artist*: T. Keber

Fig. 25.2. Hexagram of 7 from the Book of Changes; *artist*: T. Keber

Fig. 25.3. Hexagram of 2 from the Book of Changes; *artist*: T. Keber

Fig. 25.4. Alignment of the vector/axis system; *source*: Upledger Italia

Fig. 25.5. Vector/axis system with polarity and chakras; *artist*: T. Keber

Fig. 25.6. Third Space thought-form; *artist*: T. Keber

Fig. 25.7. Fascial release of intracranial structures; Courtesy of Upledger Italia

Fig. 25.8. The three cranial vault holds; *artist*: Frank Lowen, courtesy of Upledger Institute International

Fig. 25.9. Meninges; *artist*: T. Keber, adapted from Tad Wanveer image, courtesy of Upledger Institute International

Fig. 25.10. Connecting the cerebral hemispheres; Courtesy of Upledger Italia

Fig. 25.11. Corpus callosum and cerebral hemispheres; *artist*: Frank Lowen's, courtesy of Upledger Institute International

Fig. 25.12. Corpus callosum and RAS, courtesy of Upledger Italia

Fig. 25.13. Reticular formation; *artist*: T. Keber, adapted from Frank Lowen's image, courtesy of Upledger Institute International

Fig. 25.14. Brain stem and spine; *artist*: Tad Wanveer, courtesy of Upledger Institute International

Fig. 25.15. Anatomical connections with the corpus callosum; *artist*: Tad Wanveer, courtesy of Upledger Institute International

Fig. 25.16. Thoracic inlet technique for pericardium/heart meridians, courtesy of Upledger Italia

Fig. 25.17. Hand placement for pericardium meridian; *artist*: T. Keber

Fig. 25.18. Hand placement for heart meridian; *artist*: T. Keber

Fig. 25.19. Pericardium and heart; *artist*: T. Keber, adapted from a Freepik image

Fig. 25.20. Emptying and filling; *artist*: T. Keber

Fig. 25.21. Vagus nerve and respiratory diaphragm release; courtesy of Upledger Italia

Fig. 25.22. Connection of the emotional system to the digestive system; *artist*: T. Keber

Fig. 25.23. Hand placement for the respiratory diaphragm release; *artist*: Frank Lowen, courtesy of Upledger Institute International

Fig. 25.24. Vagus nerve; *artist*: T. Keber

Fig. 25.25. Third chakra and liver meridian; *artist*: T. Keber

Fig. 25.26. Seventh chakra, center, and pons; *artist*: T. Keber, adapted from Tad Wanveer's image, courtesy of Upledger Institute International

Fig. 25.27. The seventh chakra; courtesy of Upledger Italia Images in bulleted list in chapter 25:

    Center; *artist*: T. Wanveer/Älice Quaid, courtesy of Upledger Institute International

    Pons; *artist*: T. Wanveer/Frank Lowen, courtesy of Upledger Institute International

    Cerebellum; *artist*: T. Keber, adapted from Tad Wanveer's image, courtesy of Upledger Institute International

    Reticular formation; *artist*: T. Keber, adapted from Frank Lowen's image, courtesy of Upledger Institute International

    RAS; *artist*: T. Keber, adapted from Tad Wanveer's image, courtesy of Upledger Institute International

    Amygdala; *artist*: T. Keber, adapted from Frank Lowen's image, courtesy of Upledger Institute International

    Hippocampus; *artist*: T. Keber, adapted from Älice Quaid's image, courtesy of Upledger Institute International

    Hypophysis; *artist*: T. Keber, adapted from Frank Lowen's image, courtesy of Upledger Institute International

    Pineal gland; *artist*: T. Keber, adapted from Frank Lowen's image, courtesy of Upledger Institute International

    Fornix; *artist*: T. Keber, adapted from Tad Wanveer's image, courtesy of Upledger Institute International

    Thalamus; *artist*: T. Keber, adapted from Frank Lowen's image, courtesy of Upledger Institute International

    The seventh chakra and energetic system; *artist*: T. Keber

Fig. 25.28. *Rainbow*; *artist*: Augusto Giacometti; *source*: Wikimedia

Fig. 26.1. The genealogical-emotional tree; *artist*: T. Keber, adapted from the original by Gustav Klimt, Tree of Life in the *Stoclet Frieze*

Fig. 26.2. The genealogical-emotional tree; *artist*: T. Keber, adapted from the original by Gustav Klimt, Tree of Life in the *Stoclet Frieze*

Fig. 26.3. *Primavera*; *artist*: Sandro Botticelli; *source*: Wikiart

Fig. 26.4. Reproduction of *Dance*; *artist*: T. Keber, adapted from the original by Henri Émile Benoît Matisse

Fig. 26.5. Reproduction of *Office at Night*; *artist*: T. Keber, adapted from the original by Edward Hopper

Fig. 26.6. *Three Graces*; *artist*: Raffaello Sanzio (Raphael); *source*: Wikimedia

Fig. 26.7. Reproduction of *Nude from Behind*; *artist*: T. Keber, adapted from the original by Umberto Boccioni

Fig. 26.8. Reproduction of *Daydream*; *artist*: T. Keber, adapted from the original by Alfons Maria Mucha (Alphonse Mucha)

Fig. 26.9. Reproduction of *Three Tahitians*; *artist*: T. Keber, adapted from the original by Paul Gauguin

Fig. 26.10. Reproduction of *Moses (Nucleus of Creation)*; *artist*: T. Keber, adapted from the original by Frida Kahlo

Fig. 26.11. Reproduction of *Woman before the Rising Sun*; *artist*: T. Keber, adapted from the original by Caspar David Friedrich

Fig. 26.12. Reproduction of the *Stoclet Frieze*; *artist*: T. Keber, adapted from the original by Gustav Klimt

Fig. 26.13. Reproduction of *Portrait of Mrs. P. in the South*; *artist*: T. Keber, adapted from the original by Ernst Paul Klee

Fig. 26.14. Reproduction of *David*; *artist*: T. Keber, based on the statue by Michelangelo Buonarroti

Fig. 26.15. *Book of Life,* by David Kracov; *artist*: photo by Diego Maggio Parting. John Matthew Upledger and his father, Dr. John Edwin Upledger, courtesy of Upledger Institute International

Acknowledgments. Reproduction of *L.H.O.O.Q.*; *artist*: T. Keber, adapted from the original by Marcel Duchamp

Index

abandonment, 1–2
acceptance, 27, 36, 57, 262, 266–67
acoustics and acoustic signaling, 368
action, healing, 26–27
active listening, 23
adaptive unconscious, 210, 213–15
amplitude, 13, 14, 29, 30, 63. *See also* symmetry, quality, amplitude, and rate (SQAR)
amygdala, 95, 96, 98, 254, 451
"analysis creates paralysis," 215
analytical psychology, ego in, 48
andropause, 73
anger
    as grief stage, 264–65
    limbic system and, 64
    liver and, 172, 175, 181
    as spender, 92
    trapped, 174
Annica, 241
anthropology, of grief, 261–63
antireductionism, 341–45
aptonomic touch
    about, 20
    channeled energy through, 396
    observations, 20
    release of entropic energy through, 289, 290
    SER and, 20–21
Aquino, Pietro, 99–100
Arcing
    about, 32
    clinical notes, 33
    Energy Cysts and, 32–33
    evaluation illustration, 31
    therapist requirements, 32
    use of, 362
Arena, Sebastiano, 432
Aristotle, 59, 94, 153, 346
art of treatment, 415–16
Ascoltare la Vita blog, 242
Assagioli, Roberto
    Egg Diagram, 114, 156–57
    ego and, 49–51
    photosynthesis and, 153–54
    polarity and, 103, 113–14
    ten laws, 155–56
    transformation and, 155
attachment theory, 73
attention, direction of energy through, 163–64
auxology, 59
awareness
    as art, xv
    body, 22
    emotional, 97–98, 100
    freedom of listening and, 25–26
    patient, 38, 47, 72, 93, 153
    shifts in, 35
awareness field, 159

balance phenomenon, 285, 286
Banich, Marie T., 97–98
Barbagli, Marzo, 315–16
bargaining (negotiation, compromise), as grief stage, 265
Beauregard, Olivier Costa, 282
belief system, 15

Bettoschi, Gabriele, 241–42
Bianciardi, Giorgio, 388–89
bioenergetics, 59, 373
Biological Process
    first phases of, 73
    loss and separation and, 72–73
    significant losses in, 75–76
    traumatic factors in, 74
biological processes
    Cellular Memory, 57–65
    circadian rhythms, 61–63
    destructive events and, 55–57
    in Life Cycle, 54–69
    living organisms, 65–66
    reticular system, 54–55
    triune brain, 61–63
biology
    about, 66
    polarity in, 116–17
    quantum, 138–39
biophonons, 368–69
birth, 72, 170, 261, 309–10
Bowlby, John, 73–74
brain stem, 54–55, 95
brainwave synchronization/coherence, 140
Bratina, Edoardo, 305
Brunetti, Guido, 304, 344–45

Campanello, Laura, 317–18
Caressa, Devid, 337–41, 342
Carmignani, Umberto, 326–27
cell priority, 117–18
Cell Talk (Upledger), 363, 364–66
Cellular Memory
    about, 57
    auxology and, 59
    bioenergetics and, 59
    character-analytic vegetotherapy and, 59
    circadian rhythms and, 61–63
    clinical observations, 68–69
    entelechy and, 59–60
    epigenetics and, 57–58
    evolution and, 66–67
    as feedback, 57–65
    negativity retention, 76
    psychoneuroendocrinoimmunology (PNEI) and, 58
    quantum theory and, 66–67
    triune brain and, 63–65
center, 321, 450
central nervous system, 136–38
cerebellum, 257, 320, 450
cerebral cortex, 96, 256
cerebral hemispheres
    about, 133–35
    asymmetries, 135
    clinical observations, 146–47
    connection with, 166, 440–41
    corpus callosum and, 136, 441
    differences between, 135
    illustrated, 134
    left hemisphere, 134
    right hemisphere, 134–35
    symmetry, 134, 135
chakras
    aligning vectors with, 243–48
    clinical observations, 249–50
    energetic framework, human body and, 217
    fifth, 234
    first, 231
    fourth, 233
    function of, 229
    illustrated, 108
    in Indian religious tradition, 238
    lower, commentaries on, 241–43
    mapping vector/axis system with, 230, 245
    medicine, yoga and, 240–41
    meridians and, 109
    role in Western culture, 237–40
    second, 232
    seventh, 235
    sixth, 234–35
    therapeutic vibrations and, 374
    third, 232–33

two-dimensional map of, 218
vector/axis system map and, 219
vectors through, 244, 246–47
in yogic disciplines, 237–38
character-analytic vegetotherapy, 59
chemistry
   of emotions, 182
   entropy in, 281
   polarity in, 118–19
Chetta, Giovanni, 302
chiropractic, HPA axis in, 302
Chladni figures, 370–71
Cieloevento, 434
Cilento, Francesca, 213
circadian rhythms, 61–63, 64
clinical observations
   Cellular Memory, 68–69
   cerebral hemispheres, 146–47
   chakras, 249–50
   death and dying, 325–28
   ego, 52
   emotions, 101–2
   energetic framework in the human body, 226–28
   entropy and syntropy, 293–94
   final treatment, 355–58
   grief, 271–72, 326
   loss, 77–78
   mind-body-spirit continuum, 418–20
   Ode to Life, 483–84
   photosynthesis, 168–69
   polarity, 129–30
   seats of emotions, 192–94
   seven-step treatment, 456–59
   small deaths, 205–6
   stress, 89–90, 308
   Third Space, 398–403
   vibrations, 378–79
cognitive science, therapeutic vibrations and, 372
collective unconscious, 160
complex (complicated) grief, 252
compression triad, 253

conception, 72
consciousness
   alpha state of, 20
   art as expression, 416
   cellular, 117
   center of, 159
   Ego as central complex of, 48
   energy field, 84
   experimental perspective, 408–11
   Facilitator/patient relationship and, 25
   intelligence and, 149
   levels of, 38, 40, 100, 158, 160
   polarity, 113
   pure essence and, 211
conscious self, 159
conscious versus non-conscious, 23–25
constructive/destructive emotions
   about, 92
   heart and, 179
   kidneys and, 180
   liver and, 182
   lungs and, 180
   pericardium and, 178
   spleen and, 181
constructive energies, 103, 289, 395, 445
cooperating with the inevitable, 166–67
corpus callosum
   about, 136
   anatomical connections with, 443
   cerebral hemispheres and, 441
   connection with, 442–43
   fibers, 136
   RAS and, 442–43
Cosmic Spiral, 384–85
cranial vault holds, 336, 351–53
craniosacral rhythm (CSR)
   about, 29
   abrupt interruption in, 35
   amplitude, quality, rate, 30–31
   palpating, 34, 35
   Significance Detector and, 34–35, 36, 37, 38
   techniques to perceive, 12
   vault holds and, 352–53

CranioSacral Therapy (CST). *See also*
    SomatoEmotional Release
  development of, 9–13
  Direction of Energy, 11, 138
  Energy Cysts and, 13–15
  first experiences with, 4–5
  grieving family support with, 268
  as holistic treatment, 22
  for integration and release, 91–102
  Intensive, 83–84
  as life journey, 190
  meridians, 174–77
  as Ode to Life, 465–82
  patient-facilitator relationship in, 22–28
  physiology of death in, 318–21
  polarity in, 122–25
  practice development, xv–xvi
  teleonomy in, 461–62
  vibrational energy of 432 Hz grid in, 374–75
creative process, 209
creativity, evolutionary, 210–12
CST-centered visions
  For All Liverpool's Liver Birds (Curtis), 277
  balancing rock art (Grab), 420
  Big Sphere (Pomodoro), 148
  Black and White (Ray), 329–30
  Book of Life (Kracov), 491–92
  Brera Madonna (Francesca), 170–71
  A Certain Oppression (Smith), 331–32
  color production, 131
  Composition No. IV with Red, Blue, and Yellow (Mondrian), 131–32
  Concert in the Egg (Bosch), 171
  Dance (Matisse), 485
  Dancer (Whatson), 277
  David (Michelangelo), 491
  Day and Night (Escher), 102
  Daydream (Mucha), 487
  Demeter (Arp), 404
  Dragonfly and Chrysanthemums (Hiroshige), 278
  Dream of a Sunday Afternoon (Rivera), 274
  egg shape, 170

  Enjoy Your Life (Banksy), 275
  An Eye with a View (Dali), 28
  Feeling Material (Gormley), 148–49
  Guernica (Picasso), 273
  Harmony and Counterpoint series (Melotti), 380
  Hologram of Europe (Pogacnik), 195
  Kiss Me (Savethewall), 276
  Kuwait: A Desert on Fire (Salgado), 329
  mandala (Brunt), 404
  Montreal mural (Malland), 274
  Moses (Kahlo), 488
  Nude, Baie des Anges (Brandt), 330–31
  Nude from Behind (Boccioni), 487
  Office at Night (Hopper), 486
  Our Present Image (Siqueiros), 273–74
  Over the Town (Chagall), 45
  Portrait of Félix Fénéon (Signac), 296
  Portrait of Mrs. P. in the South (Klee), 490
  Primavera (Botticelli), 485
  Rainbow (Giacometti), 459
  Seers (Schiele), 53
  Self-Portrait (Warhol), 333
  Separation (Munch), 79
  Shell (Weston), 331
  The Song of Love (Chirico), 45
  Starry Night (van Gogh), 295
  Stoclet Frieze (Klimt), 489–90
  The Tetons and the Snake River (Adams), 330
  There Is Always Hope (Banksy), 273
  The Three Ages of Woman (Klimt), 79
  Three Graces (Sanzio), 486
  Three Tahitians (Gauguin), 488
  Tranquility (Koentjoro), 332
  Transfer (Magritte), 53
  Untitled work (Basquiat), 276
  Untitled work (Haring), 275
  Water Lilies (Monet), 295
  Woman before the Rising Sun (Friedrich), 489
  Yesterday, Today, Tomorrow (Clerc), 206
  Zenith (Paladino), 359

curandera, 412
curriculum vitae (CV)
    Education and Training, 477–78
    Freedom, 482
    Life Cycle, 471–82
    Passions and Hobbies, 481
    Personal Information, 471–75
    Personality and Social Skills, 479–80
    vital energy continuum exercise, 470–71
    Working Experience, 476–77
cymatics, 369–71

D'Alisa, Pamela, 204
Damasio, Antonio, 214–15
death and dying. *See also* seven-step treatment; small deaths
    assistance, as most difficult task, 312
    clinical observations, 325–28
    CST-centered visions, 329–33
    emotional level of, 173
    experience for the living, 269
    fear of, 310, 313–15
    feelings and emotions and, 313–18
    loss and, 71, 73
    mourning after, 261–62
    observations, 318
    personal growth exercises and, 322–24
    physiology, in CST and SER, 318–21
    scenarios a Facilitator might expect, 313
    stereotypes about, 315–16
    therapist focus and, 310–11
De Fanis, Francesca, 346
denial (rejection), as grief stage, 264
depression
    as grief stage, 265–66
    liver and, 181
    separation from mother figure and, 74
    transformation from, 276
Descartes, René, 93–94, 99
destructive emotions, 92
destructive energies
    Energy Cysts, 173
    polarity and, 103–32

    regenerative power, 163
    transformation of, 395
destructive events, influence of, 55–57
Di Corpo, Ulisse, 389
Di Muro, Carmen, 105–6
Direction of Energy
    about, 11, 138, 142
    exercise, 143–44
    hand placement, 143
    implementation of, 142
    objectives, 142
    self-listening exercise, 144–45
    technique, 143
    three cranial vault holds, 143
direct route, 95
DNA, 58, 75, 311
Driesch, H., 60

Early Declaration of Treatment, 316
Earth's polarity, 120–21
ecopsychology, 203–4
Education and Training, CV, 477–78
egg, 115, 170–71
Egg Diagram, 114, 156–57
ego
    about, 46–47
    in analytical psychology, 48
    center and, 321
    characteristics of, 51
    clinical observations, 52
    in Gestalt psychology, 49
    Higher Self and, 46, 47, 51
    non-conscious versus, 47–48
    personal self objectives and, 51
    in psychosynthesis, 49–51
    rejecting, 310
    self-preservation and, 50
    tools for not feeding, 46–47
eidetic intuition, 210–11
Einstein, Albert, 212, 284
Eliade, Mircea, 239
"embodied cognition," 343
embrace, 73

embryology, polarity in, 114–16
emotional intelligence, 94, 213
emotions
   acquiring awareness of, 98
   clinical observations, 101–2
   communication between viscera and, 182–83
   constructive and destructive, 92
   CST and SER and, 91
   defining, 93–99
   experiencing, 100
   feelings versus, 99–100
   held in viscera, treating, 183–88
   in history, 93–95
   importance of being conscious of, 100
   internal organs and, 93
   intuition and, 212–13
   LEAS and, 97
   molecules of, 177–78
   negative, options, 164
   neuroscience and, 95–99
   organs and, 175, 199
   processing, 91–102
   seats of, clinical observations, 192–94
   of small deaths, 198–200
   Therapeutic Imagery and Dialogue and, 100, 101
   trauma and, 98
empathy, 310, 428–31
emptying and filling technique, 395
energetic framework in the human body
   about, 207
   chakras and, 217
   clinical observations, 226–28
   creative process, 209
   illustrated, 208, 340
   intuition and, 210–13
   intuitive intelligence and, 213–15
   misalignment, rebalancing, 220
   polarity and, 215–17
   principles of, 215–17
   vector/axis system and, 215–17
   vectors, 212

energetic touch and mobilization, 222–23
"energetic vectors," 340
energetic visualization and mobilization, 221–22
energies
   constructive, 103, 289, 395, 445
   destructive, 103–32, 163, 173, 395
   direction through attention, 163–64
   entropic, 289–90
   judging, avoiding, 162
   latent, accessing, 154–55
   melding in Higher Self, 165
   as mutable forces, 162
   therapeutic, 290–91
   transformation of, 161–62
   use of, 162
energy continuum, 8
Energy Cysts
   about, 13, 104
   Arcing and, 32–33
   arc of movement of, 173
   cell vibrations and, 117
   characteristics of, 14–15
   development of, 13
   dissipation of, 174
   emission of, 14
   energy vortex emanation from, 33
   as entropic dysfunctions, 289–90
   entropic energy release, 279
   formation of, 125
   localization of, 200
   manifestation of, 18
   meridians and, 173–74
   as physical points, 362
   in practice, 104
   reactions freezing in, 167
   release of, 13, 14
   treatment of, 13–15, 200
   vibrations, 32
   vortexes of, 362–63, 375
   wave expansion generated by, 221
energy meridians, 109–10
energy vortexes, 361, 362–63

entanglement
  global, 406
  quantum, 67, 283, 284, 423
  therapeutic side of, 291–92
entelechy, 59–60
entropic phenomenon, 285, 286
entropy
  about, 279–80
  chemistry and, 281
  in Facilitator's practice, 288
  illustrated, 284
  philosophy and, 281
  physics and, 281–82
  physiology and, 281
  psychotherapy and, 282–83
  quantum physics and, 283–85
  thermodynamics and, 280
epigenetics
  about, 57–58
  in homeostatic process, 58
  therapeutic vibrations and, 373
  trauma and, 74–75
everything flows (*panta rhei*), 493–94
evolution, 6–7, 66–67, 93, 113
exercises
  Arcing, 33
  balancing the vector/axis system, 43
  curriculum vitae of the vital energy continuum, 470–71
  Direction of Energy, 143–44
  energetic touch and mobilization, 222–23
  energetic visualization and mobilization, 221–22
  genealogical-emotional tree, 466–69
  meridian emptying and filling technique, 187–88
  mind-body-spirit continuum, 454–55
  nonverbal SER technique, 306–7
  perceiving vibrations and harmonizing energy, 375–76
  personal growth, 322–24
  polarity and transformation, 125–26
  principles for the final treatment, 417
  realigning vectors using the Third Space, 397
  respiratory diaphragm release, 350
  self-assessment, 85–87
  self-listening Direction of Energy, 144–45
  Significance Detector, 36
  SQAR, 30
  Therapeutic Imagery and Dialogue, 39–40
  thoracic inlet release, 350
  visualization, assessment and mobilization of vector through chakras, 244, 246–47
extropy, 287–88

Facilitators
  active listening, 23
  emotions and, 92
  entropy and syntropy in practice, 288–89
  healing implementation needs, 26
  Higher Self, 25
  reality emergence during sessions and, 25
  in separation and/or loss situations, 72
Fantappié, 285
fascia
  about, 122–23
  description of, 124–25
  direction in human body, 123
  restrictions, graphical representation, 124
fascial release of intracranial structures
  first vault hold, 351–52, 439
  illustrated, 438
  second vault hold, 352, 439
  seven-step treatment, 438–39
  third vault hold, 353–54, 439
fear
  of death and dying, 310, 313–15
  kidneys and, 172, 175
  limbic system and, 64
feelings
  attentive listening of, 163–64
  death and dying and, 313–18
  emotions versus, 99–100
Fey, Ange, 316
fifth chakra, 234

fifth diaphragm, 253
final treatment. *See also* seven-step treatment
   about, 334–35
   antireductionism and ontology and, 341–45
   clinical observations, 355–58
   fascial release of intracranial structures, 351–53
   fundamental principles of, 417
   intuitive analogy, 336–37
   observations, 345, 353–54
   respiratory diaphragm and thoracic inlet release, 348–51
   techniques, 347–53
   uniting CNS, RAS, limbic system, three brains, 335–41
first chakra, 231
fornix, 255, 452
fourth chakra, 233
fractals
   about, 382–84
   butterfly-shaped structures, 387
   chaos and, 388–89
   defining, 384
   in human body, 389
   in neuronal ramifications, 386
   in organic structure of plants, 388
   syntropy and, 389
Francis, Patrick, 411–12
Fredrickson, Barbara, 98–99
Freedom, CV, 482
freedom of listening, 25–26

Galimberti, Umberto, 259
Garaventa, 260
Gardiner, Howard, 210
Gardini, Simone, 74
Gazzola, Flavio, 342–43
genealogical-emotional tree
   about, 466
   fruits, 468
   illustrated, 467, 469
   roots, 468

geology, polarity in, 120
geometry, polarity in, 120
geophysics, polarity in, 120
Gestalt psychology, 48, 103, 113
gesture, healing, 26–27
Giudice, Emilio del, 141–42, 176–77
Goethe, J. W. von, 60
Goleman, Daniel, 191, 430–31
gratitude, 312, 462–64, 465
gray matter, 137–38
Greggio, Fausto Bersani, 281
grief
   anatomy and physiology of, 252–63
   anthropology of, 261–63
   celebration of life through, 271
   clinical observations, 271–72, 326
   complex (complicated), 252
   CST and SER support, 269
   CST-centered visions, 273–78
   definitions of, 251–52
   Kübler-Ross's stages of, 263–67
   micro, 252
   mild, 252
   neurobiology of, 258–59
   reducing to individual phenomenon, 262
   revelation and, 7–8
   serious, 252
   suffering from loss and, 263
   therapeutic intervention in process, 267–70
   transformation through, 271–72
   traumatic, 251
   Western philosophy of, 259–61
grieving process
   about, 267–68
   experience of death and, 269
   gradual processing and, 267–68
   happiness as birthright and, 270
   key points in intervention, 270
   specificity of environment and, 268
   support with CST and SER, 268
   therapeutic intervention in, 267–70
Guardini, Romano, 104–5

half mourning, 252
Haramein, Nassim, 390–91
heart
    about, 174, 179
    destructive/constructive emotionality, 179
    emotions and, 199
    hand placement for meridian, 184, 445
    pericardium and, 178–79
    seven-step treatment and, 444–45
    treating, 184
Heidegger, Martin, 314
Higher Self
    characteristics of, 51
    conscious/non-conscious, dialog between, 23–25
    conversation with, 14
    ego and, 46, 47, 51
    as healing space, 164
    identification with, 164–65
    listening to voice of, 25
    melding of energies in, 165
    patient-Facilitator relationship, 25
    sharing impulse of, 165
    transpersonal self as, 51
    will to meet, 155–56
higher unconscious, 158–59
hippocampus, 255, 451
holistic vision, 464–65
Holmes, Thomas, 80–83
Holmes and Rahe Stress Scale, 80–83, 86, 197, 298
Hologram of Europe (Pogacnik), 195
homeostasis, 13, 17, 65, 66, 167, 198, 301, 387
horror vacui, 346
HPA axis
    about, 298–99
    in chiropractic, 302
    in clinical psychology, 301–2
    in cognitive psychotherapy, 300
    function of, 299
    in osteopathy, 300
    response to stress, 301
HPA organs, 299

Husserl, Edmund, 211
hypophysis, 236
hypothalamic-pituitary-adrenal (HPA). *See* HPA axis
hypothalamus, 236, 452

"I"
    apparent duality of, 160
    conscious, 159
    indivisible, 160–61
    true, 159–60
I Ching (Book of Changes), 433–34
imagination, 165–66
indirect route, 95
indivisible "I," 160–61
inevitable, cooperating with, 166–67
Inner Physician, 14, 46. *See also* Higher Self
integrated perspective, 188–91
Interview for Recent Life Events (IRLE), 86
intuition
    about, 210
    eidetic, 210–12
    emotion and, 212–13
    neurobiology of, 214
intuitive intelligence, 213–15

Jenny, Hans, 370, 371
Jewish mysticism, 337–41
Jodorowsky, Alejandro, 431
Jung, Carl Gustav, 48, 60, 113, 238–39, 412, 423

Kelly, Kevin, 287–88
kidneys
    about, 174, 180
    destructive/constructive emotionality, 180
    emotions and, 199
    hand placement for meridian, 185
    illustrated, 180
    treating, 185
Kübler-Ross, Elisabeth, 263, 267, 317
Kübler-Ross's stages of grief
    about, 263–64
    acceptance, 266–67

anger, 264–65
bargaining (negotiation, compromise), 265
denial (rejection), 264
depression, 265–66
kundalini, 231

labor/delivery, 73
Lane, Richard D., 97
Leadbeater, Charles Webster, 239, 303
LeDoux, Joseph, 95–97
Leibniz, G. W., 60
Levels of Emotional Awareness Scale (LEAS), 97
Levi-Montalcini, Rita, 251
Licata, Ignazio, 286–87
life changes, constructive, 3
life change units (LCUs), 196, 297
Life Cycle
    about, xv–xvi
    biological life processes in, 54–69
    curriculum vitae, 471–82
    introduction to, 17–18
    moving ahead in, 6
    phases, 2
limbic system, 63–64, 258
Lipton, Bruce, 393, 394
listening
    active, 23
    attentive, 163–64
    consciously, 407–8
    freedom of, 25–26
    to non-conscious, 166
    self-listening and, 144–45
liver
    about, 174, 181
    destructive/constructive emotionality, 182
    emotions and, 199
    hand placement for meridian, 186
    illustrated, 182
    meridian, illustrated, 447
    treating, 186
living organisms, 65–66
locus coeruleus, 256
logos, 110

Lorenz, Konrad, 462–64
Losa, Gabriele Angelo, 385–86, 393
loss
    in Biological Process, 72–73
    clinical observations, 77–78
    as consequence of possession and belonging, 73–74
    death and, 71
    experience of, 70
    objectives, 71
    objectivity and subjectivity in, 200–202
    as opportunity, 2–3
    rites of passage and, 71
    separation as, 71–73
    small deaths and, 196, 198, 203–4
    subjective, 71
    suffering from, 263
    as transformation opportunity, 311–12
Lowen, Alexander, 59
lower unconscious, 157–58
Lucarelli, Giovanni, 209
lungs
    about, 174, 179
    bereavement and, 179–80
    cross-sectional view, 179
    destructive/constructive emotionality, 180
    emotions and, 199
    hand placement for meridian, 185
    treating, 185

MacLean, Paul D., 63–65, 96
Maggio, Diego (author), 1–8
magnetic field lines, 119, 120–21
Mancuso, Vito, 346–47, 407–8, 425
Mandelbrot, Benoit, 385–86, 387
Mandelbrot set, 388
Manzelli, Paolo, 138–39, 390
Mapelli, Mario, 260–61
Marx, Karl, 112
Mastrobisi, Giorgio Jules, 212
Matthew, John, 7–8
Mayer, Giulia, 429–30
Mazzocchi, Alberto, 314–15

medulla oblongata, 255–56
Melottie, Fausto, 380
meninges, 439
menopause, 73
meridians
   of CST, 174–77
   dysfunctional, 173–74
   emptying and filling technique, 187–88
   Energy Cysts and, 173–74
   flow, assessing, 183
   hand placements for, 183–86
   palpation of, 173
micro-grief, 252
middle unconscious, 158
mild grief, 252
mind-body-spirit continuum, 405–20, 448–53, 454–55
Minotti, Roberto, 283–84
Mistretta, Rosa, 384–85
molecules, polarity, 118–19
Montalto, Pasquale Angelo, 151–52
Moonboulevard blog, 242–43
music therapy, 367

natural science, 66
negentropy, 284, 285. *See also* syntropy
neocortex, 64
nervous system, 136–38
neurobiology
   about, 258
   of grief, 258–59
   of intuition, 214
neuroscience
   current research in, 20
   in defining emotion, 93
   emotions and, 95–99
   synergy and, 426–28
non-conscious
   concept, 47
   conscious versus, 23–25
   ego versus, 47–48
   listening to, 166
nonverbal SER, 305–7

number 7, 431–34
nutrition, 88

objective loss, 71
objectivity and subjectivity
   in biophilosophy, 202–3
   in loss, 200–202
O'Connor, Max T., 287
Ode to Life, xv–xvi, 8, 312, 465–84
Oliveri, Diana, 117–18
ontology, 342
oocyte, 115–16
open-system human being
   CST and SER and, 465–82
   systemic perspective, 464–65
   teleonomy and, 461–64
orogeny, 120
osteopathy, HPA axis in, 300

Pagliaro, Gioacchino, 291–92
Palmas, Claudia, 391–92
palpation, 348–49
panta rhei (everything flows), 198, 493–94
Pascal, Blaise, 313
Pasin, Chiara, 326
Passions and Hobbies, CV, 481
patient-Facilitator relationship
   about, 22–23
   characteristics of, 27
   conscious and non-conscious, 23–25
   ego and, 46
   Third Space and, 23–25
Perceived Stress Scale (PSS), 86
perceptive realization, 392–93
pericardium
   about, 174, 178
   destructive/constructive emotionality, 178–79
   emotions and, 199
   hand placement for meridian, 183–84, 445
   heart and, 178–79
   seven-step treatment and, 444–45
   treating, 183–84

Perls, Fritz, 49, 103, 113
personal growth exercises, 322–24
Personal Information, CV, 471–75
Personality and Social Skills, CV, 479–80
Personal Self, 161
Pert, Candace, 58, 177–78, 182, 240–41
phenomenology, 211–12
philosophy
    Eastern, 107–10
    entropy and, 281
    polarity in, 107–12
    Western, 110–12
phonons, 368–69
photosynthesis
    clinical observations, 168–69
    cooperation with the inevitable, 166–67
    effectiveness of, 154
    interconnected steps, 154
    latent forces, 154
    objective of, 154, 155
    polarity and interactions in, 152–54
    poliversion and, 152–54
    practical method, 154
    transformation and, 150–51, 167
physics
    entropy in, 281–82
    polarity in, 119
    quantum, 12–13, 67, 283–85, 393, 405
    vectors in, 41
physiology
    of death, CST and SER and, 318–21
    entropy and, 281
    of grief, 252–58
pineal gland, 237, 452
Planck, Max, 67
Pogacnik, Marko, 188–89
polarity
    about, 103–4
    in ancient Egypt, 111
    aspects of, 106–22
    in biology, 116–17
    cell, 117–18
    in chemistry, 118–19

    clinical observations, 129–30
    conclusions on, 125
    conflict and synthesis and, 153
    contemporary perspectives on, 104–6
    in CST and SER, 122–25
    Earth's, 120–21
    of the egg, 115
    in embryology, 114–16
    exercise, 125–26
    in geology, 120
    in geometry, 120
    in geophysics, 120
    Neoplatonic principle of, 111–12
    oocyte and, 115–16
    in philosophy, 107–12
    in photosynthesis, 152–54
    in physics, 119
    in psychology and psychotherapy, 112–14
    relevance, 106
    toroid and, 122
    vector/axis system and, 216–17
poliversion, 152–54
pons, 319, 450
post-traumatic stress disorder (PTSD), 83–84, 259, 263
Preparata, Giuliano, 140–41, 176–77
Pressurestat Model, 11
proprioceptors, 224
psychoacoustics, therapeutic vibrations and, 373
psychology/psychotherapy
    entropy in, 282–83
    HPA axis in, 300, 301–2
    polarity in, 112–14
psychoneuroendocrinoimmunology (PNEI), 58
psychophysics, therapeutic vibrations and, 373
psychosynthesis, ego in, 49–51
PTSD self-assessment questionnaire, 85–87
puberty, 72

quality, 13, 29, 30. *See also* symmetry, quality, amplitude, and rate (SQAR)
quantum biology, 138–39

quantum electrodynamics (QED), 138, 140–42, 176
quantum entanglement, 67, 283, 284, 423
quantum interdisciplines, 139–40
quantum medicine (QM), 367
quantum physics, 12–13, 67, 283–85, 393, 405
quantum theory, 66–67

Rahe, Richard, 80–83
Rasini, Vallori, 202–3
rate, 13, 29, 30. *See also* symmetry, quality, amplitude, and rate (SQAR)
Ravasi, Gianfranco, 432–33
receptive mindfulness, 46
reflection, 172
reptilian brain, 63
respiratory diaphragm release
  about, 446–47
  hand placement for, 349
  illustrated, 446
  objectives for, 350–51
  palpation, 348
  technique for, 350
  therapeutic pulse, 349
reticular activating/alarm system (RAS)
  about, 12, 54–55
  activation of, 55, 136
  connection with, 442–43
  corpus callosum and, 442–43
  seventh chakra and mind-body-spirit continuum, 451
  shock and, 297
reticular formation, 451
reticular system, 54–55
Rispoli, Luciano, 426–28
rites of passage, 71

Sacchetti, Aldo, 139–40
sadness, 172, 175, 179–80, 200, 254, 264–65
Saint Francis of Paola, 414
Saint Giuseppe Moscati, 413
Saint Nicholas, 414–15
Sartre, Jean-Paul, 314

Scheler, Max, 314
Schneerson, Rebbe Rav Menachem Mendel, 341
Schopenhauer, Arthur, 423
second chakra, 232
sedimentology, 120
separation
  in Biological Process, 72–73
  experience of, 70
  Facilitator's objectives and, 72
  going through, 1–2
  as loss, 71–73
  stress and, 70
serious grief, 252
seven (7), number, 431–34
seven-step treatment
  about, 421–23
  alignment of vector/axis system, 436–37
  allegoric symbolism of, 431–34
  approach to, 421–22
  clinical observations, 456–59
  connection with cerebral hemispheres, 440–41
  connection with corpus callosum and RAS, 442–43
  empathy and, 428–31
  fascial release of intracranial structures, 438–39
  heart and pericardium meridians, 444–45
  phases of, 435–53
  preparing for, 417
  respiratory diaphragm and vagus nerve, 446–47
  seventh chakra and, 448–53
  steps illustration, 422
  structure, 421
  synchronicity, 423–24
  synergy and, 424–28
seventh chakra
  about, 235, 453
  characteristics of, 235
  connecting with, 448
  illustrated, 449
  mind-body-spirit continuum and, 448–53

sharing impulse, 165
Shem Ha Meforash, 338
Sierra, Ramona, 188–89
Significance Detector
   clinical notes, 36–37
   implementation of, 36
   reasons for manifestation, 36
   Still Point versus, 34–35
   unsolicited image and, 34
Silvestrini, Paolo, 423–24
Simone, Matteo, 84
sixth chakra, 234–35
skin, 20
"Skull Motion," 10
small deaths
   about, 173, 198
   clinical observations, 205–6
   emotions of, 198–200
   as necessary losses, 203–4
   types of, 196
SomatoEmotional Release (SER). *See also*
      CranioSacral Therapy (CST)
   about, 12
   aptonomic touch and, 20–21
   assessment techniques, 19
   clinical analysis of patients, 19
   development of, 12–13
   emotions and, 91
   Energy Cysts and, 13–15
   eurythmy of, 18
   grieving family support with, 268
   implementation of, 18
   for integration and release, 91–102
   methodology and objective, 18, 19
   nonverbal, 305–7
   as Ode to Life, 465–82
   physiology of death in, 318–21
   polarity in, 122–25
   refinement of, 12–13
   teleonomy in, 461–62
   Treatment Protocol, 83–84
   vibrational energy of 432 Hz grid in, 374–75

SomatoEmotional Release and Beyond
      (Upledger), 224
sphenobasilar joint, 11
spinal cord, 236
spleen
   about, 174, 181
   destructive/constructive emotionality, 181
   emotions and, 199, 200
   illustrated, 181
   meridian, hand placement, 186
   treating, 186
Steiner, Rudolf, 239–40
Still, Andrew, 9–10, 17
Still Point, 34–35
Stranieri, Daniela, 241
stress
   assessment scales, 85
   clinical observations, 89–90
   HPA axis response to, 301
   pathologies connected to, 83–85
   separation and loss and, 70
stressors
   about, 80
   clinical observations, 308
   discourse on, 87–88
   Holmes and Rahe Stress Scale, 80–83, 86, 197, 297–98
   life factors and, 87–88
   major, 297–98
   measuring, 80–90
   occurring together, 83
subjective loss, 71
superconscious, 158–59
Sutherland, William G., 9–11, 17
symmetry, 13, 30, 173, 286. *See also* symmetry, quality, amplitude, and rate (SQAR)
symmetry, quality, amplitude, and rate (SQAR)
   about, 29
   Arcing technique and, 33
   assessment, 31, 44, 68
   definitions, 30–31
   evaluations, 29
   implementation of, 30

synchronicity, 423–24
synergy, 426–28
syntropic phenomenon, 285, 286
syntropy
   about, 285
   as constructive energy, 289
   in Facilitator's practice, 288–89
   fractals and, 389
   illustrated, 284

techniques, foundational
   Arcing, 31–33
   Significance Detector, 34–37
   symmetry, quality, amplitude, and rate (SQAR), 29–31
   Therapeutic Image, 37–38, 39–40
   vector/axis system, 40–44
teleology, 462
teleonomy, 461–62
Teodorani, Massimo, 405–7
Terzani, Tiziano, 408–11
thalamus, 95, 96, 257, 452
thanatology, 316–17
"theory of everything," 390–91
therapeutic energy, 290–91
Therapeutic Imagery and Dialogue
   about, 37–38
   clinical notes, 40
   dialogue, 38–39
   emotions and, 100, 101
   implementation of, 39–40
   initiation of, 38
   objectives, 39
   solicited and unsolicited images and, 38
therapeutic pulse, 349
therapeutic vibrations, 374–75
thermodynamics, 280
third chakra, 232–33
Third Space
   about, 23, 128, 305, 381
   clinical observations, 398–403
   fractals and, 382–89
   illustrated, 24

   introduction to, 392–93
   in patient-Facilitator relationship, 23–25
   perceptive visualization of, 382
   thought-forms, 383, 393–94, 437
   toroidal magnetic field and, 389–92
   vectors and, 396–97
third ventricle, 254
thoracic inlet release
   hand placement for, 350
   objectives for, 350–51
   palpation, 348–49
   technique for, 350
   therapeutic pulse, 349
thought-forms
   concept, 303
   effect of, 303–4
   identifying, 384, 395
   Third Space and, 303–5, 383, 393–94, 437
three cranial vault holds, 143
toroid, 122, 389–92
toroidal magnetic field
   about, 389–90
   of da Vinci's *Vitruvian Man*, 392
   as energetic space, 389–92
   illustrated, 391
traditional Chinese medicine (TCM), 175–76
training objectives, 27
transformation
   being and becoming and, 151–52
   of destructive energy, 395
   of energies, 161–62
   loss and, 311–12
   photosynthesis and, 150–51, 167
   through grief, 271–72
Transpersonal Self, 159–60
transpersonal will, 161
trauma
   emotions and, 98
   epigenetics and, 74–75
   points of view on, 84–85
   radicalized, 328
   unresolved, 83

traumatic grief, 251
triune brain, 63–65
Tulli, Roberto, 241

unconscious
    adaptive, 210, 213–15
    collective, 160
    higher, 158–59
    lower, 157–58
    middle, 158
unsolicited image, 34
Upledger, John E.
    about, xv–xvi, 9–13, 15–18, 493–94
    "analysis creates paralysis" and, 215
    art of treatment and, 416
    author and, 4–6, 7
    death and dying and, 319–20
    emotions and, 92, 93
    non-conscious and, 47–48
    observations to a new method, 223–24
    photos, xvi, 8, 493
    polarity and, 103–4
    on PTSD, 83–84
    spiritual heritage, 128
    vector/axis system and, 41
    on "the whole," 464–65
Upledger, John Matthew, xv, 7–8, 493, 494

vagus nerve, 257–58, 320, 446–47
vagus system, 253–54
Valcarenghi, Marina, 198–99
Valentino, Virginia, 259
Valesini, Simone, 213–14
Vannini, Antonella, 285–86, 389
vector/axis system
    about, 40–41
    alignment (7-step treatment), 436–37
    assessing with, 207–28
    balancing, implementation of, 43
    chakras and, 219, 437
    clinical notes, 44
    diagram, 42
    direct and energy force and, 42

    energetic framework and, 215–17
    energetic imbalance in, 41
    mapping, 218
    mapping with chakras, 230, 245
    objectives, 43
    polarity and, 216–17, 437
    realigning, 220–21
    realigning with chakras, 248
    after realignment, 247
    vector visualization, 41–43
vectors
    aligning, 221–23
    aligning with chakras, 243–48
    aligning with Third Space, 397
    assessment and rebalancing techniques on, 223
    landmarks in the human body, 217
    misalignment of, 220, 247
    Third Space and, 396–97
    using, 218–21
    visualization, assessment, and mobilization of, 244, 246–47
    visualization of, 41–43, 396
Venuti, Pasquale, 386–87
vibrations
    about, 360–62
    acoustics and acoustic signaling, 368
    bioenergetics and, 373
    chakras and, 374
    clinical observations, 378–79
    cognitive science and, 372
    cymatics, 369–72
    epigenetics and, 373
    432 Hz versus 440 Hz, 364–67
    introducing in therapeutic applications, 372–74
    music therapy and cosmology, 367
    observations, 376–77
    perceiving, and harmonizing energy, 375–76
    phonons and biophonons and, 368–69
    psychoacoustics and, 373
    psychophysics and, 373

quantum medicine (QM), 367
   therapeutic, 374–75
   in Therapeutic Imagery and Dialogue, 361
   as universal language, 363–64
   voice and, 360–61
viscera
   about, 172
   clinical observations, 194
   communication between emotions and, 182–83
   emotions held in, treating, 183–88
   treating, 183
Visceral Manipulation (VM), 123
visualization
   energetic, 221–22
   exercises, 221–22, 244, 246–47
   interactive, practicing, 396–97
   of Third Space, 382
   of vectors, 41–43, 396
Vitruvian Man (da Vinci), 16

Wallis, Christopher, 243
white matter, 137
will
   free, respecting, 310–11
   to meet Higher Self, 155–56
   transpersonal, 161
   wise, 156–61
Winnicott, Donald, 201–2
Working Experience, CV, 476–77
A Work of Mind and Body (Caressa), 337–41

yin and yang, 107, 110, 176

Zilio, Federico, 343–44

Upledger Institute International

The mission of Upledger Institute International is to provide world-class CranioSacral Therapy (CST) education while supporting the overall therapeutic philosophies of CST developer Dr. John E. Upledger. For more than thirty-five years, Upledger Institute International has been training manual therapists in evidence-informed and evidence-based disciplines. Our disciplines and techniques have been shown to increase the effectiveness of client treatments, thus helping our alumni rapidly expand their therapy practices. Supporting more than 132,000 manual therapists in 122 countries, Upledger Institute International continues the work developed by renowned health care innovator Dr. John E. Upledger by providing acclaimed health care education. His development of CST and SomatoEmotional Release (SER) earned him an international reputation and established him as a leader in integrative, whole-person, manual therapy education, clinical services, and ongoing research.

To find a practitioner or to learn more about Upledger Institute International and their courses and products, visit **Upledger.com**.

BOOKS OF RELATED INTEREST

Craniosacral Chi Kung
Integrating Body and Emotion in the Cosmic Flow
by Mantak Chia and Joyce Thom

The Reflexology Manual
An Easy-to-Use Illustrated Guide to the
Healing Zones of the Hands and Feet
by Pauline Wills

Trigger Point Therapy for Myofascial Pain
The Practice of Informed Touch
*by Donna Finando, L.Ac., L.M.T., and
Steven Finando, Ph.D., L.Ac.*

Acupressure Self-Care Handbook
Healing at Your Fingertips
by Roger Dalet, M.D.

The Book of Tapping
Emotional Acupressure with EFT
by Sophie Merle

Total Reflexology of the Hand
An Advanced Guide to the Integration of
Craniosacral Therapy and Reflexology
by Martine Faure-Alderson, D.O.

The Biodynamics of the Immune System
Balancing the Energies of the Body with the Cosmos
by Michael J. Shea, Ph.D.
Foreword by Bill Harvey

The Secret of Resilience
Healing Personal and Planetary Trauma through Morphogenesis
by Stephanie Mines, Ph.D.
Foreword by Cherionna Menzam-Sills, Ph.D.

INNER TRADITIONS • BEAR & COMPANY
P.O. Box 388
Rochester, VT 05767
1-800-246-8648

www.InnerTraditions.com
Or contact your local bookseller